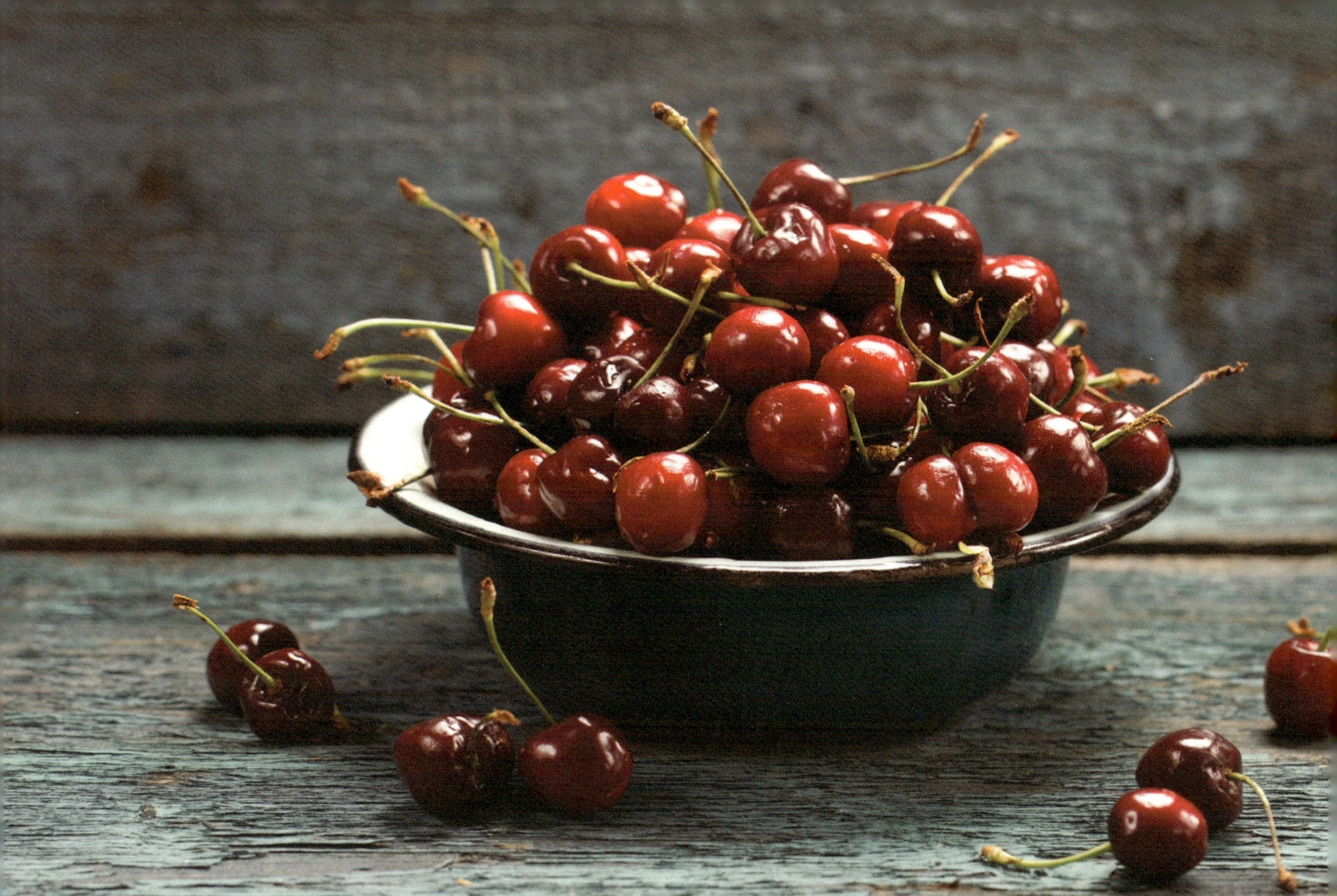

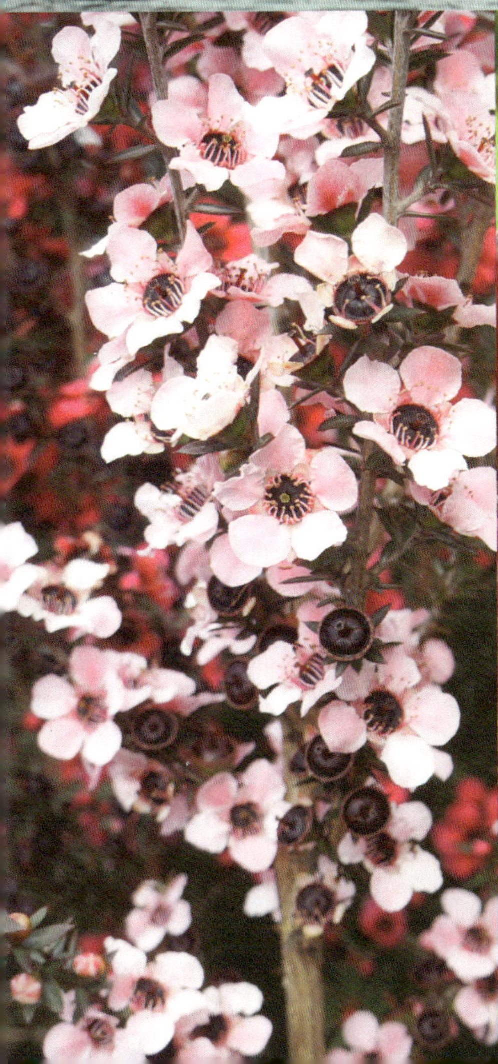

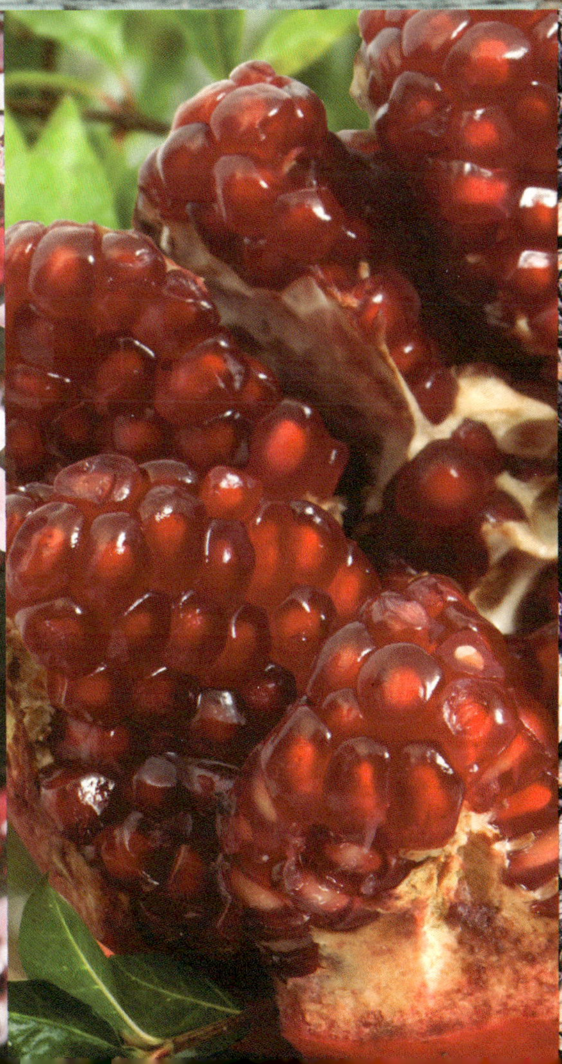

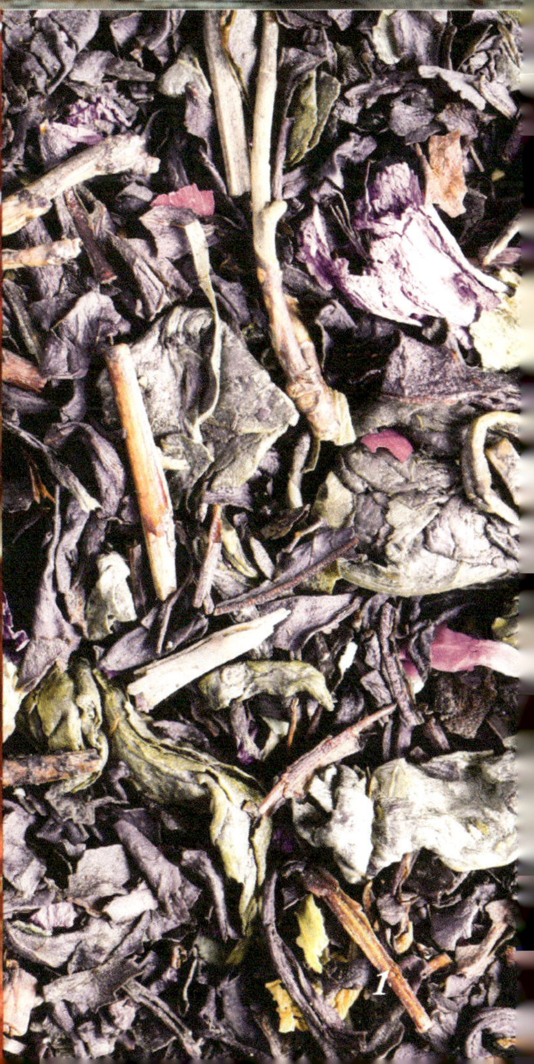

TESTIMONIALS

I became an active alternative healer by accident 20 years ago, when both of my children were diagnosed by the medical community with an 'incurable' illness. As their mother, I of course immediately rededicated my life to studying all possible solutions.

During my journey into alternative medicine I tried very many approaches, often with minimal results. However, after years of searching I was able to find solutions for healing my children and have been able to help many others as well.

I met Firozé quite a few years ago and a large part of our connection was the shared joint passion of alternative means for healing. As I learned the history of Firozé's grandmother's body of work, I was full of admiration and respect. Firozé graciously shared some of the recipes with me, especially when I was taking care of my mother who was on a rapid decline.

My mother had a pulmonary embolism, which left five blood clots lodged in her lungs causing continual coughing and difficulty breathing. She was in agony as she couldn't sleep, had continual incontinence from coughing and [she] was so sore. I had an exceptional relationship with Mom's doctor, Dr. Dean Smith, in Myrtle Beach, SC. He was actually open to our alternative healing practices and called me to ask if I had anything to help Mom as the normal medical practices were not working.

I did not have a solution so I called Firozé and she gave me a recipe for removing blood clots from the lungs, which also had the ability to stop the coughing. I made it immediately and Mom was taking it every hour initially. Amazingly, after only a few days her coughing started to diminish and we continued treatment for the next few weeks until it actually stopped as the blood clots dissolved. Dr. Smith was amazed and I even gave him the recipe, as he is a believer.

I have used this recipe over and over again as several of my friends and colleagues ended up with bronchitis, chest colds, flus and various lung ailments. It has never failed to work its miracle. My lawyer was so ill and sore from coughing endlessly causing lack of sleep and pain. I made it for him and within days he was able to sleep and heal.

I cannot wait to get Firozé's complete book and try the many other recipes. I am a believer and know it will shorten the process of many trial-and-error attempts one faces when seeking an alternative option. I wish I had known Firoze when I was on my exhaustive search to heal my children. It would have saved years of suffering and thousands of dollars seeking a cure. After the experience of my friends and family, Firozé's book will be our 'go to' source for all that we face in the years to come.

Gratefully,
Dawn Longhi, Austin, TX

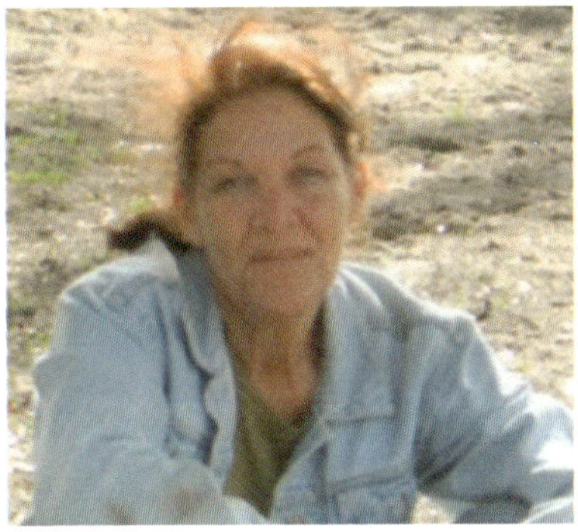

Firozé was the first person to introduce me to turmeric, a spice I had never heard of until that day. Her Turmeric Elixir has worked miracles in my life. I had been battling with a chronic cough, as well as mucus in my lungs, for more than a year and no medication cleared it. After about ten days of taking Firozé's Turmeric Elixir, my cough had stopped, and I felt I was able to breathe better. On my last visit with my doctor he took x-rays, and was amazed to see how clear my lungs were. In turn, I am amazed to find myself with more energy and stamina, as well as [a] clear lungs. Thank you for this gift of well being Firozé.

- Woody Wolverton,
FORMER TOWN COMMISIONER of Longboat Key, FL

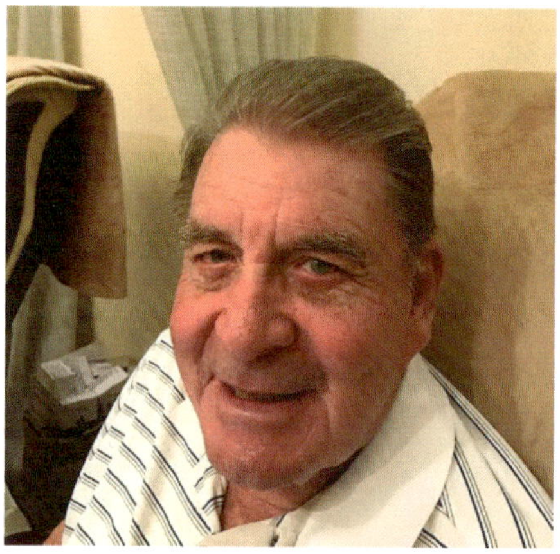

Firozé may look like she catwalked off the pages of Vogue, but don't be fooled. When she dispenses her grandmother's healing potions and salves she's more like an old-time witch doctor. The Turmeric Elixir she prescribed for my throat not only eased my symptoms, but was also absolutely delicious.

- Debra Scott, East Hampton, NY

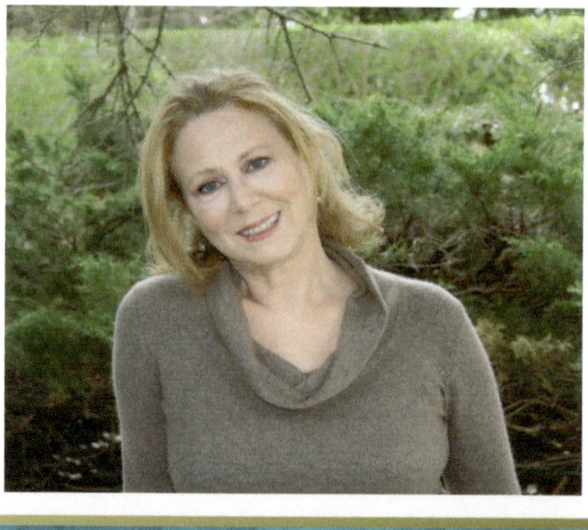

At fifty plus, bad habits have started catching up with me: sun, coffee, red wine, reading screens in the dark - bad for the skin, the teeth and the eyes, respectively. A casual encounter with Firozé put me back in control.

A super-logical ex-banker, I often put on sunscreen although I was always too harried to bother with a cover layer of makeup. Still, a quarter-sized sunspot appeared on my cheek. It defied laser treatment, and I resigned myself to its position on my face. When Firozé, at a social encounter, caught me with her deep, wise eyes and knowingly told me lemon would make that spot disappear, I read it almost like a dare. Put on a drop on that cheek before bed, and sleep with it on, she assured me. Don't go out in the sun with lemon on your skin, she warned. I could just apply lemon. If expensive laser treatments failed, how could lemon overcome? Fast, cheap and easy,it worked. Poof!

So I moved on to other 'Firozé advice.' When I eat a banana I rub the inside of the peel on my teeth, which have become whiter. So easy. So fabulous.

I continued down my list. My sun spot faded, my teeth whiter, I tried Firozé's recommendation for bleary eyes: aloe juice blended with walnuts. Ever lazy, though now way less skeptical, I bought Aloe juice at Trader Joe's, added lemon, and admittedly just drank it while munching walnuts. My body now craves this combination, and I use fewer expensive Genteal eye drops for relief.

Firozé's knowledge from the ages reached me as older age began to show. I am grateful for Firozé's wisdom, and thrilled she wrote a book. Mostly I am relieved I was smart enough to trust in her, and her heritage.

With appreciation, Firozé. To natural health and well-being!

- Jill Carrie Schachter

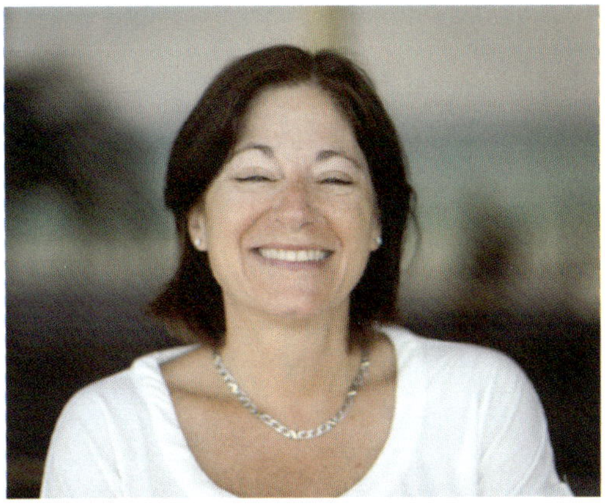

I have known Firozé for a few years and I've delighted in her sharing of her grandmother's remedies and potions, as well as the benefits they offer. I'm very much into organic, environmentally safe remedies, and I consider myself part of the movement to live a cleaner, more sustainable lifestyle.

One remedy I used whose results really impressed me was with turmeric paste. When my back was ailing me, pretty debilitating pain, couldn't leave the house, Firoze recommended I take an egg and separate the yolk from the white, mix the yolk with a tablespoon of turmeric, making it into a paste, then brush it on the ailing area, wait a few minutes and then cover with saran wrap, and hold it in place with an ace bandage.

I felt the inflammation subsiding quickly as the pain was mostly gone within 2 days. Very impressive! Firozé told me her grandmother used this remedy for fractures and bone breaks.

I am so excited for Firozé's upcoming book, such amazing beneficial ancient remedies!

- Martha Smyth

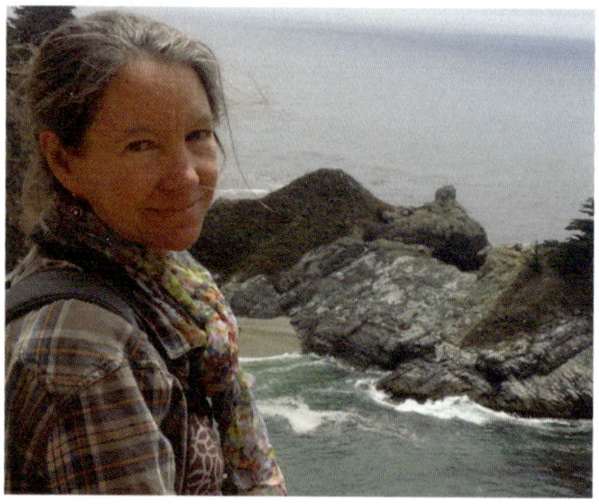

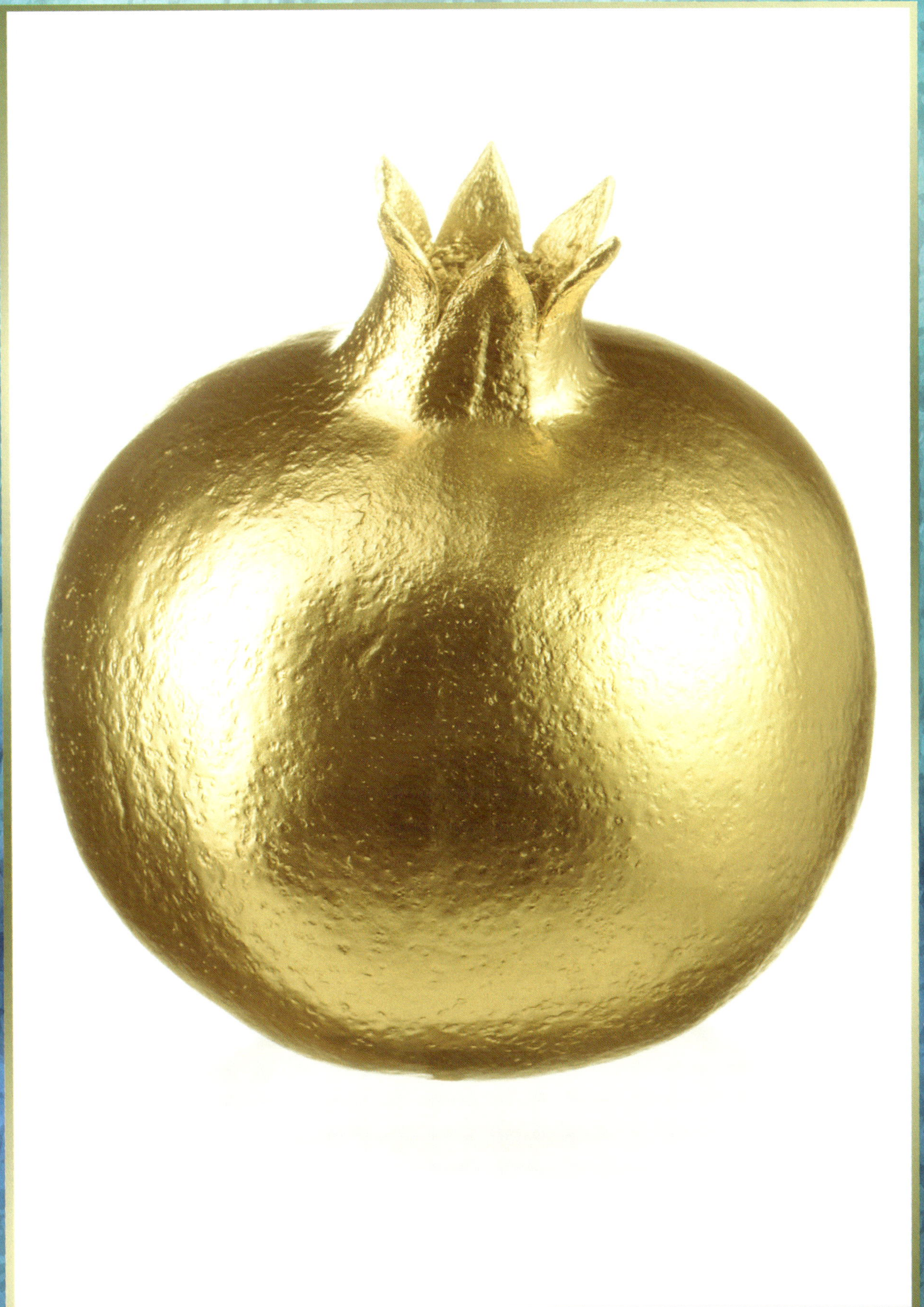

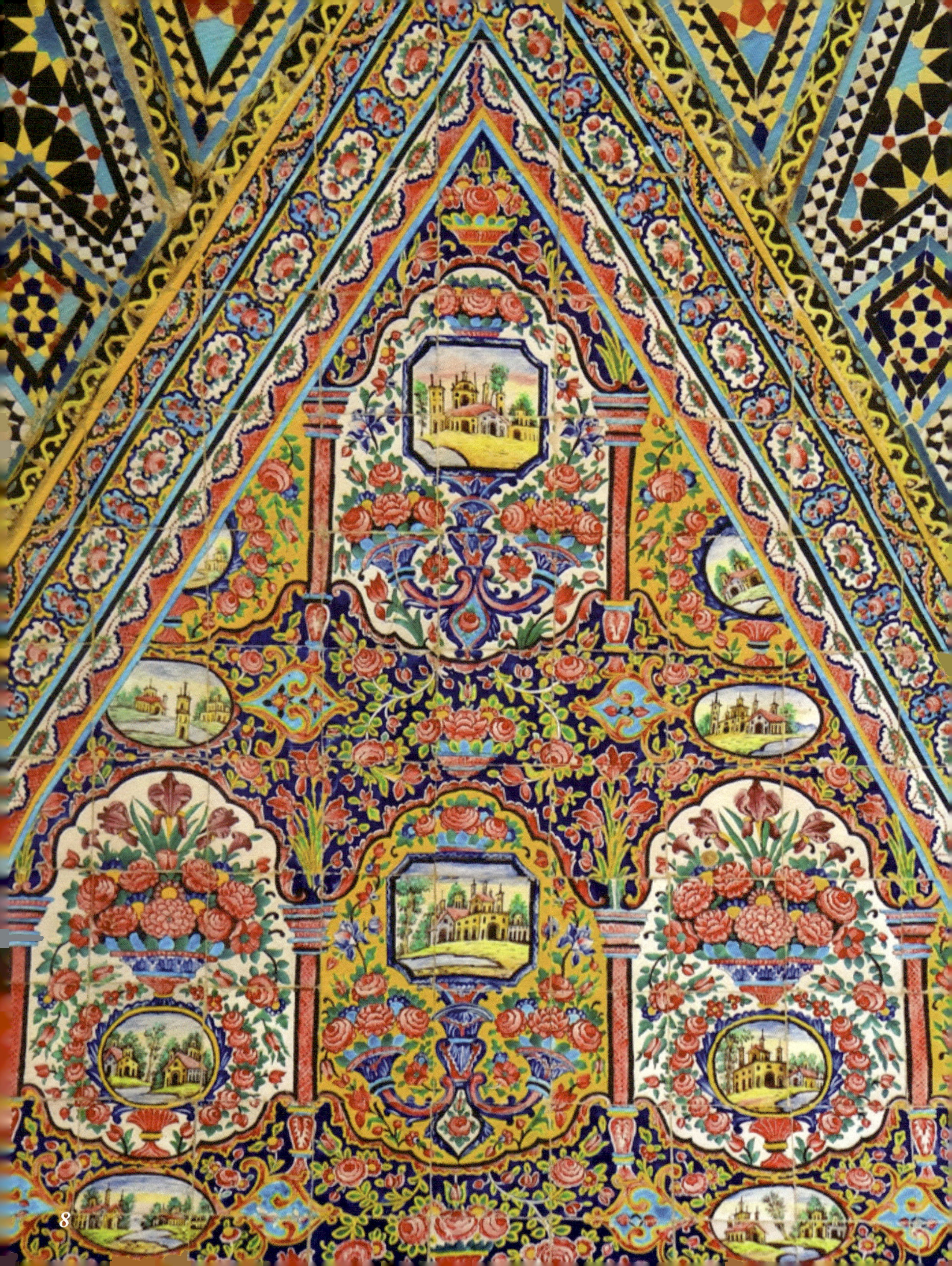

DEDICATION

I owe a debt of gratitude to people who have been life teachers along the way, who have supported me in every step of my evolution and encouraged me to share my grandmother's wisdom and heritage. This gratitude extends to the wise women who came before Mamanjoon, pioneers who passed recipes down from one woman to another through generations. This published and illustrated book continues the chain, ensuring the known remedies are preserved, not lost, and spreading them from Ancient Persia to you.

I have so many people to thank for the birth and manifestation of this book. First my Mamanjoon for being my wise generous grandmother, my mother who held dear her notes and recipes and all the people in my life who were an inspiration in my creativity who encouraged me with love and last but not certainly least, and perhaps most important, Gratitude to God Source First Eternal. This book has been the work of three years in the making with many friends and strangers assisting me on my path of co-creation.

These recipes are a small part of Persian history that started with Abū Bakr Muhammad ibn Zakariyyā al-Rāzī (known outside of Iran as Al-Razi (854 CE – 925 CE). He was a Persian polymath, physician, alchemist, philosopher and important figure in the history of medicine. A comprehensive thinker, Razi made fundamental and enduring contributions to various fields, which he recorded in over 200 manuscripts, and is particularly remembered for numerous advances in medicine through his observations and discoveries. Al-Razi was said to be compassionate and devoted to the service of his patients, whether rich or poor.

So I dedicate this book to Mamanjoon's legacy, to all the people I love and to those many people who can benefit from the use of her wisdom to reap and gain health and beauty.

Table of Content

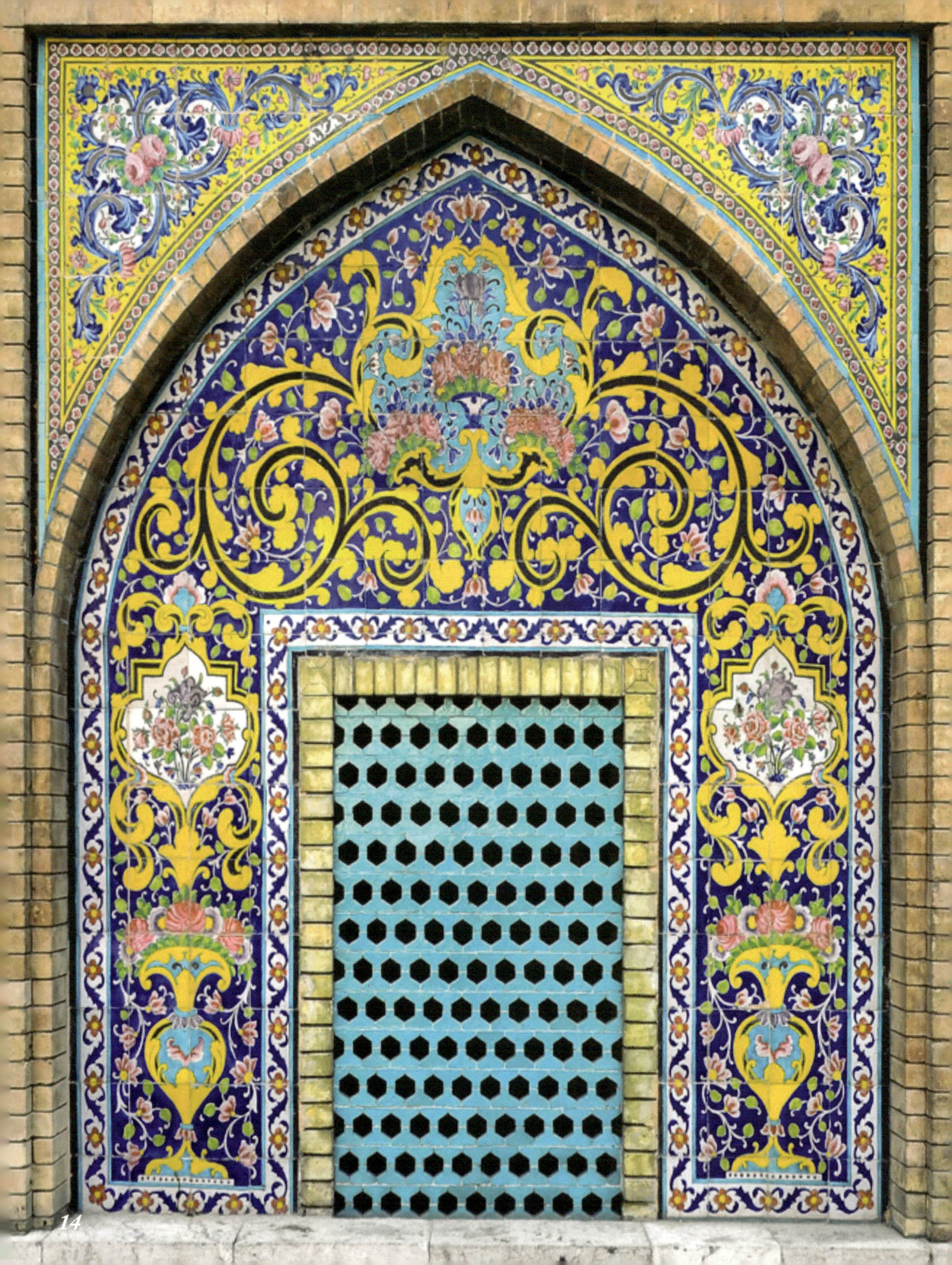

INTRODUCTION

For many years doing nails, facials and makeup, whenever a client complained of an ailment or beauty concern, I was always at the ready to suggest a natural remedy. Without realizing it at the time, I was following in my grandmother's footsteps. A natural healer, Mamanjoon had inherited her recipes and gifts from a long line of wise women before her.

Mamanjoon was both an extraordinary healer and expert in natural beauty therapies, concocting all sorts of time-tested potions to rejuvenate a youthful appearance. Fortunately I feel her abilities were passed down to me in my DNA. I was an alchemist from a young age. As a child I would mix ingredients to see what concoctions I could come up with.

I remember in 1983 when I opened my first salon in New York on East 65th Street. I started making one of her recipes at home and pouring it into antique Egyptian-looking bottles. It was an old recipe made from cucumbers and glycerin that is a great whitening, softening and spot-removing hand lotion. I couldn't wait for my clients to try it. And they loved it. Filled with fresh botanicals, it worked better than any of the dead products found on the market.

It was a natural evolution that I soon developed my own line of organic nail treatments and polishes, which became well known to beauty editors and my celebrity clientele. Over the years, as I continued to dole out Mamanjoon's prescriptions, recipes, and teas, my grateful clients would admonish me to write a book and share her secrets with everyone. So after many years of hearing that over and over again I finally sat down to tell the story of Mamanjoon and share her secrets before they are lost forever.

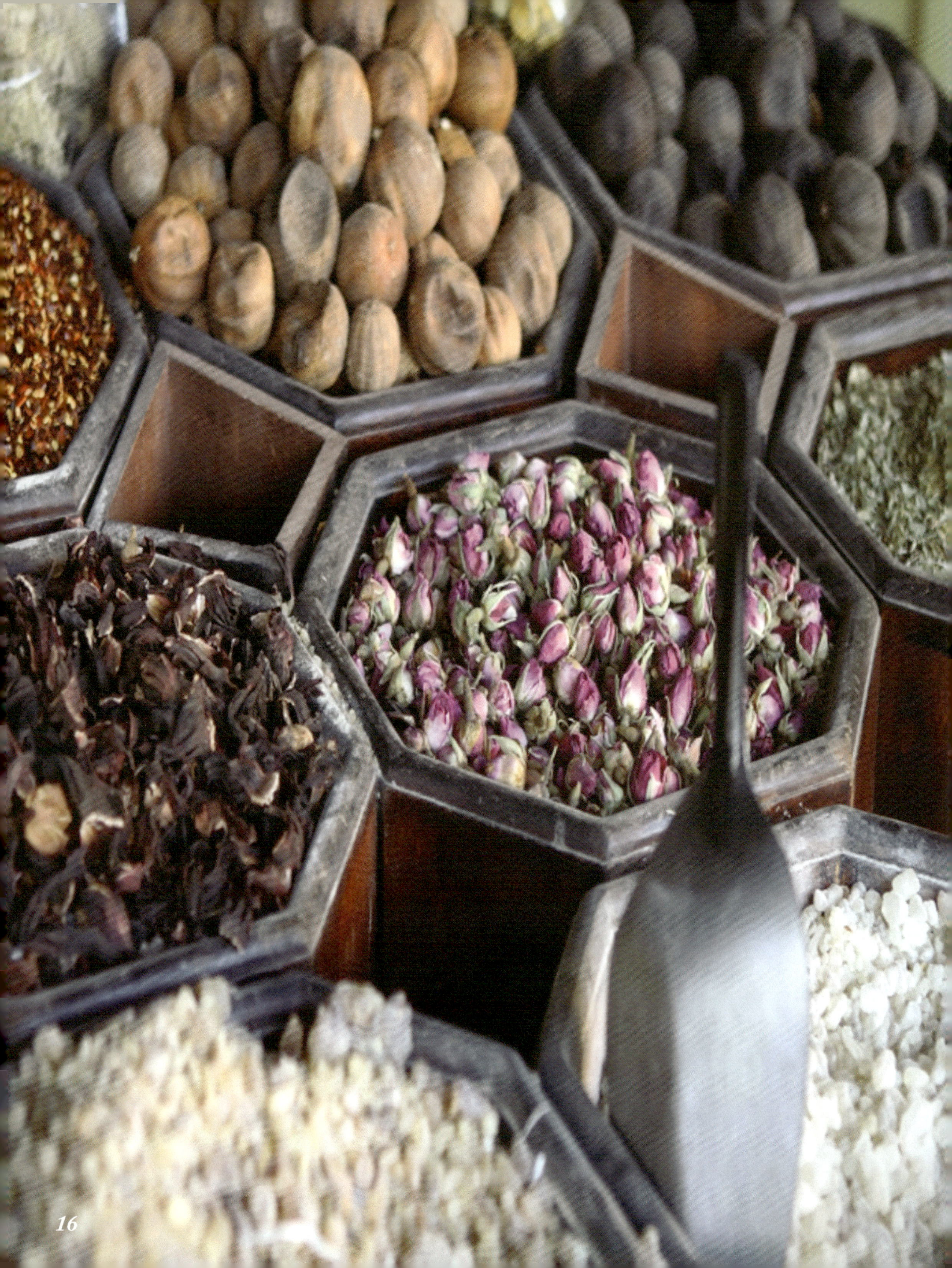

GROWING UP WITH MAMANJOON

Through the filter of many years, I can still recall images of my grandmother's garden in Tehran. As a child I was seduced by the invigorating scent of jasmine as I climbed down the big granite stairs and ducked under the arbor with its tangle of drooping grapes to find my way to her pond with its scampering goldfish. My brother and I would reverently enter the cellar through its garden door. It was our "treasure room," and was filled with the aroma of the old and the new. Though dark, we could see the trunks and big glass jars full of all sorts of mysterious potions.

Each year before the start of autumn and summer my grandmother would gather a group of women in the garden to peel tomatoes, clean grapes, and chop up an abundance of flowers, fruits and herbs. Their efforts would produce all sorts of purees, pickles and jams to be stored away for winter.

Mamanjoon seemed to always be in the midst of brewing a secret tincture, colorful tea, murky oil, or funny gelling paste that would be administered as soon as someone in the family, friend or neighbor came down with a cough or other ailment. Besides her homespun medical knowledge, she also held in her treasure trove of healing salves secrets to a youthful complexion and everlasting beauty. Mamanjoon, herself, everyday drank a cleansing water and lemon infusion first thing in the morning and a tea brewed from turmeric root and sweetened with honey and lemon, throughout the day. She lived till she was 102.

Mamanjoon was strict but very gentle and loving. She would regale us with stories that each had a special hidden meaning. In private, she always told me that women were unique beings and thus we have to brush up on all our God-given talents and never sit idle. She taught me the domestic arts: needlework, knitting, and how to crochet clothes for my only doll.

She was a young woman when she lost her husband and decided never to marry again. In 1918 she was the first woman in Iran to open a school for girls. Very forward-thinking, she spoke three languages, loved literature, philosophy and poetry and was a poet in her own right. Alas, she was never published.

It wasn't until I became an adult that I was able to fully comprehend the great wealth of knowledge that my grandmother possessed. Or understand the value of collecting her recipes and handing them down to others, as they had been handed down to her and me. With great thanks to those who have encouraged me, but mostly to Mamanjoon, I humbly offer this book of my grandmother's healing recipes.

Note: There are some ingredients that are so hard to come by (think scorpions!), that I thought of leaving those recipes out. But then I realized the importance of documenting these nearly lost recipes for posterity. For all I know enterprising women or men will figure out a suitable replacement!

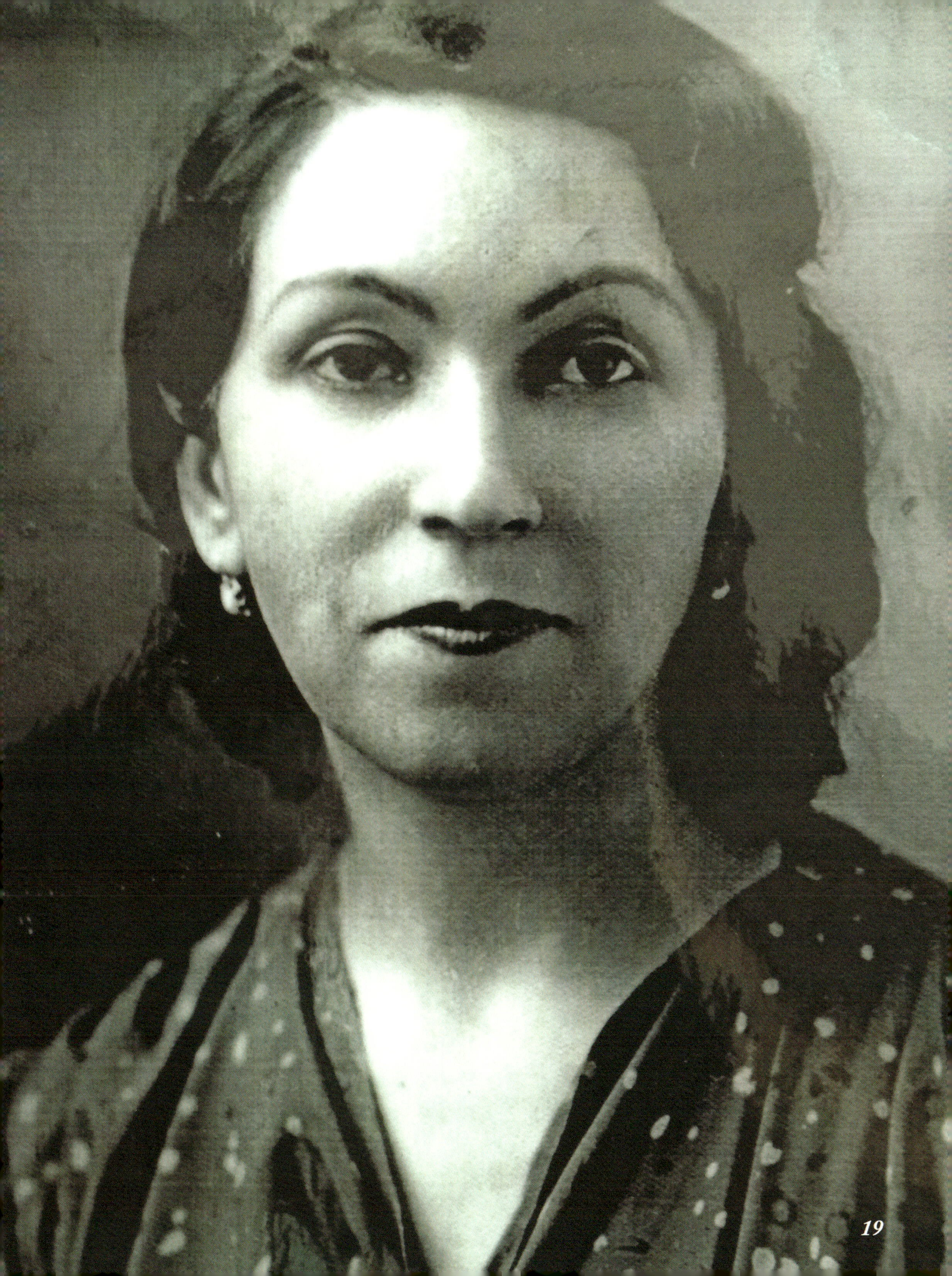

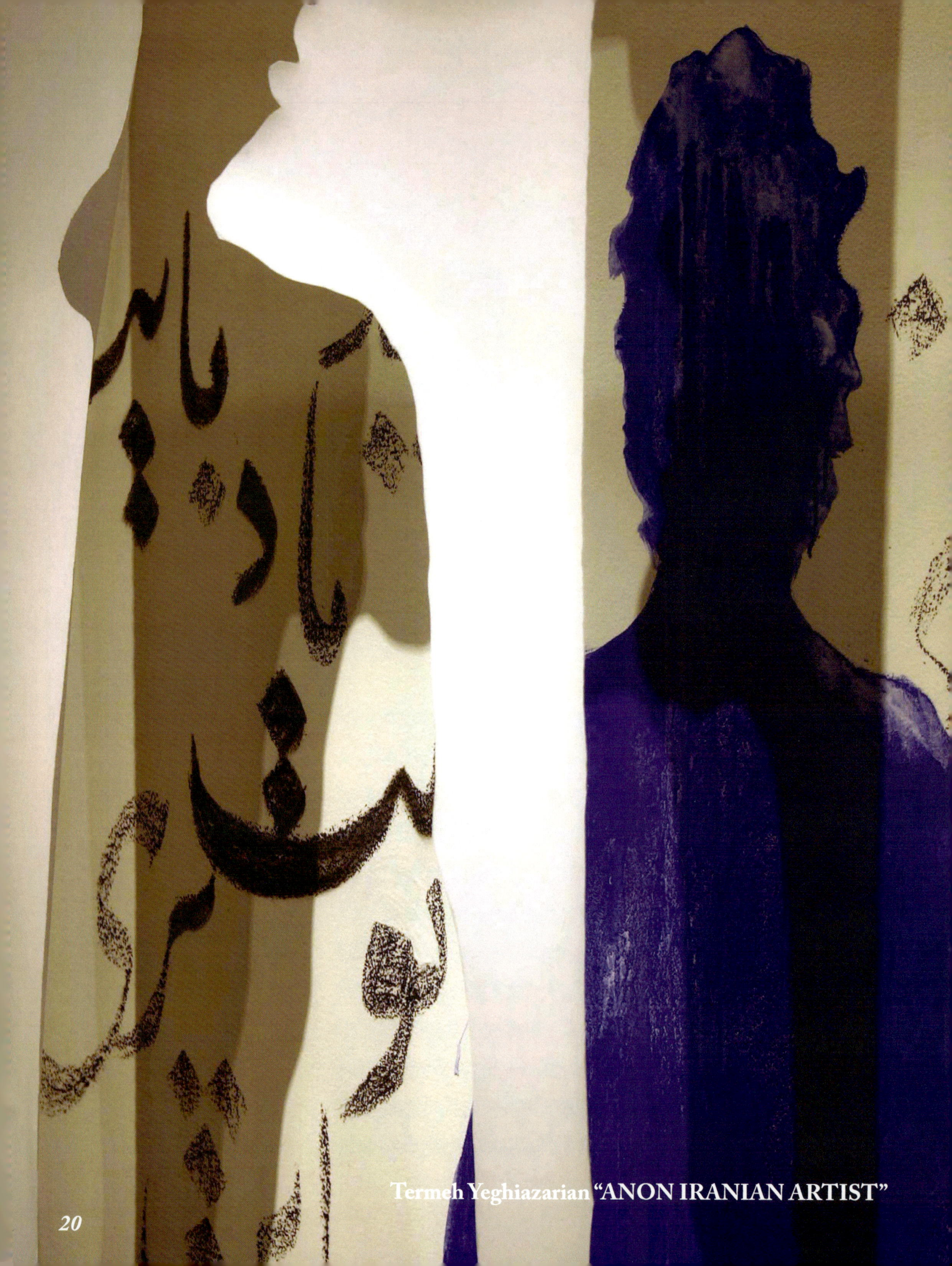

Termeh Yeghiazarian "ANON IRANIAN ARTIST"

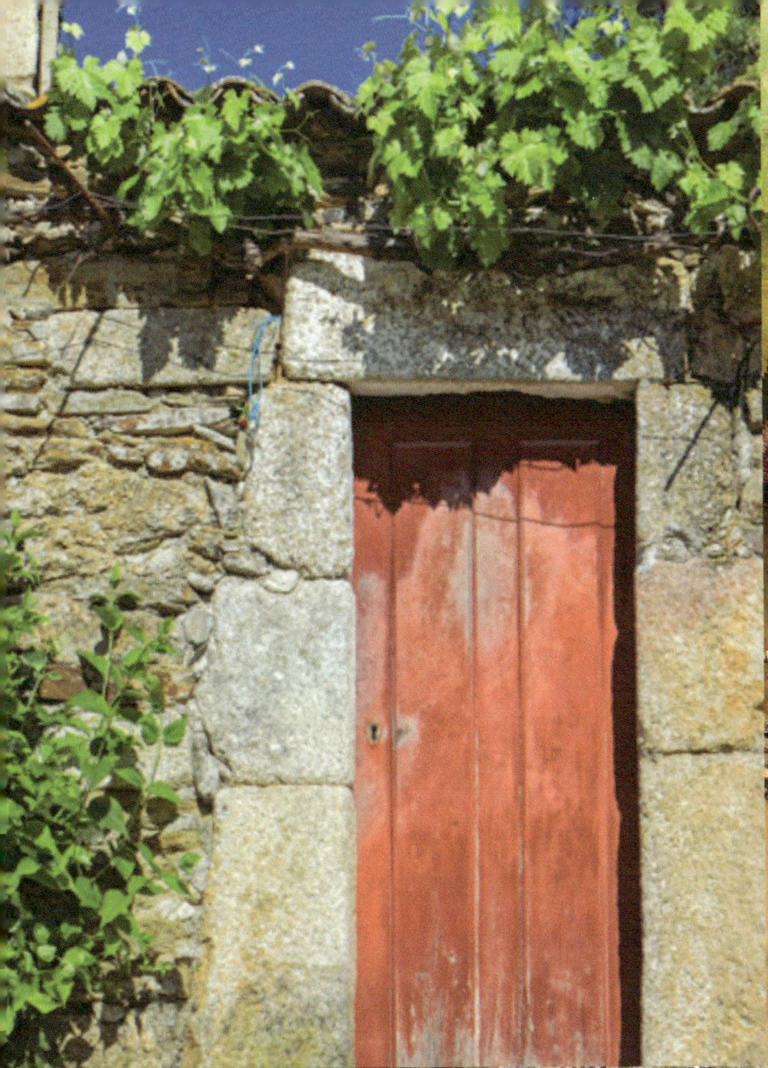

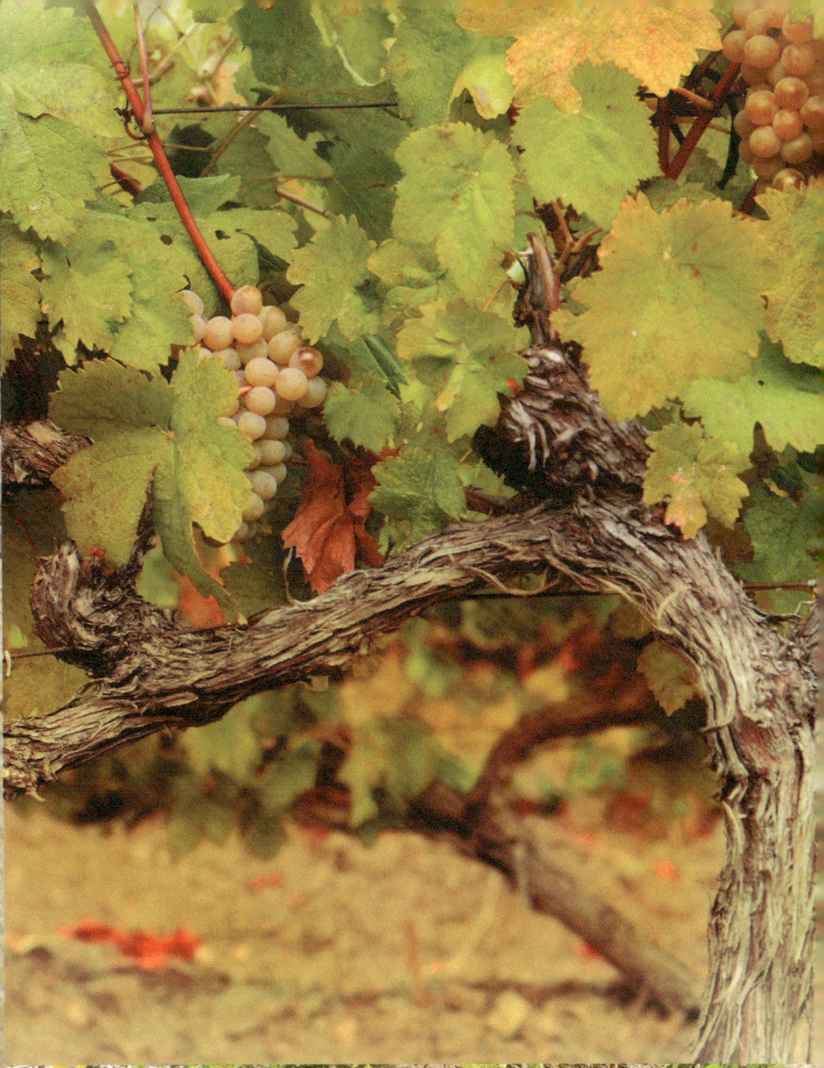

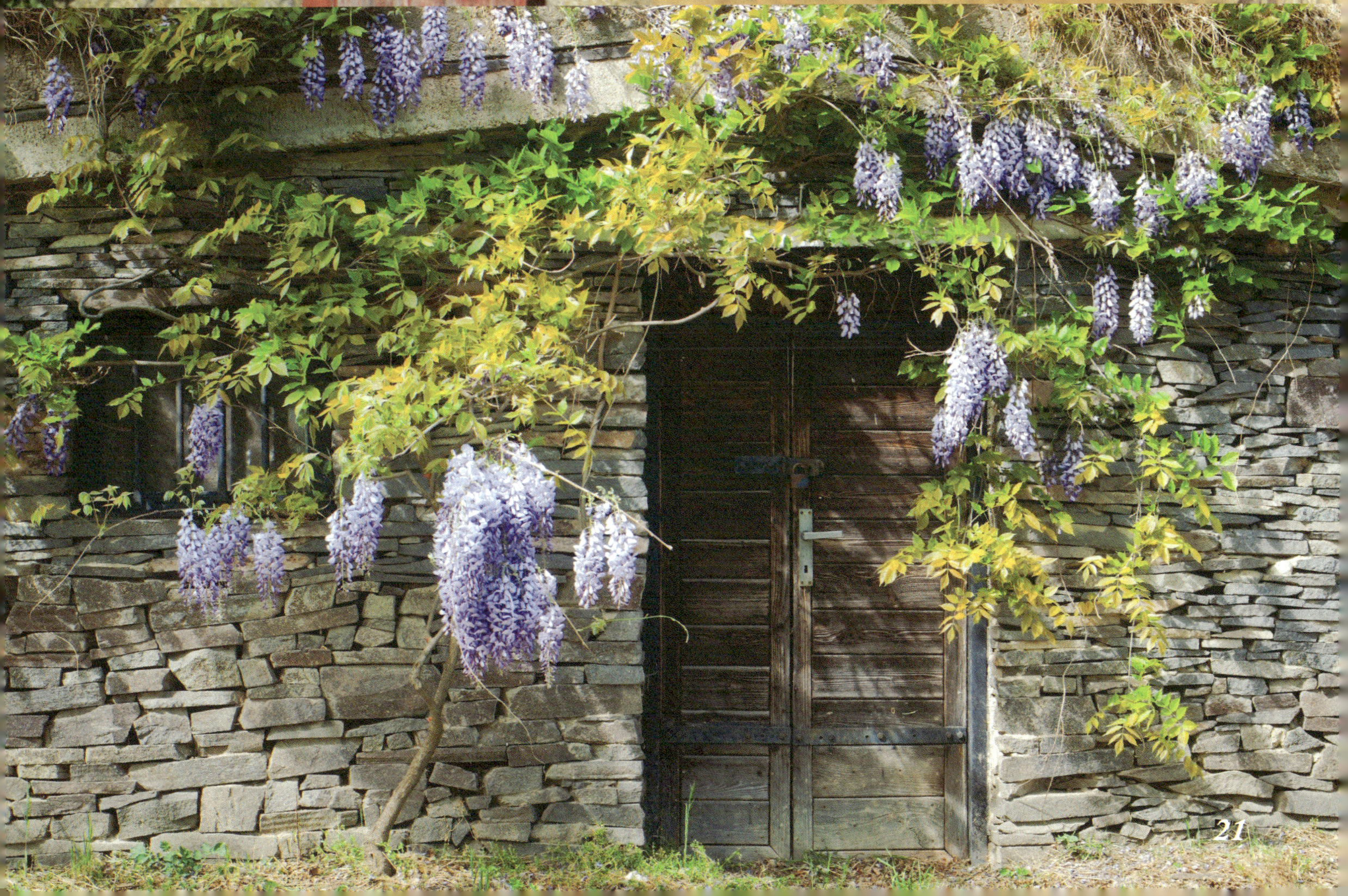

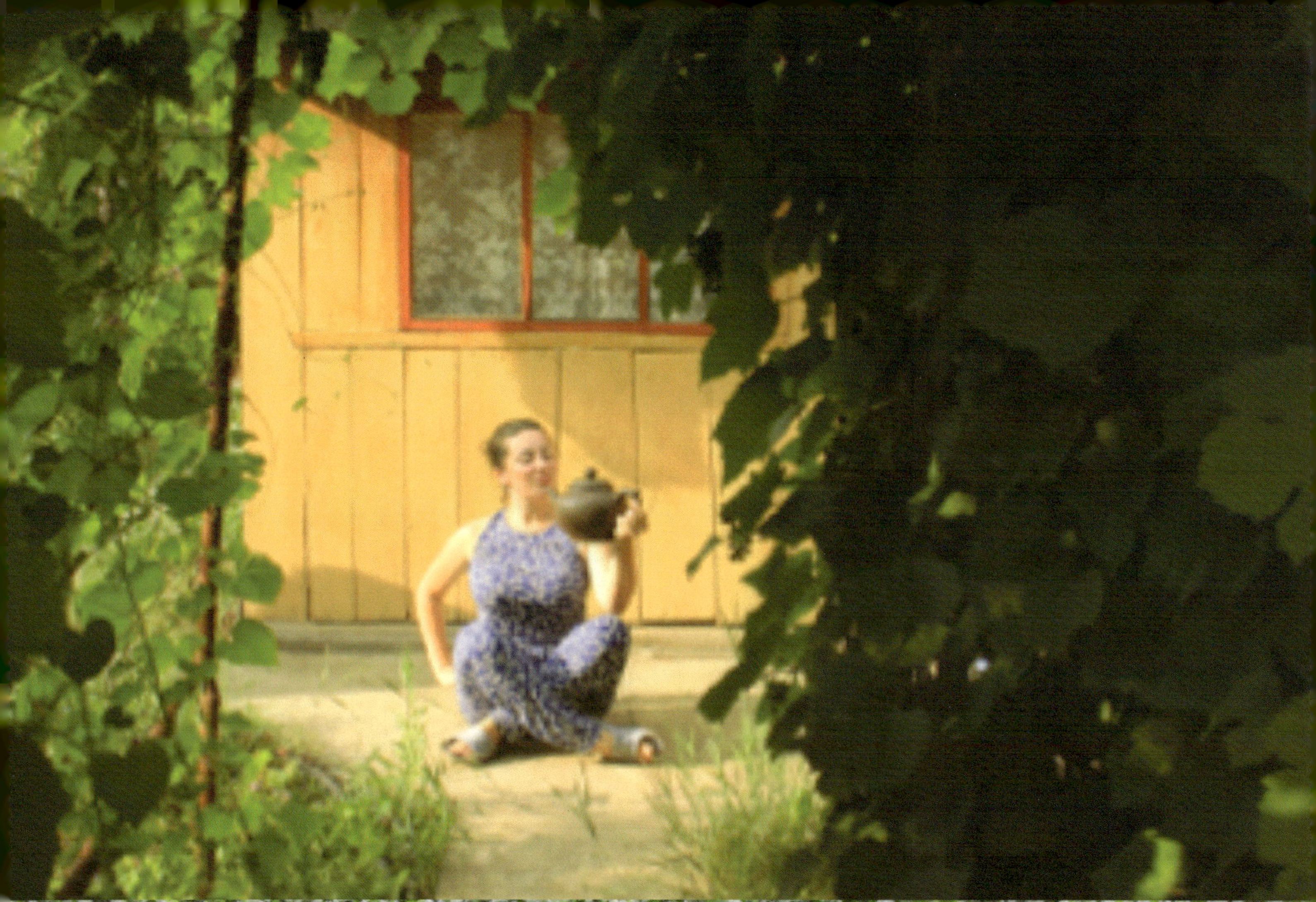

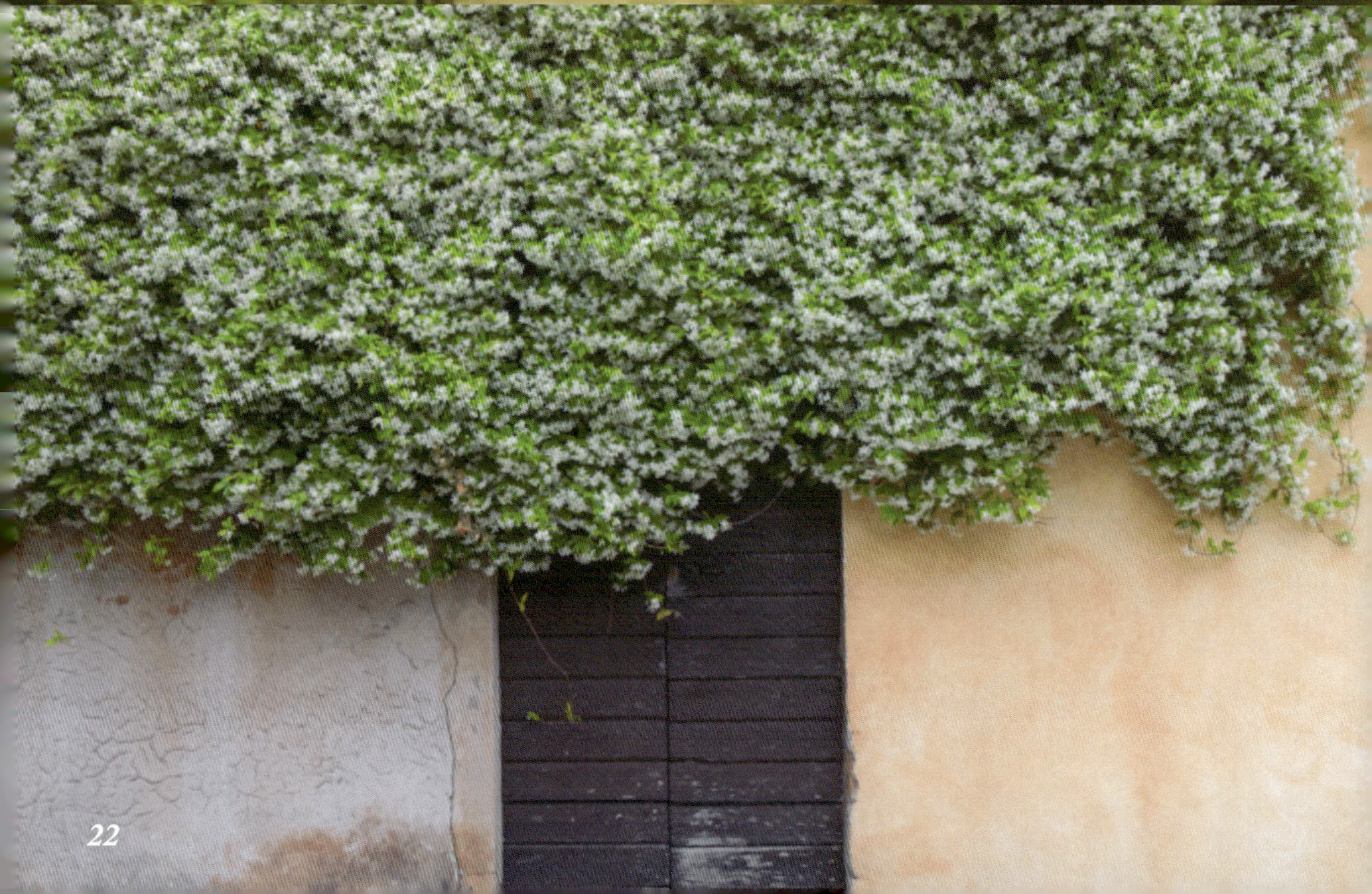

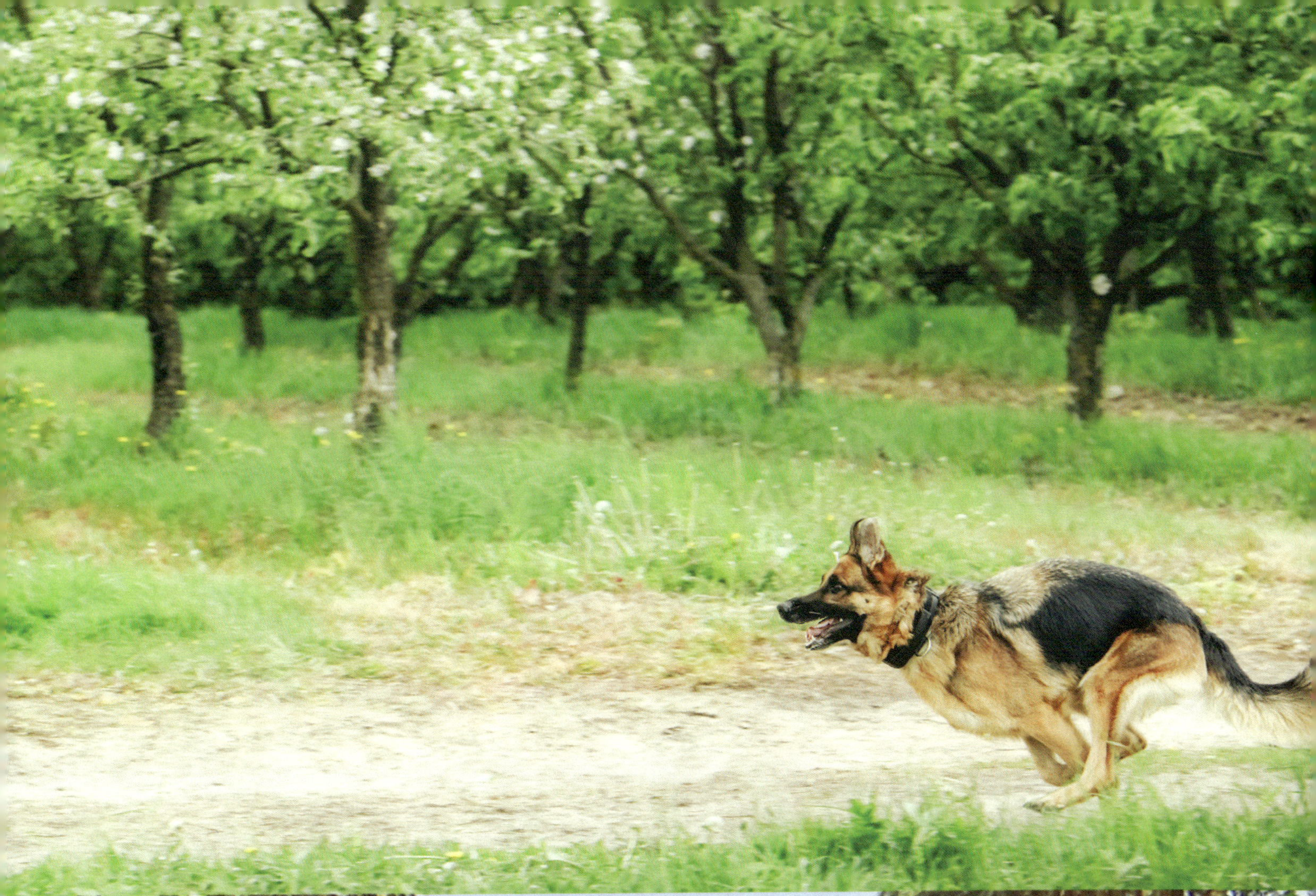
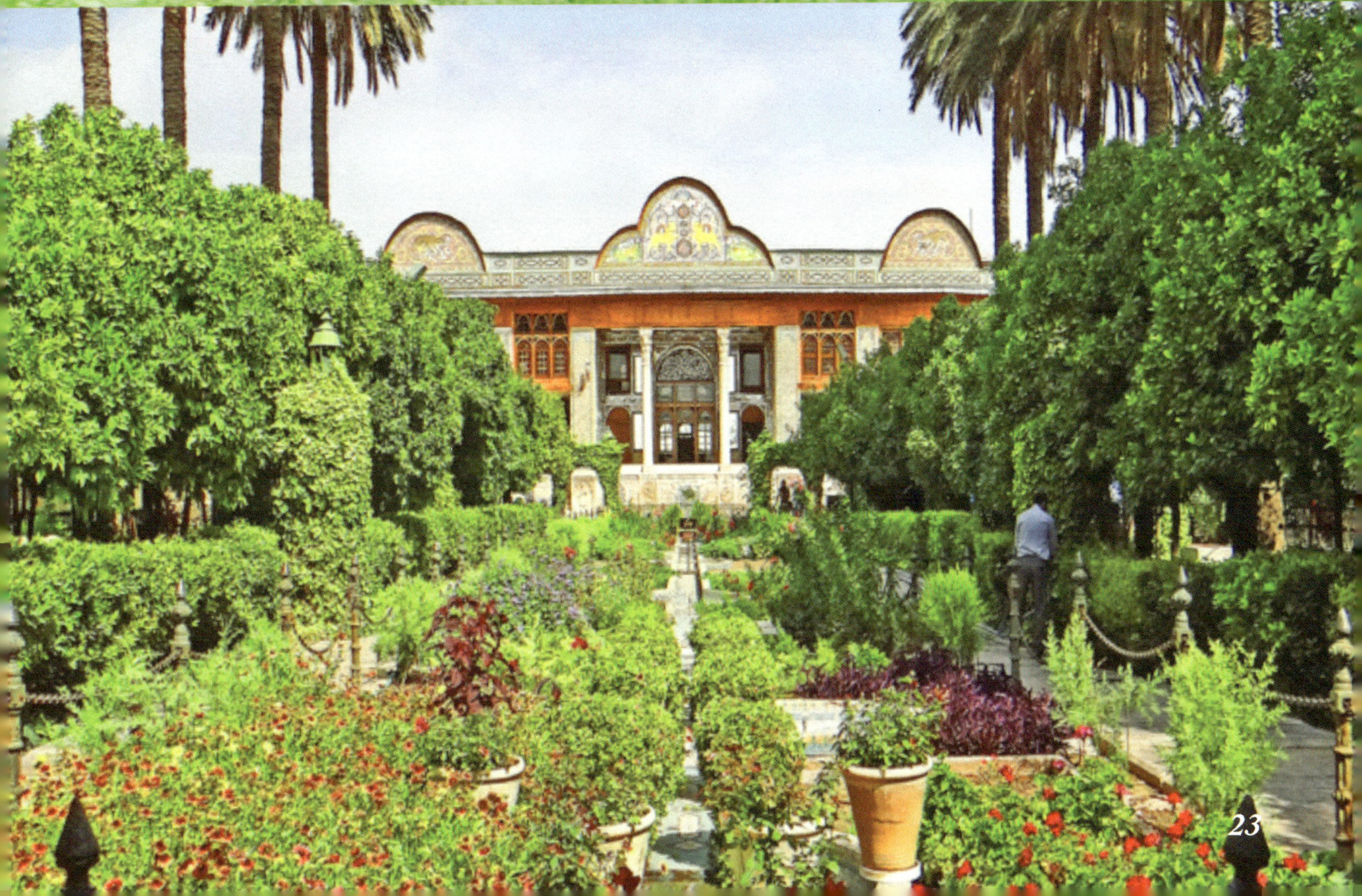

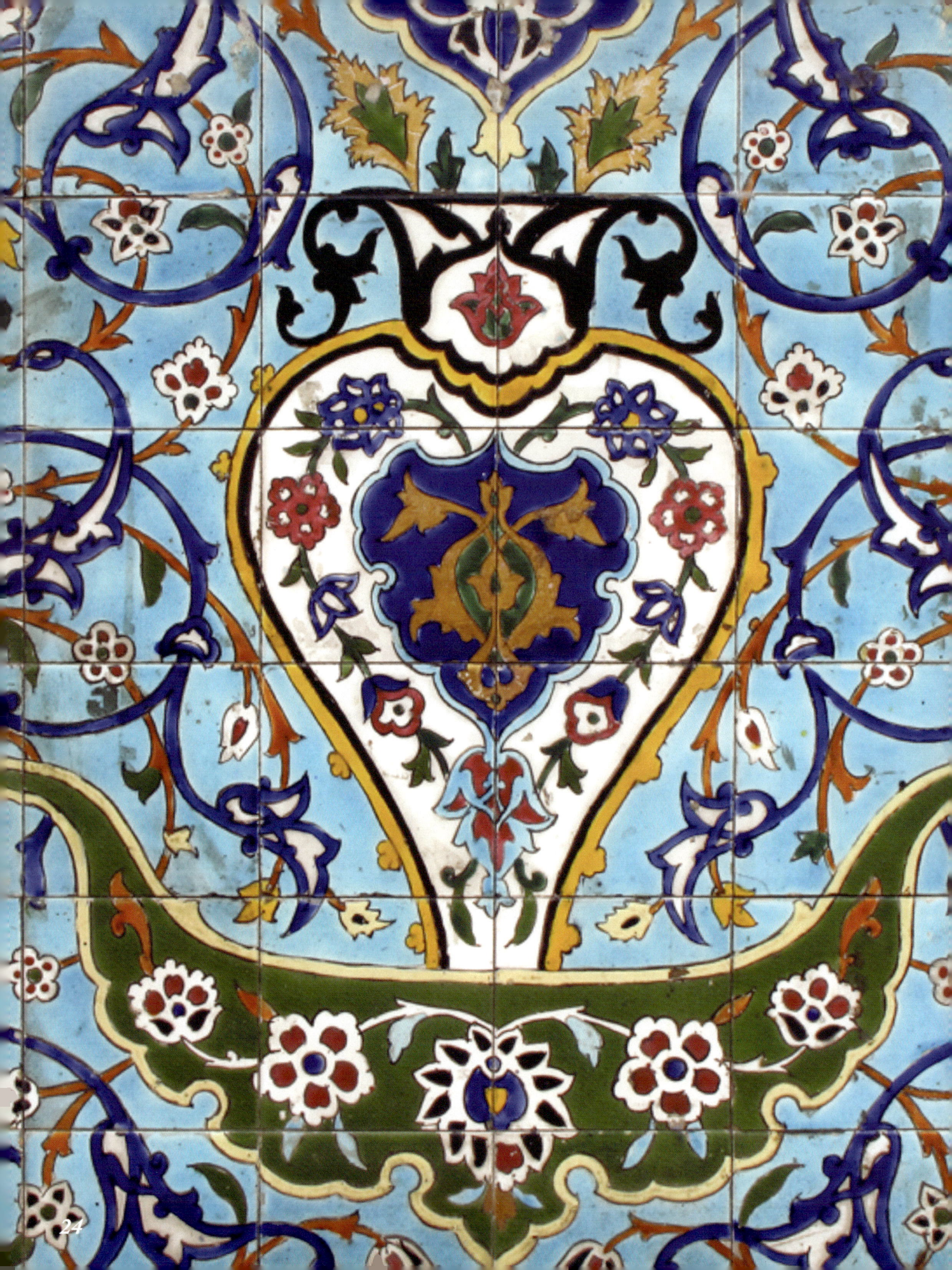

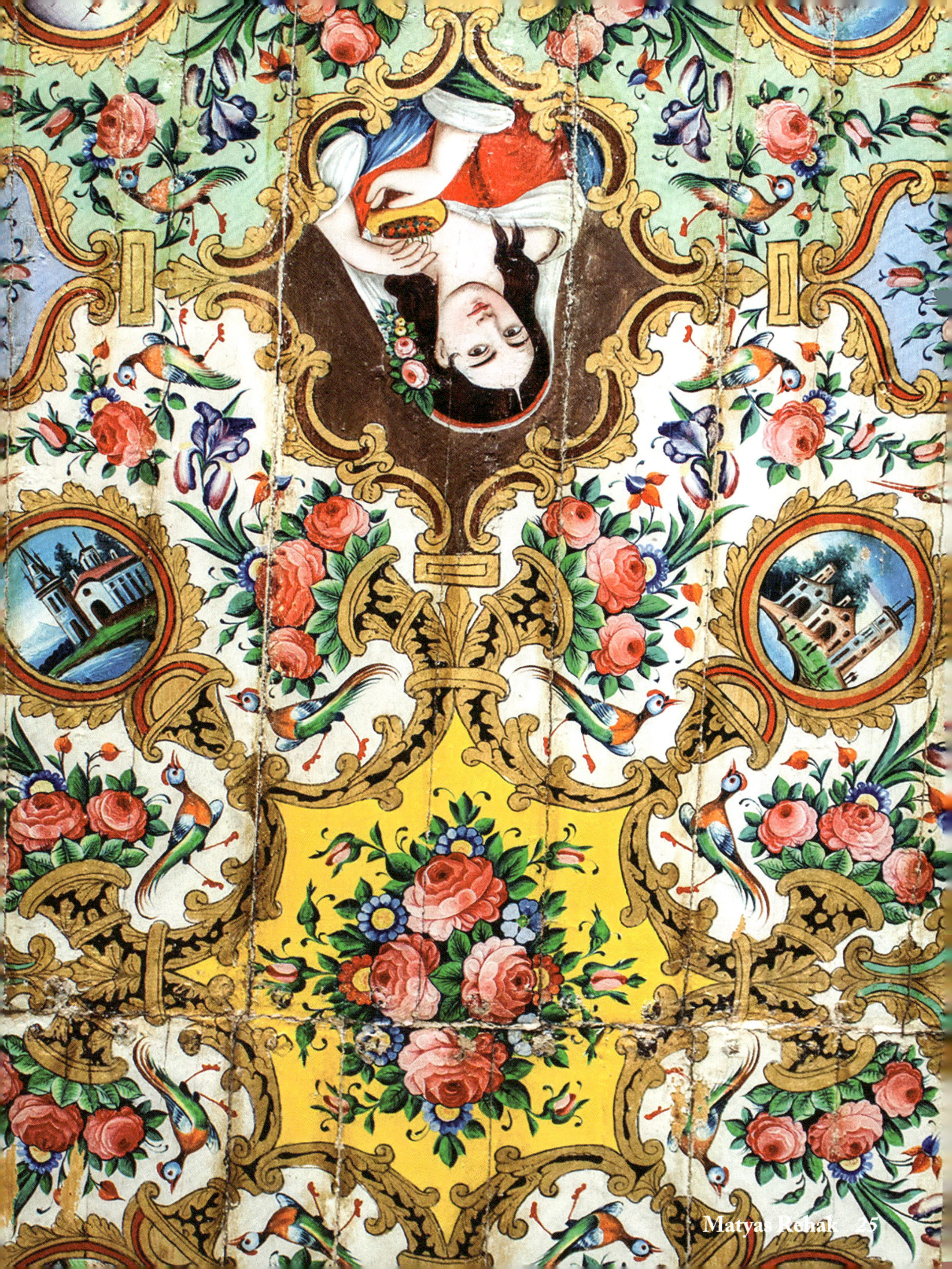

Matyas Rehak

THE STORY OF THE GOLDEN OIL

As a child Mamanjoon told me a story. It was summer day and a young neighbor's son came over to my grandmother's house to play with her children. The family had a German shepherd that was very close to my Aunt, Nana. As the kids played in the garden and the young boy wrestled with Nana, the dog mistakenly thought that he was trying to hurt her. So he attacked the boy and took a big chunk out of his ankle. When the gardener rushed to get Mamanjoon, she immediately sent him off to get her magic oil from the (zirzamin), the cellar room where she stored all her potions.

He ran back carrying the big dark lapis blue bottle, a bottle of orange Mercurochrome (a disinfectant to clean wounds used back then) and bandages. Mamanjoon kissed the boy and held him a while to calm him down from his hysterical crying and reassured him that everything would soon be all right. She proceeded to clean the wound – the calf muscle was apparently hanging from the cut. She placed the muscle back in place and gathered the skin together. The gardener very carefully dripped the golden oil into her left palm and she rubbed it all over the wound, while holding it in place with the other hand. Together she and the gardener wrapped the bandage around the boy's calf. She then gave him some fresh lemonade and sent him off.

So you ask what was the golden oil that was kept in the lapis blue jar? Well, it was castor oil into which were infused scorpions that had been caught in the garden. It turns out that scorpion oil has amazing healing abilities. The story goes on. Mamanjoon sent the butler to the boy's house to ask his mother if he could sleep over for a night or two as other family children were coming over and they would have great fun. On the third day Mamanjoon called the feisty young boy and removed the bandage to check on the wound. The skin was firmly attached, the calf muscle in place and there remained only a faint pink line to show where the horrible wound had been. And he was in no pain or distress.

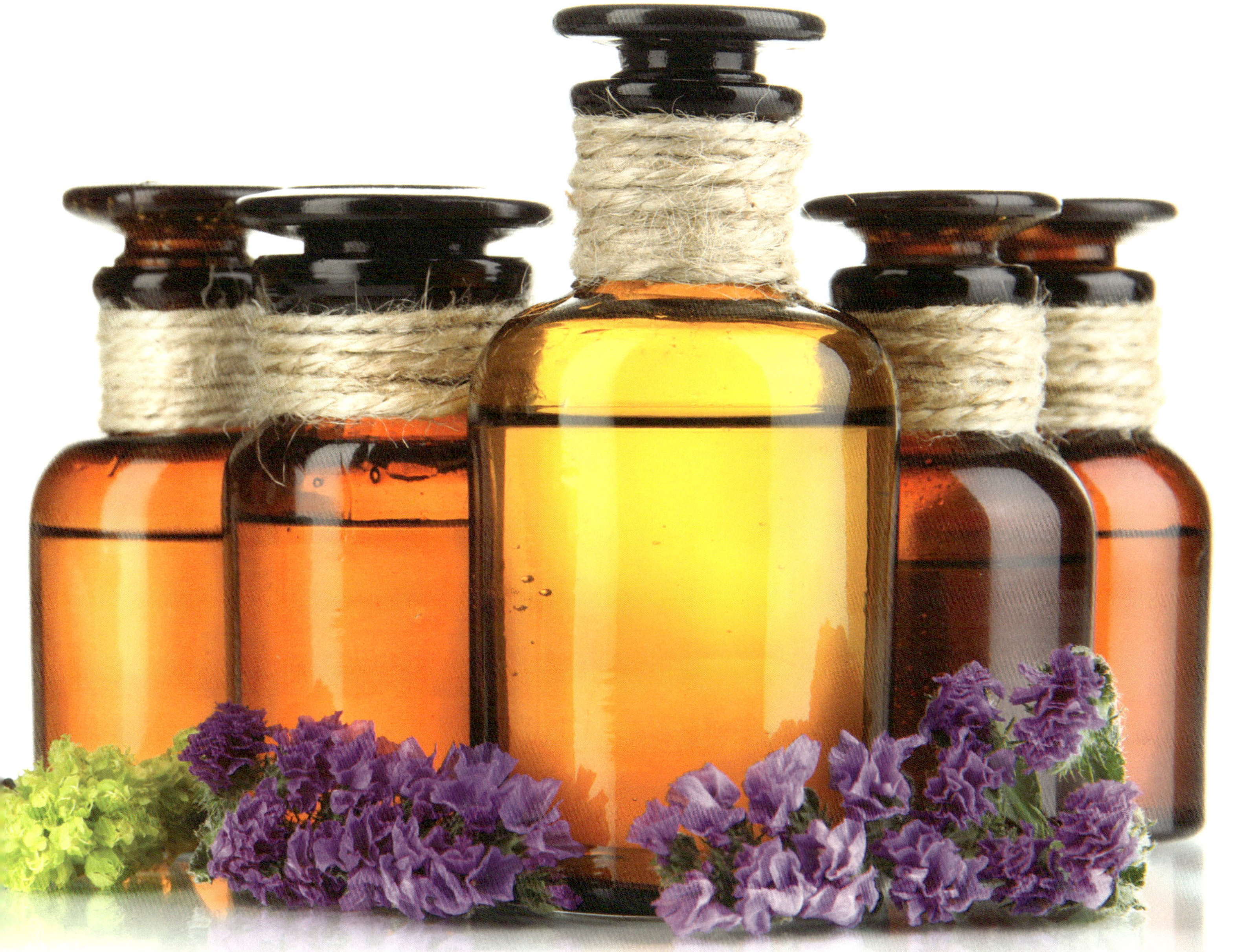

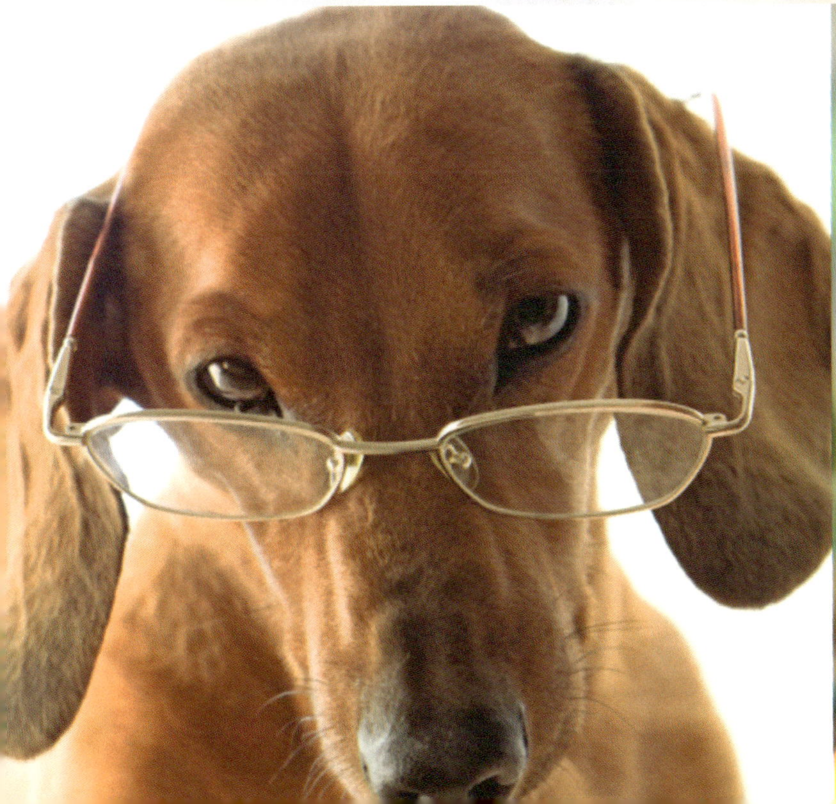

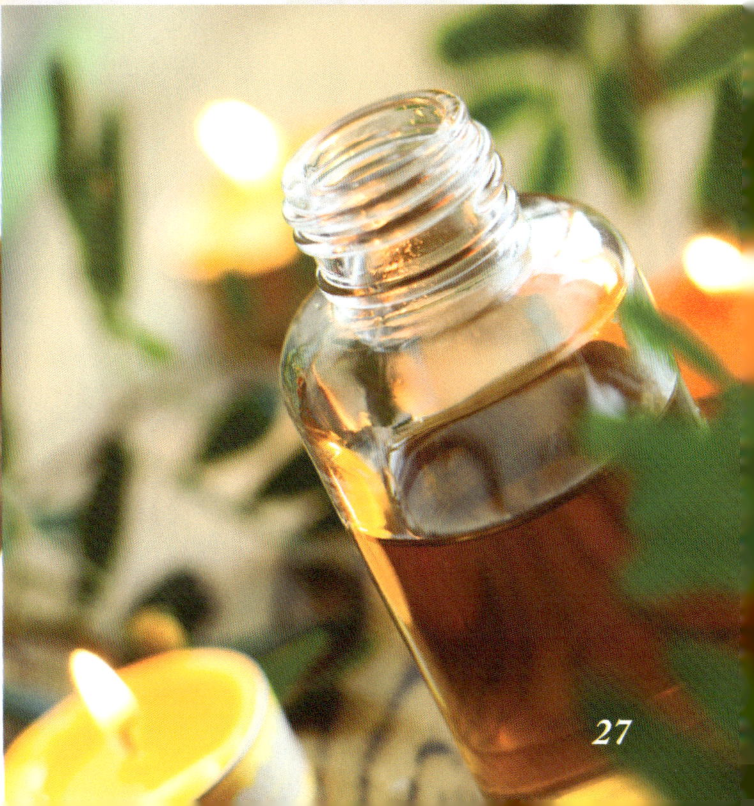

THE HEAVENLY SPICE

Mamanjoon called turmeric the spice from the heavens. I could write a book alone on just on turmeric's healing benefits internally as well as its topical use.

Turmeric is one the most thoroughly researched plants in existence today. Its medicinal properties and components (primarily curcumin) have been the subject of over 5,600 peer-reviewed and published biomedical studies to date.

The bright yellow root has been used in folk medicine for centuries and has now become valued by the medical community. There have been thousands of studies proving how the powerful spice works for so many conditions including cancer, high cholesterol, blood pressure, diabetes, arthritis and depression. It is great for bones and joints and has anti-inflammatory properties. It's even used in beauty treatments to alleviate psoriasis and remove dark spots. As a mouthwash it freshens the breath.

Turmeric is also a natural liver detoxifier and a kidney cleanser, and it speeds metabolism and aids in weight management. It's about as close to a panacea as you can get. It is said: If you use turmeric before meals it acts on the throat and lungs. If you use it during the meal it acts on the digestive system. If you use it after a meal it acts on the colon and kidneys.

The root of this miraculous spice is sold in ethnic markets and health food stores, and the powder is found in the spice section of your local supermarket.

TURMERIC WARNING
Do not consume turmeric if you suffer from bile disease because turmeric causes muscle contraction in the gallbladder.

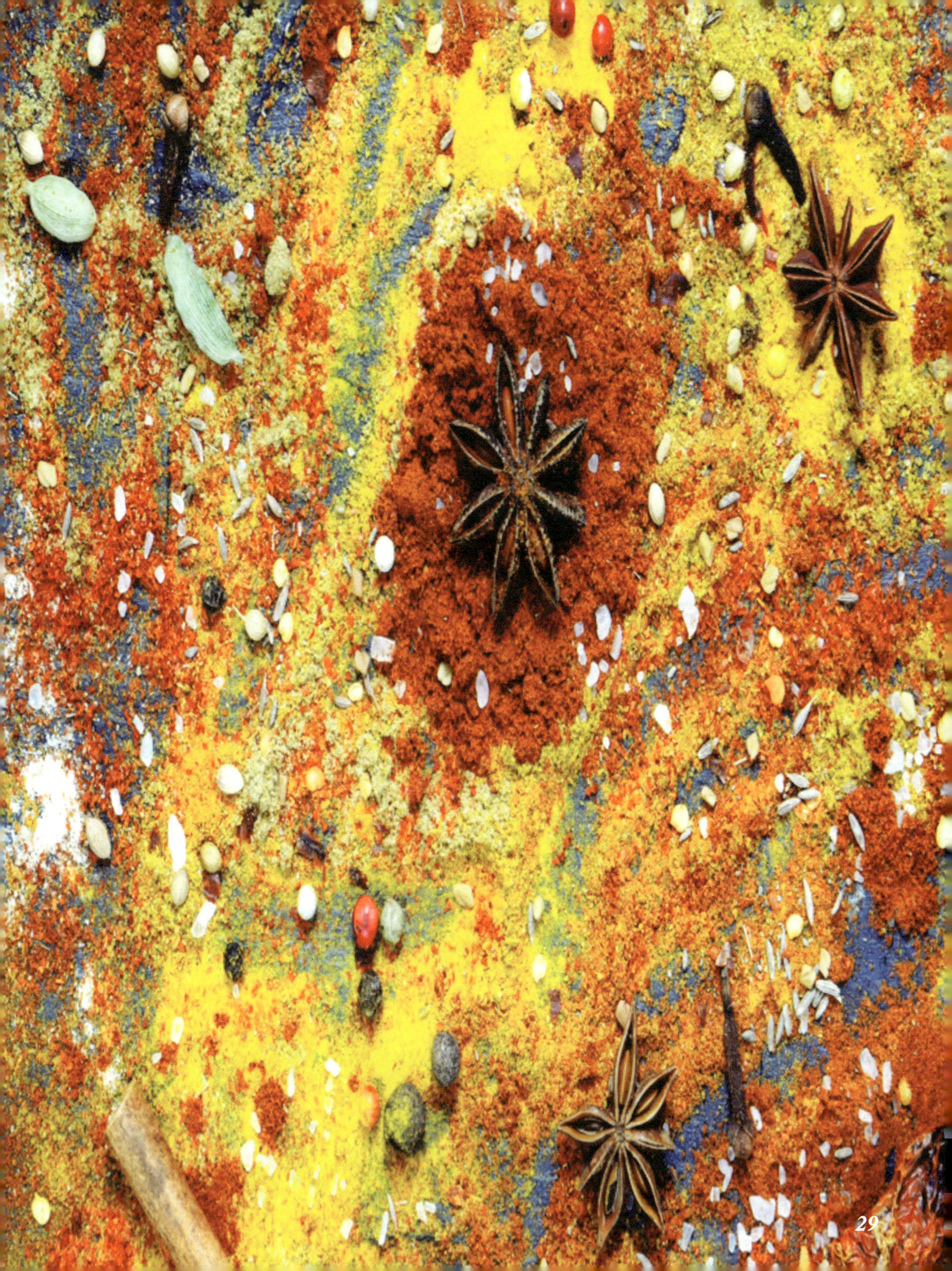

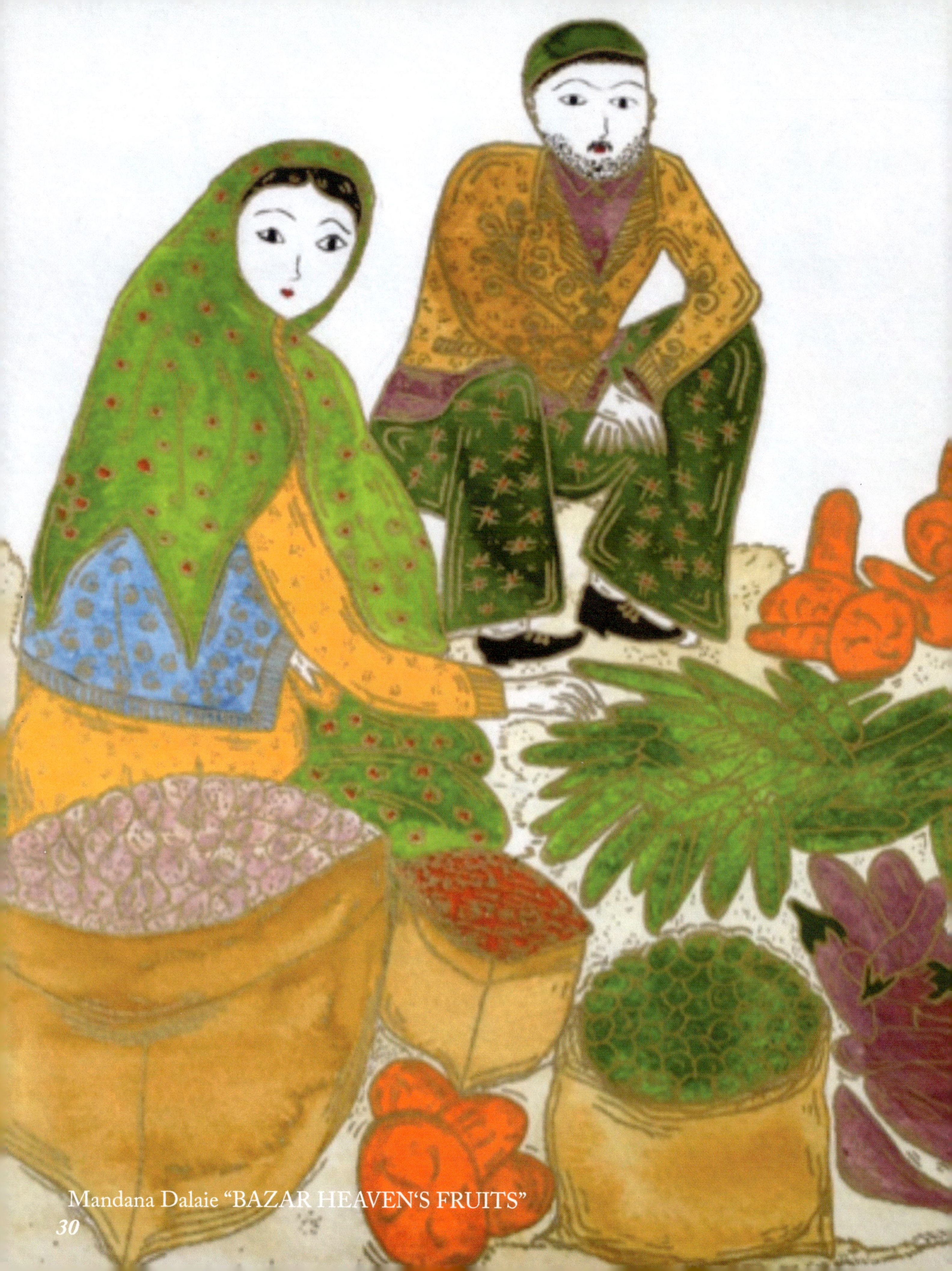

Mandana Dalaie “BAZAR HEAVEN‘S FRUITS”

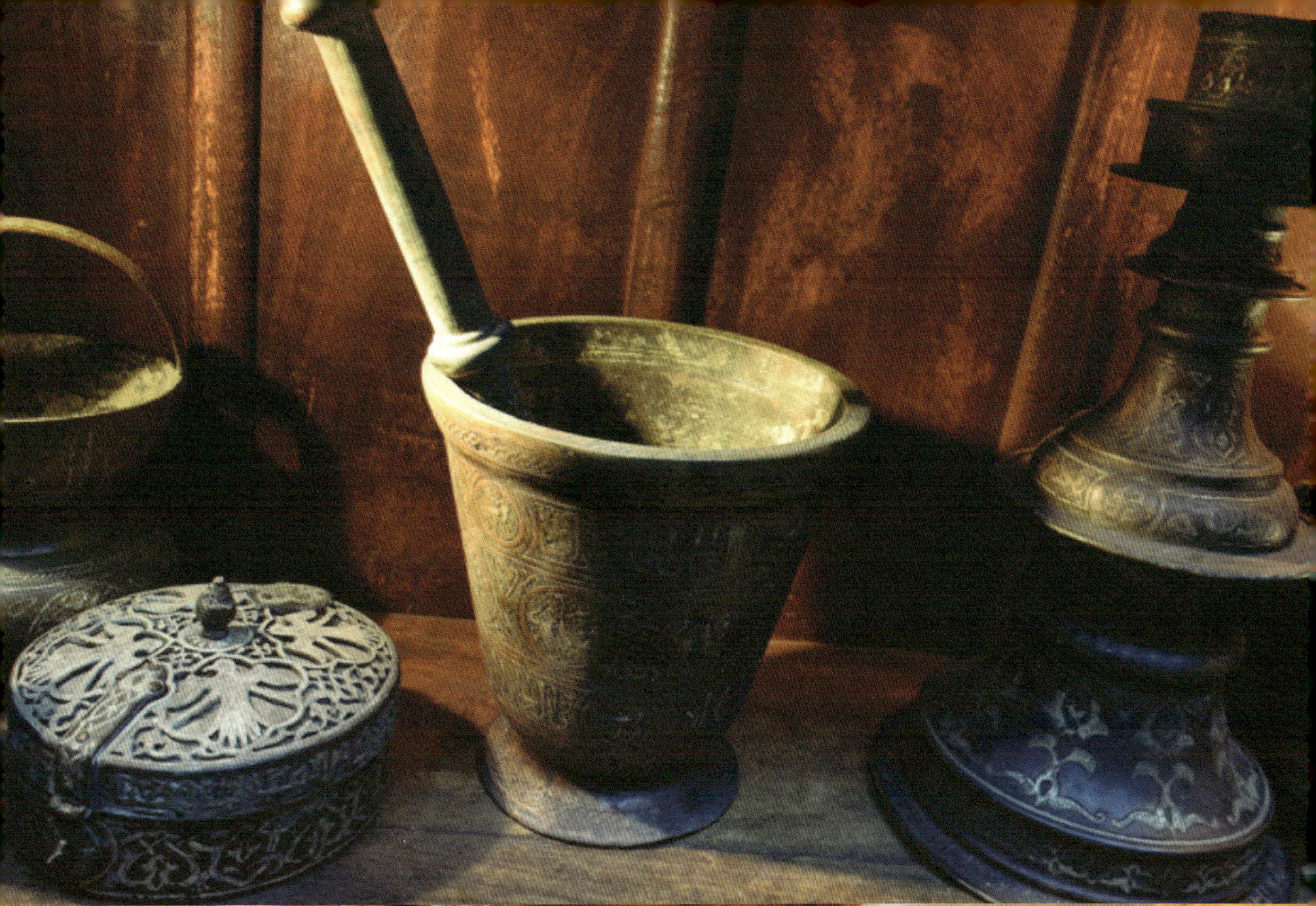

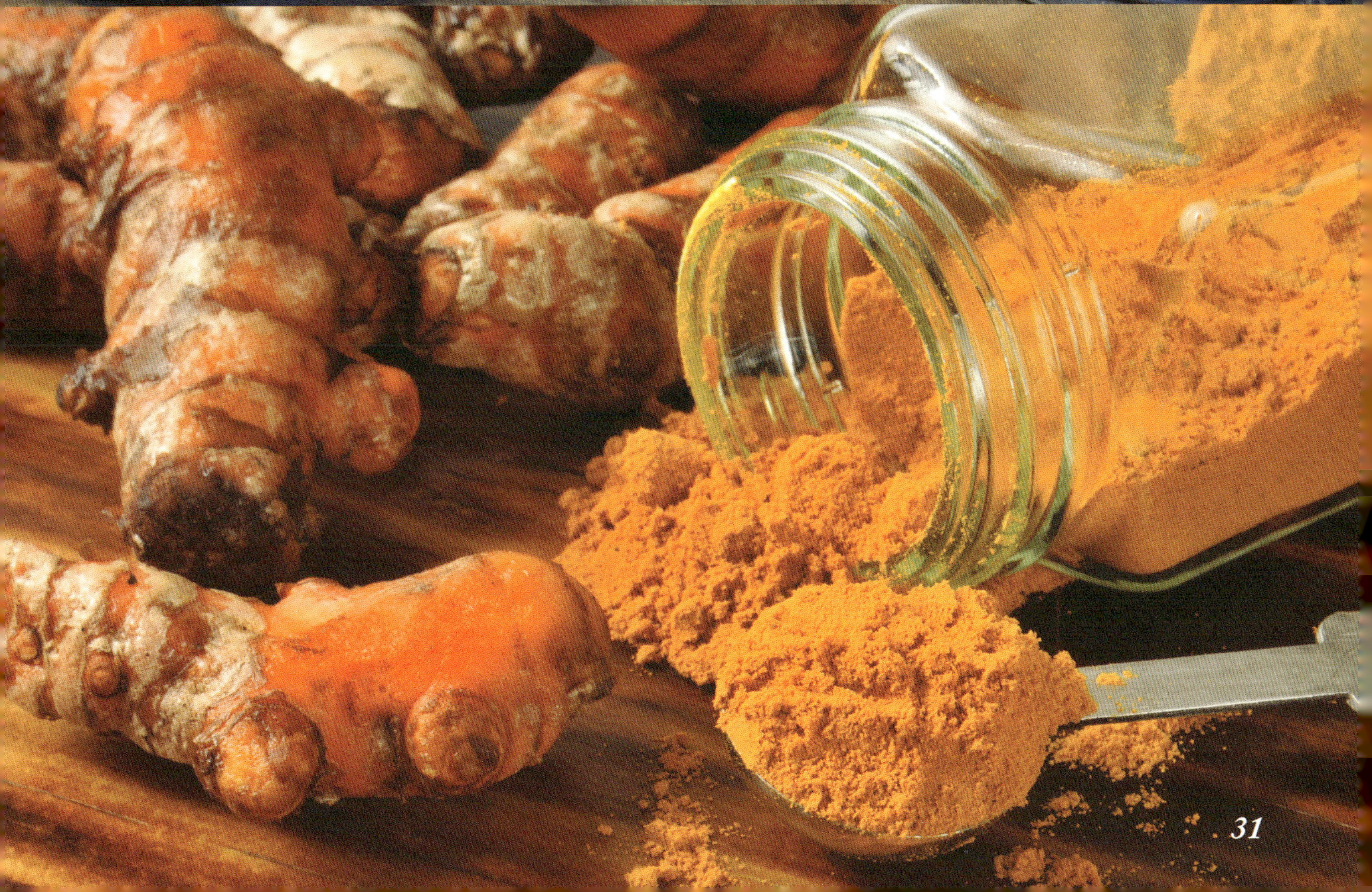

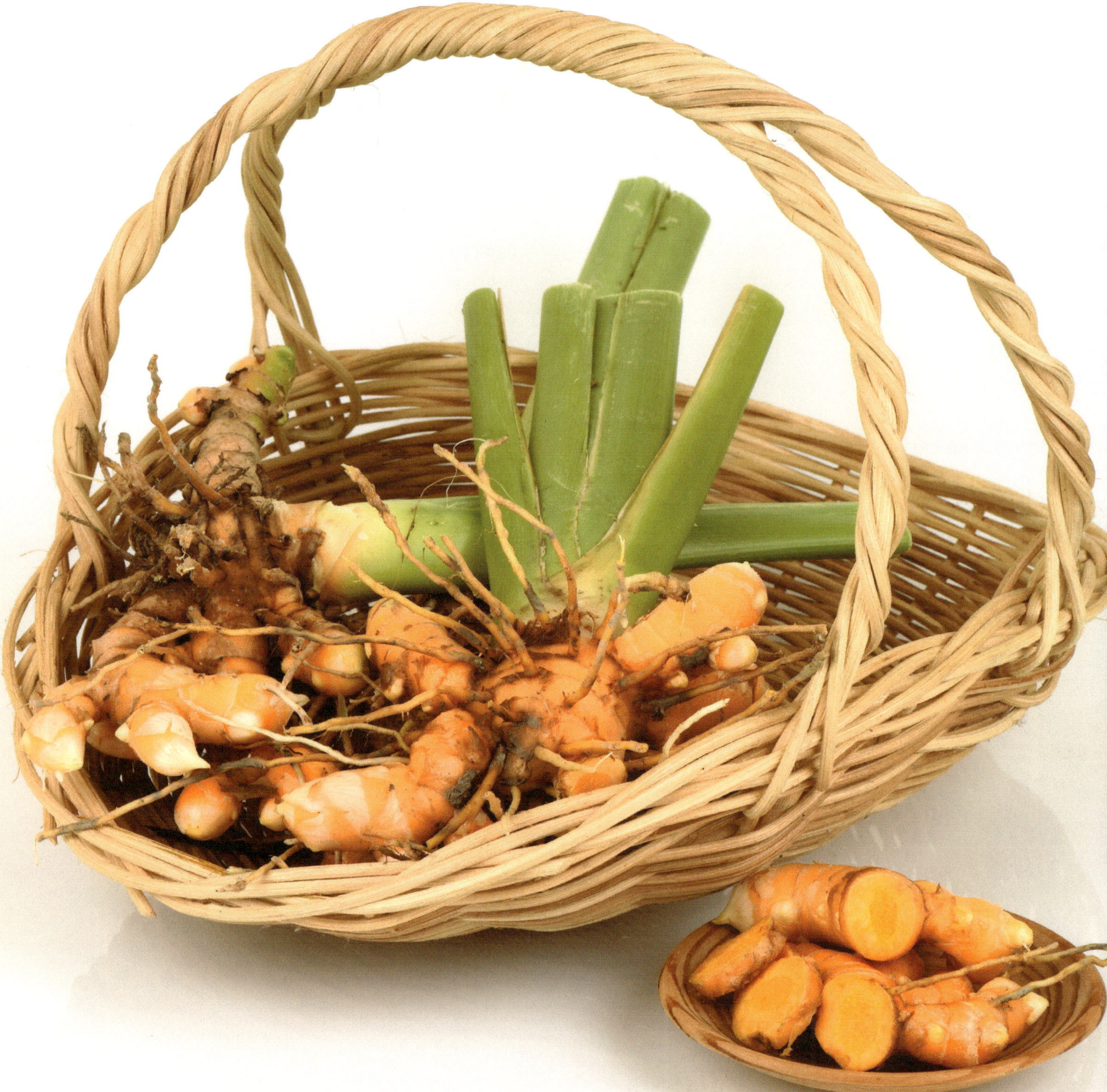

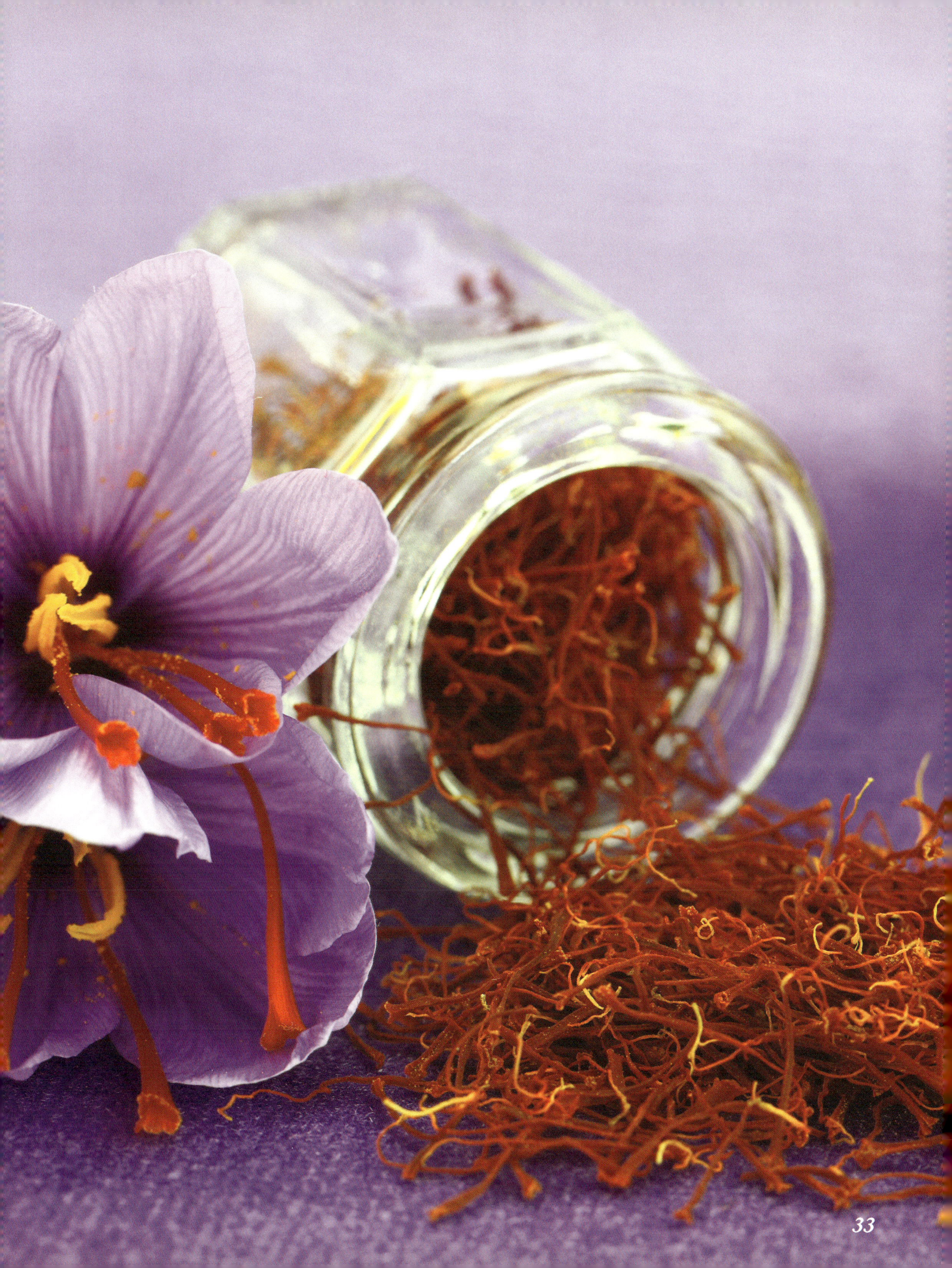

TONICS

CINNAMON ELIXIR

Arthritis cure

2 Tablespoons cinnamon powder (Ceylonese or Vietnamese)
1 Tablespoon raw honey
Pinch of saffron
8 oz of hot filtered water

Mix well and drink in the morning upon rising (30 minutes before breakfast) and in the evening before bed.

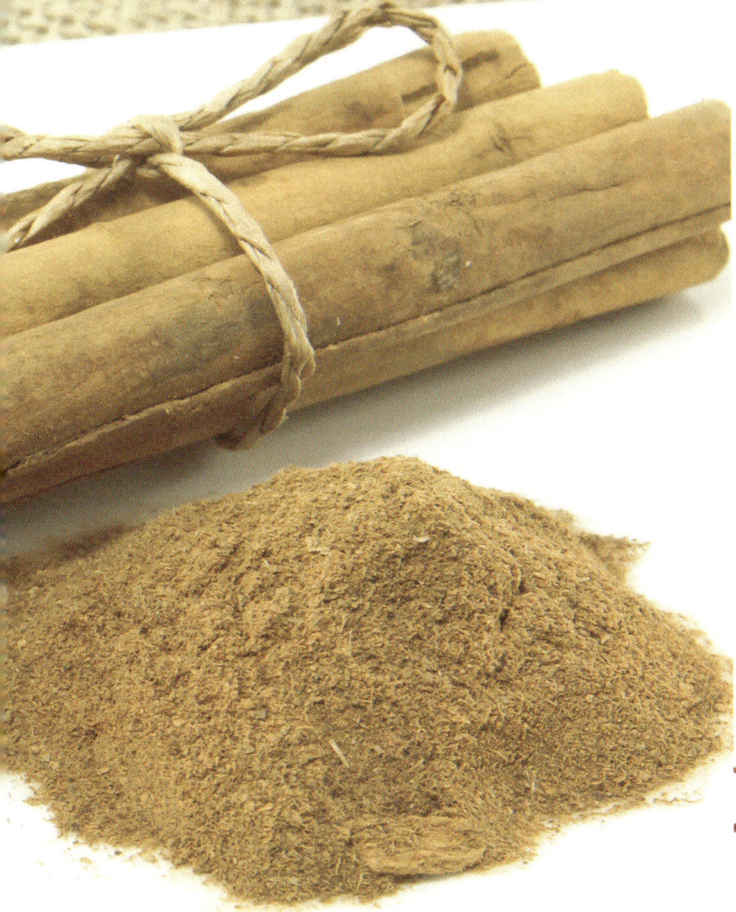
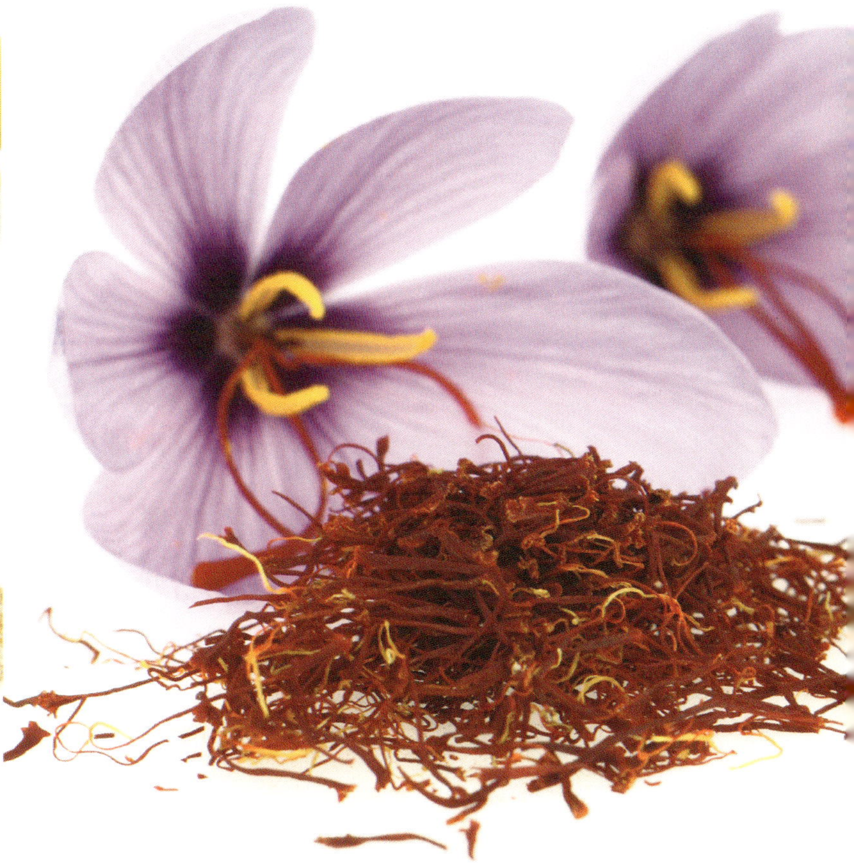
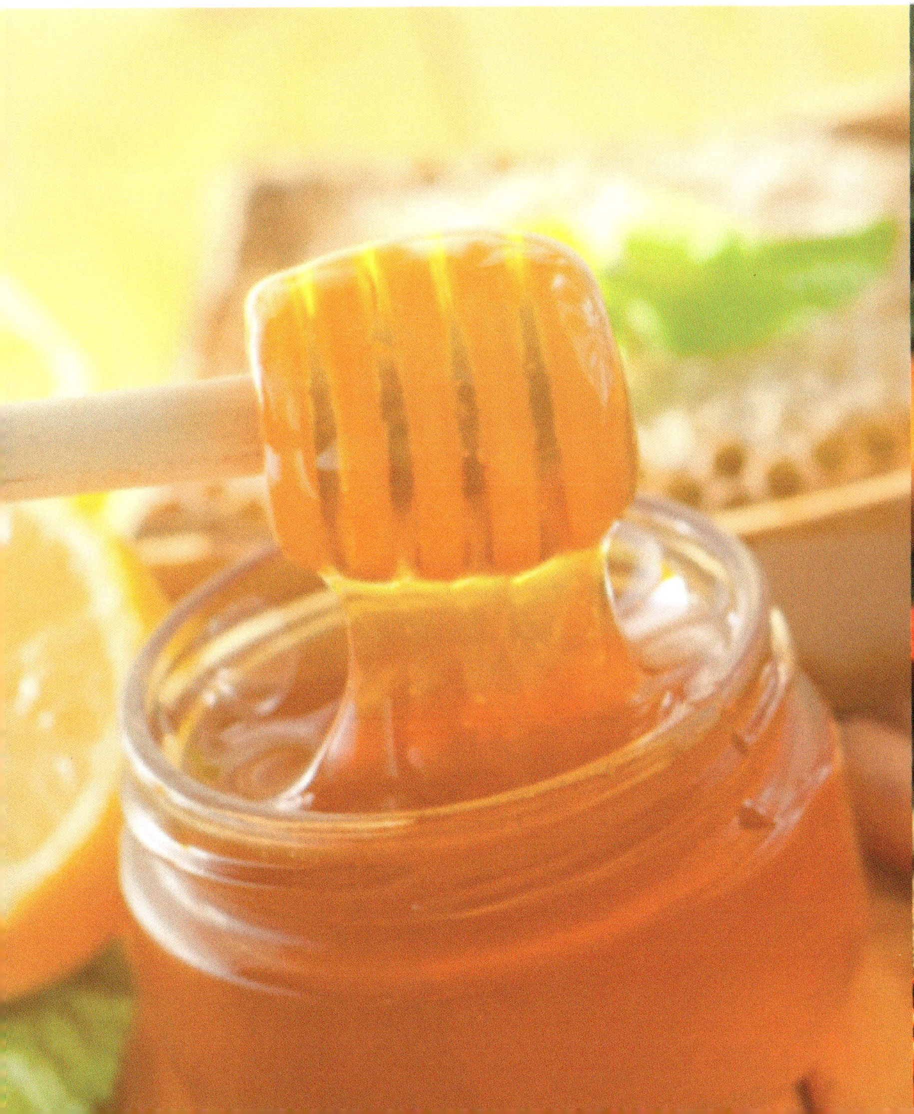
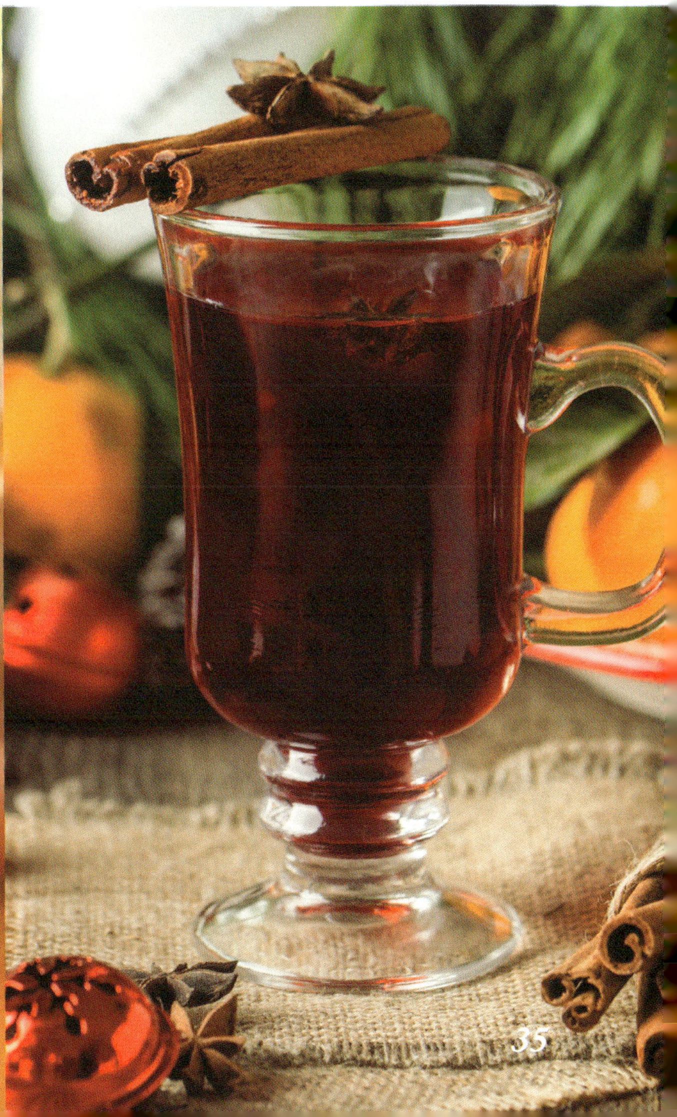

GOLDEN MILK

5 Tablespoons of turmeric powder
1 Tablespoon of raw honey
1/4 oz of water
Glass of raw cow or goat milk or almond milk

Put saucepan on low heat with water and add turmeric, use wooden spoon to stir until it becomes a paste. Let cool, then store in a glass bowl or mason jar in the fridge.

On daily basis put a teaspoon of turmeric paste in a small saucepan and heat with milk of choice (preferably raw unpasteurized), then add raw honey.

Drink three or four times a day for detoxing body, to build the Immune system and to get rid of allergies or sinus issues.

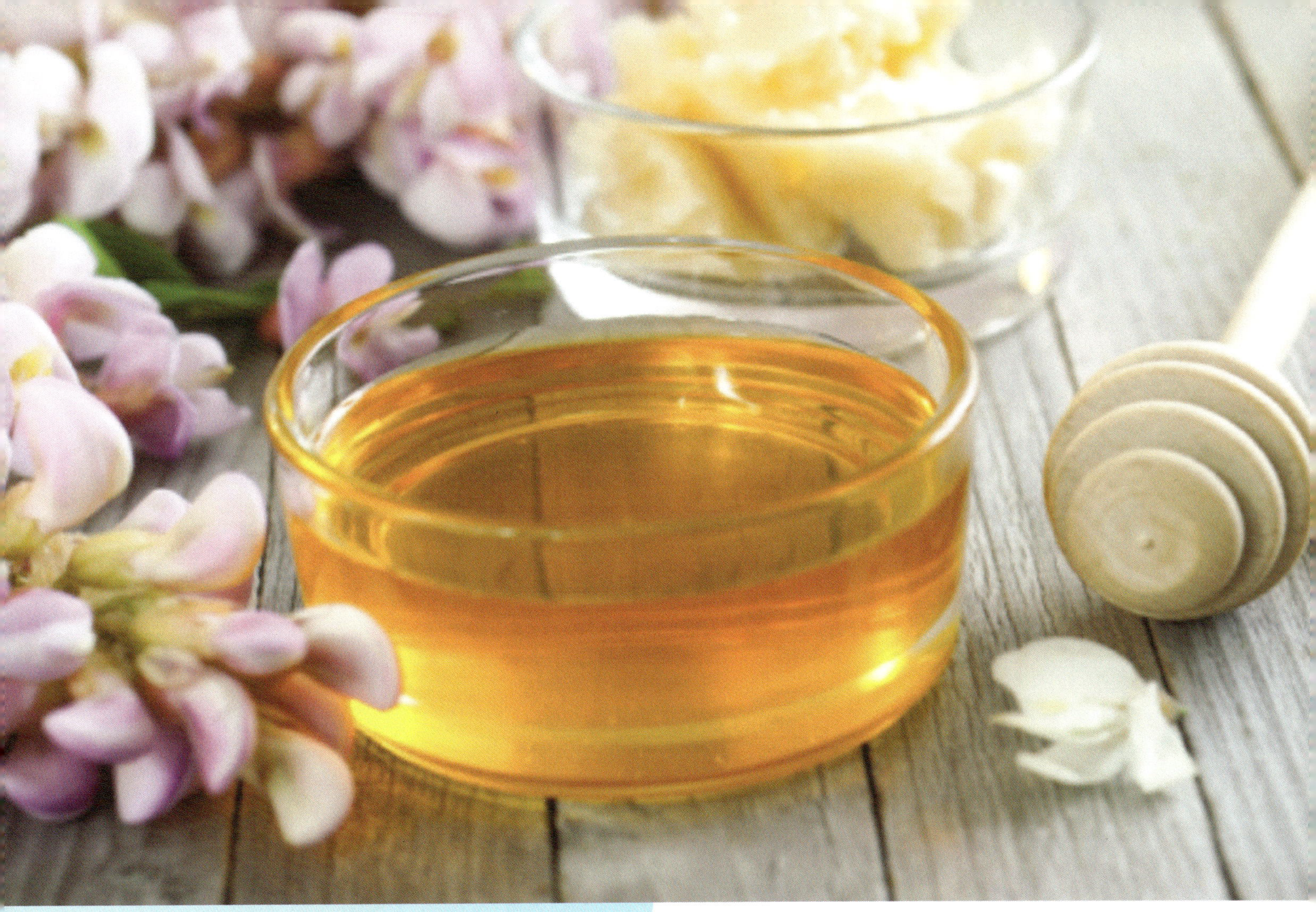

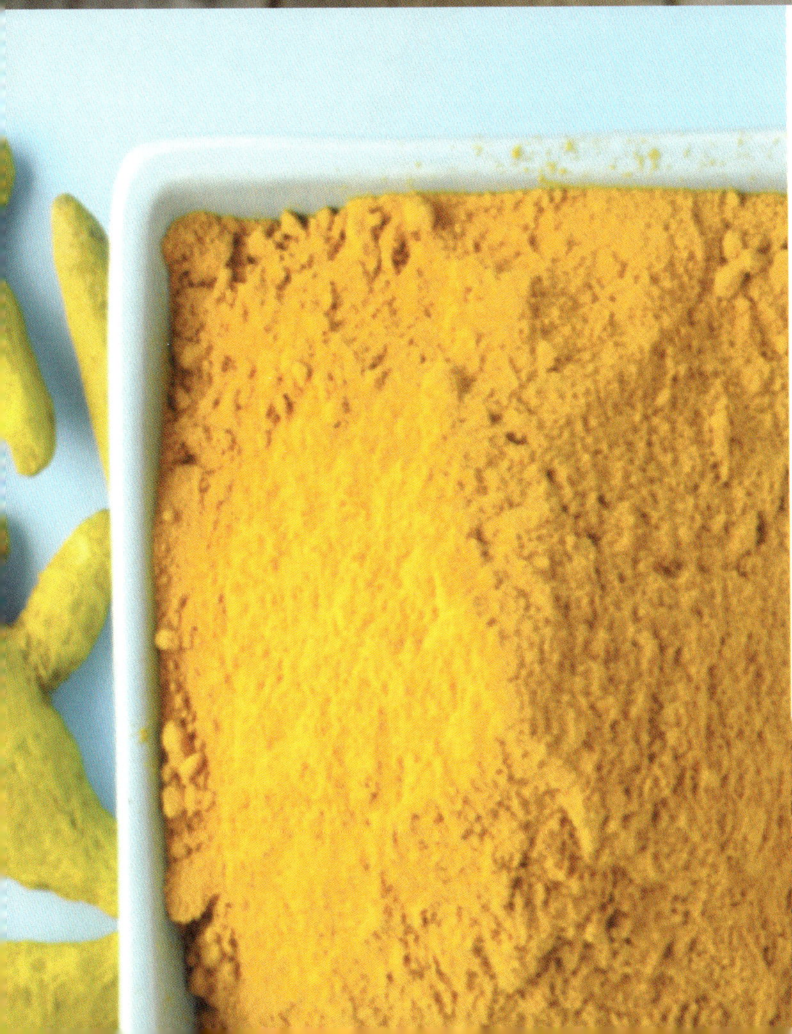

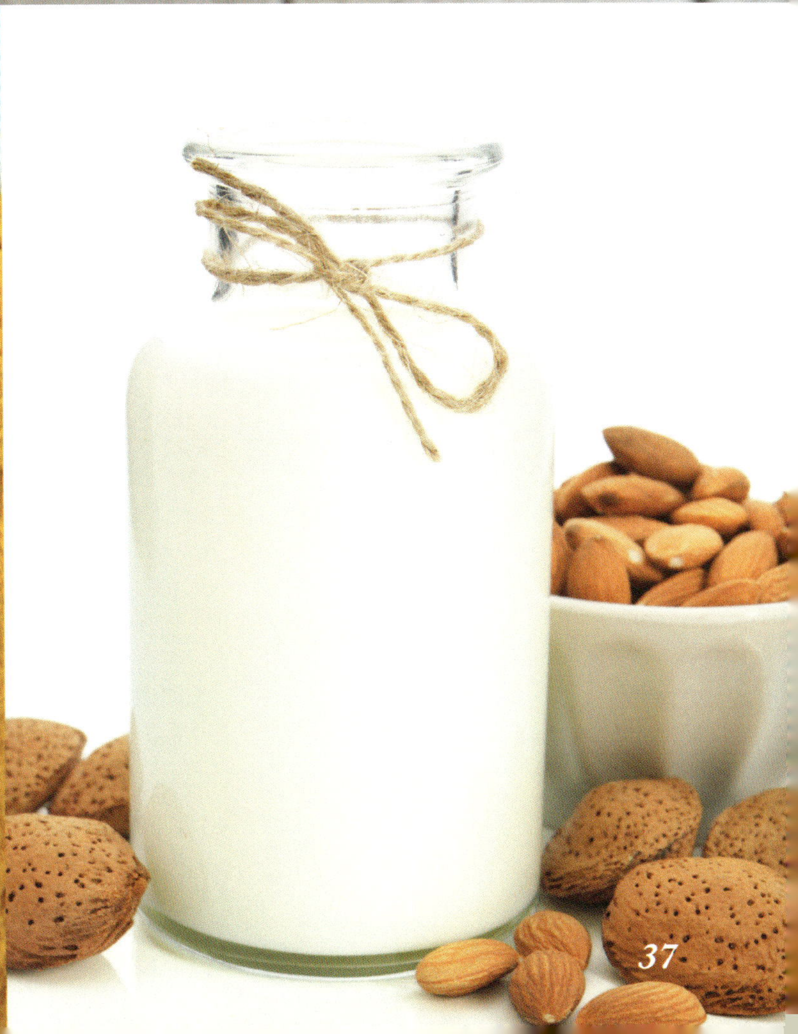

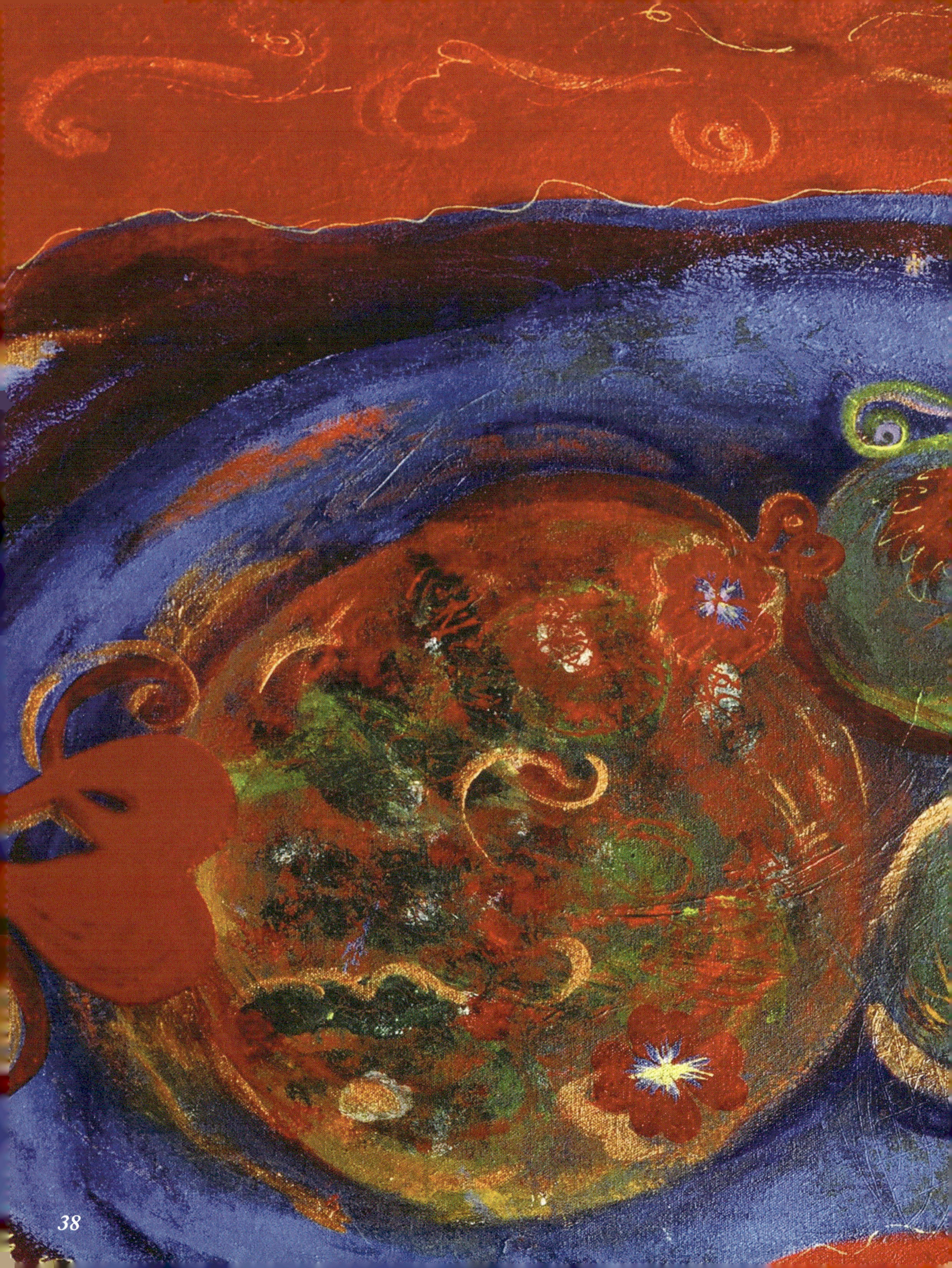

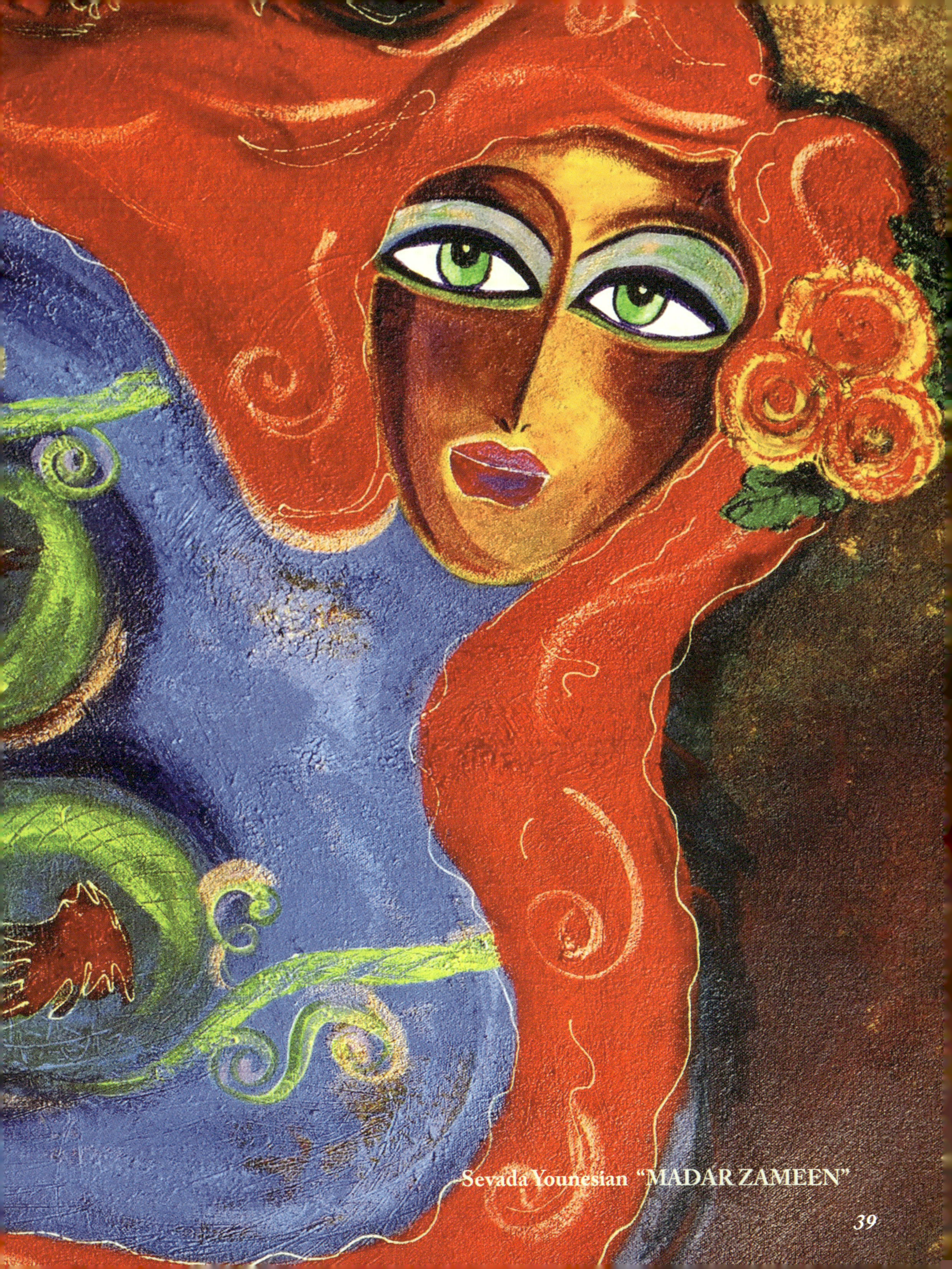

Sevada Younesian "MADAR ZAMEEN"

SPICY WINTER TONIC

Antibiotic/Antiviral/Antifungal/Anti-Parasitic

You'll want to keep this immune-strengthening tonic on hand all winter. A powerful combination of natural and fresh healing components, it has helped millions of people throughout the ages to fight countless chronic conditions and diseases.

Wear gloves during the preparation, especially when handling hot peppers, because it is difficult to get the tingling off your hands! Be careful, its smell is very strong, and it may stimulate the sinuses instantly.

- *24 oz apple cider vinegar (always use raw, unfiltered, organic (e.g.Braggs)*
- *¼ cup finely chopped garlic*
- *¼ cup finely chopped onion*
- *2 fresh chili peppers (the hottest you can find – be careful cleaning (Wear gloves!!!)*
- *¼ cup grated ginger*
- *2 Tablespoons grated horseradish*
- *2 Tablespoons turmeric powder or 2 thumb-size pieces of turmeric root*

Combine all ingredients in a bowl except the vinegar. Transfer the mixture to a Mason jar. Pour in some apple cider vinegar and fill it to the top. (It is best if two-thirds consists of dry ingredients, the rest with vinegar. Close tightly and shake. Keep jar in a cool dry place for two weeks, shaking well several times a day. After two weeks squeeze well (using rubber gloves) and strain the liquid through a plastic strainer or gauze. Add the rest of the dry mixture to a soup or stew for an extra boost of nutrition.

Your master tonic is ready.

Caution: the flavor is very strong and hot!

Gargle and swallow. Do not dilute it in water as it will reduce the effect.

Take 1 tablespoon every day to strengthen the immune system and fight cold. Increase the amount every day until you reach a dose of 1 small glass per day (the size of a liquor glass). If you struggle against more serious disease or infection, take 1 tablespoon of the tonic 5-6 times a day. It is safe for pregnant women and children (use small doses!) because the ingredients are all-natural and contain no toxins.

You do not need to keep the tonic in your fridge. It will last for at least a year in a cool dark cupboard.

Tip: You can also use it in the kitchen – mix it with some olive oil and use it as a salad dressing or in your stews.

Extra Tip: Eat a slice of orange, lemon or lime after you take the tonic to ease the burning sensation and heat.

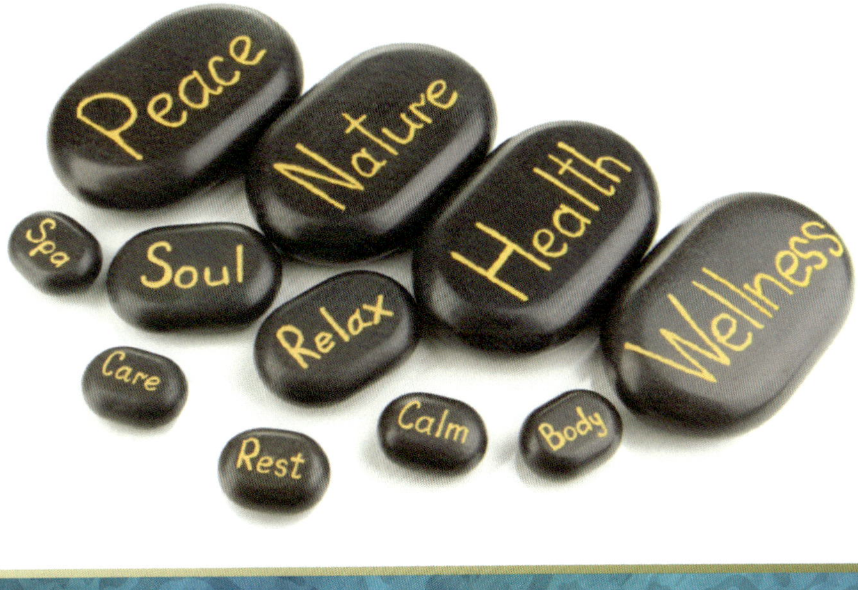

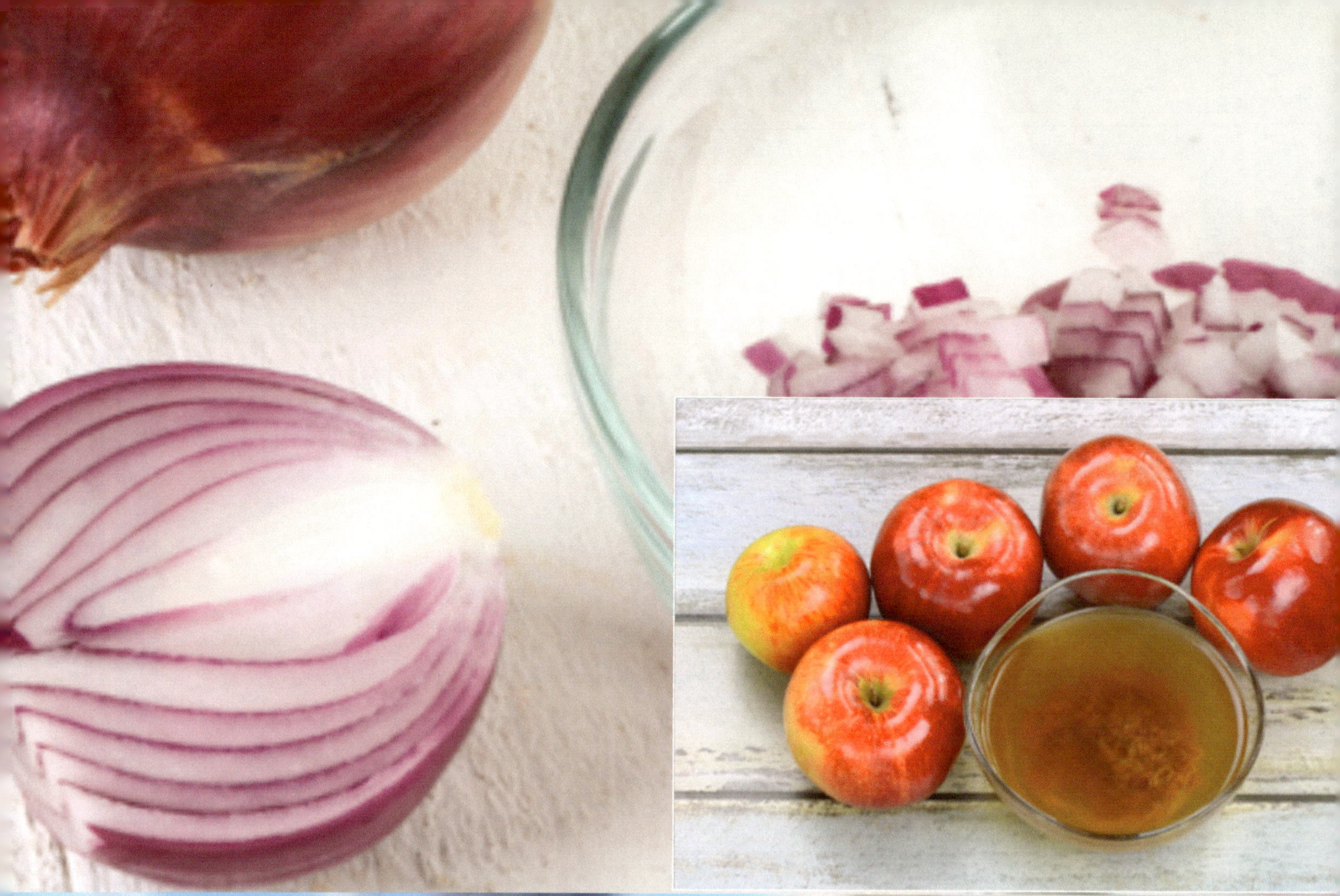

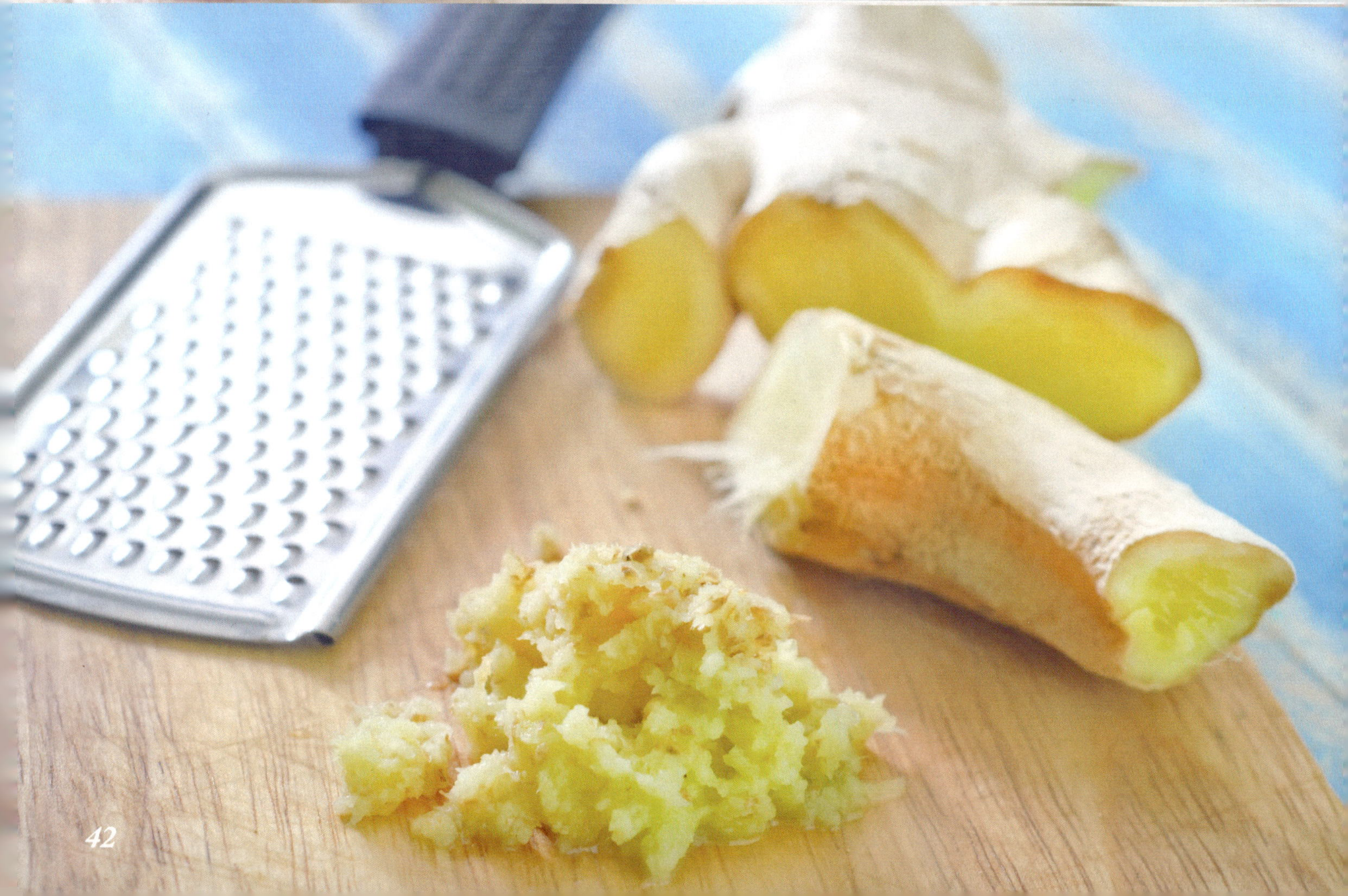

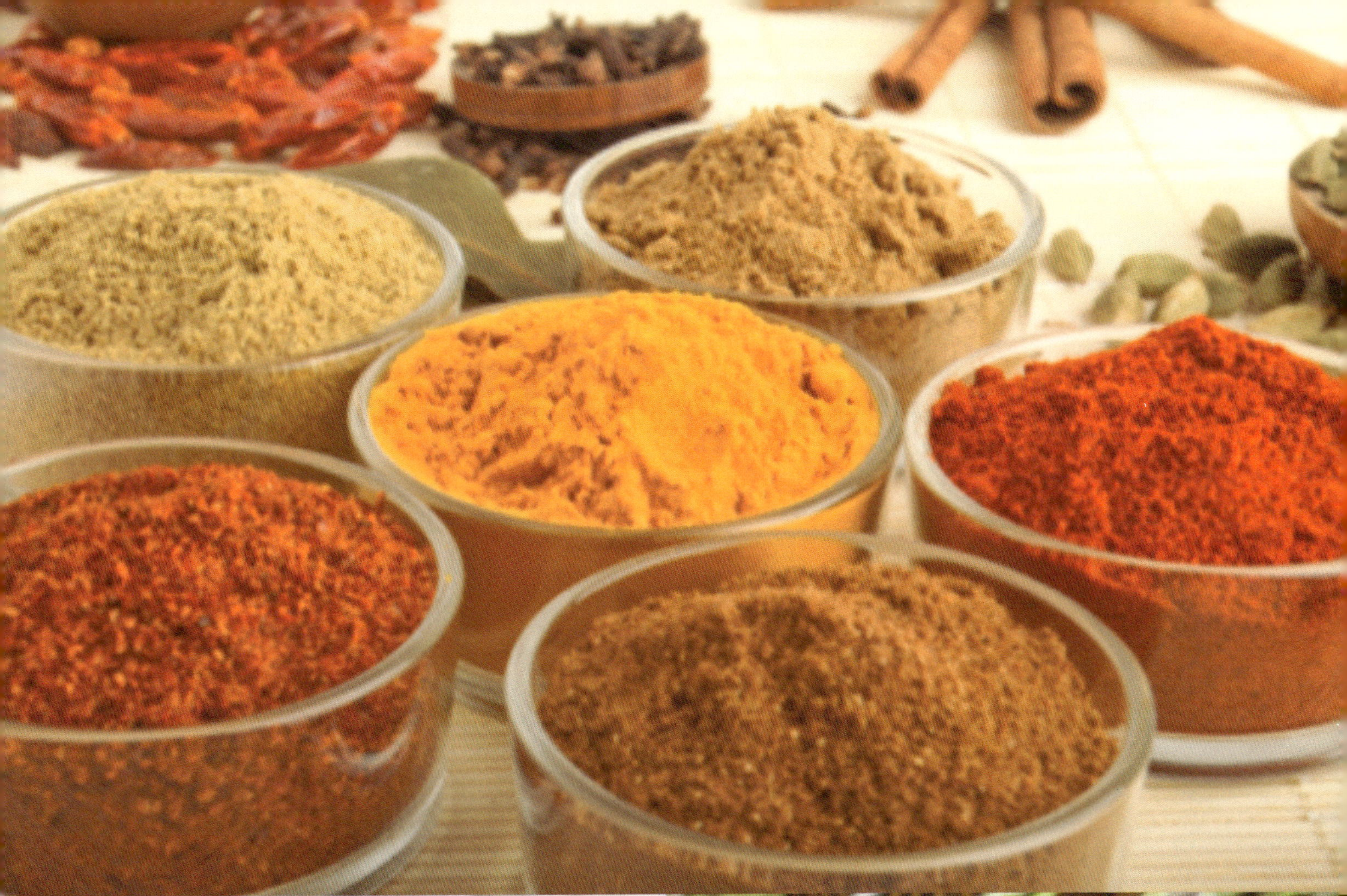

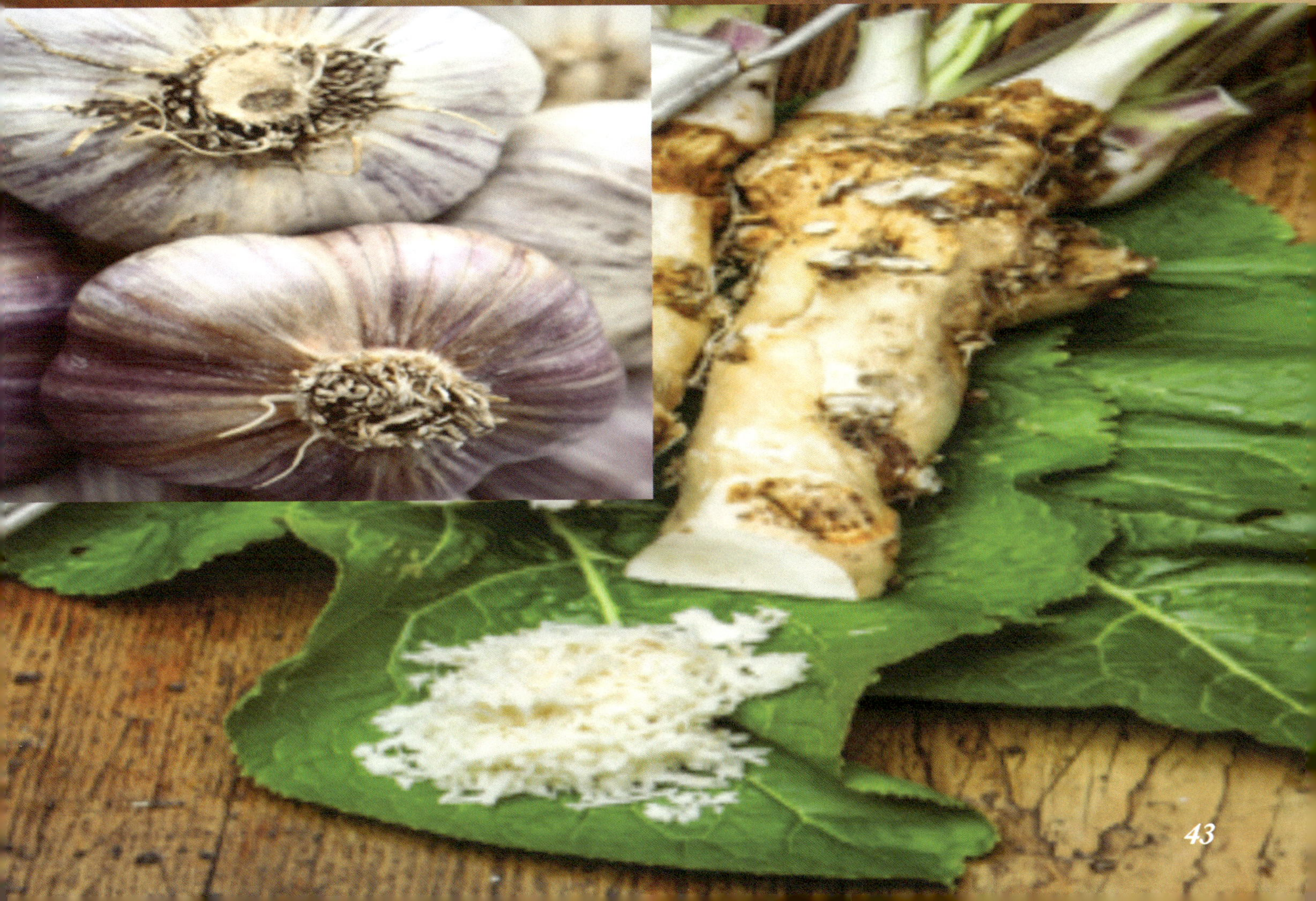

TURMERIC JUICE

To build a strong immune system

5 inches turmeric root (2 Tablespoons of ground turmeric)
5 Tamarinds (an acidic tree pod) sometimes it is hard to get fresh tamarinds. You can use powdered turmeric
2 organic lemons
Raw honey
Peel tamarind

Crack and open tamarind to access the inner fruit.

Boil turmeric in big pot of water till the water turns bright orange (20 – 30 minutes)

Put tamarind in a pot with about an inch of water and stir till it "melts" into a jam.

Take the cooled turmeric water and pour it into the blender with the turmeric.

Pour tamarind into a strainer over a bowl. Press it so that the soft fruit strains through.

Add to turmeric mixture with lemon juice and blend again.

Add honey to taste.

Store in glass jar in fridge up to 3-4 days and drink daily.

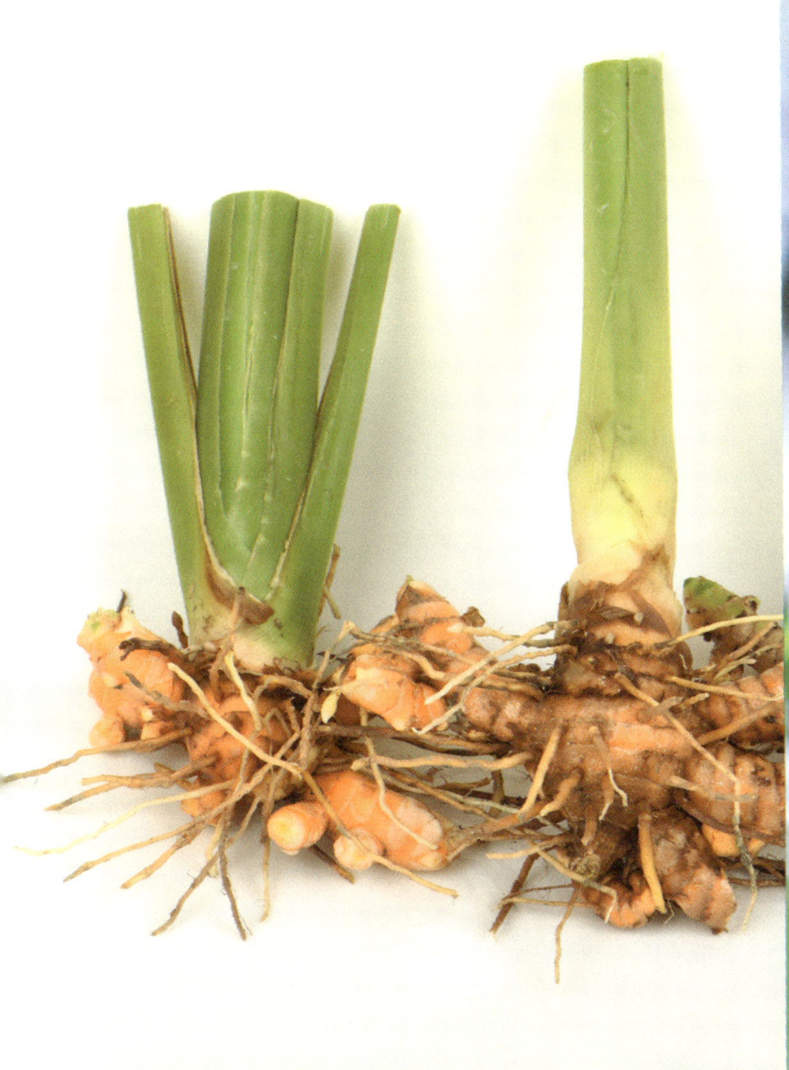
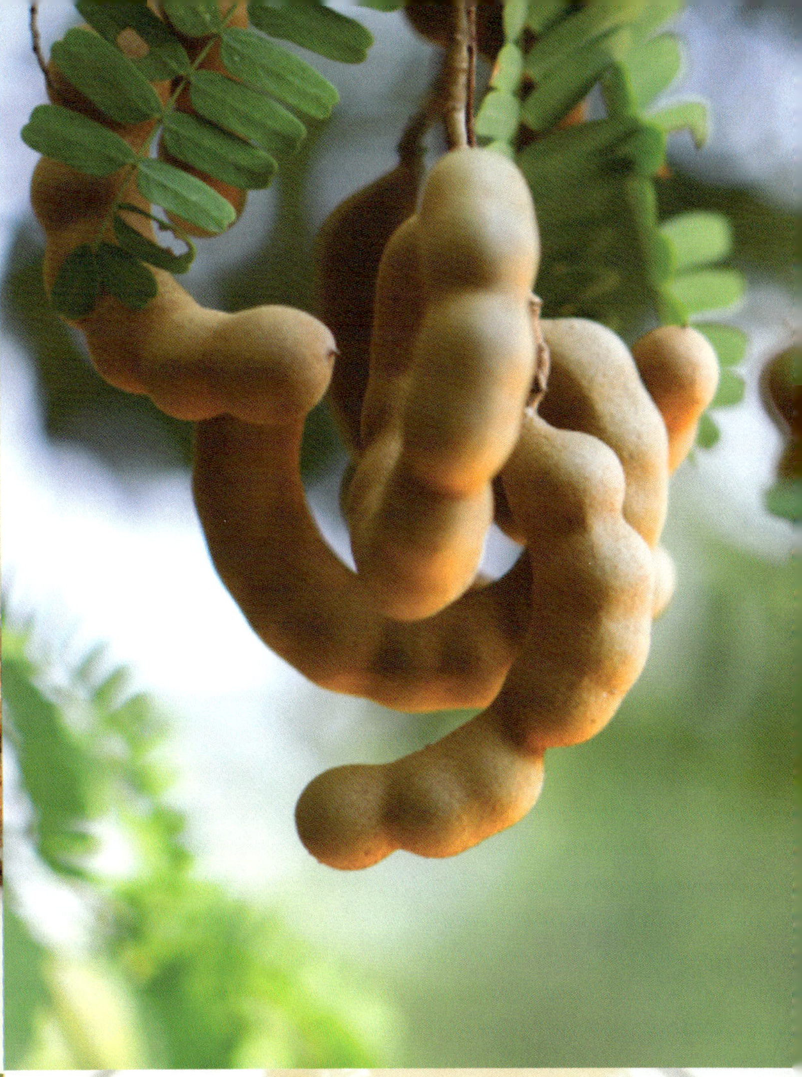
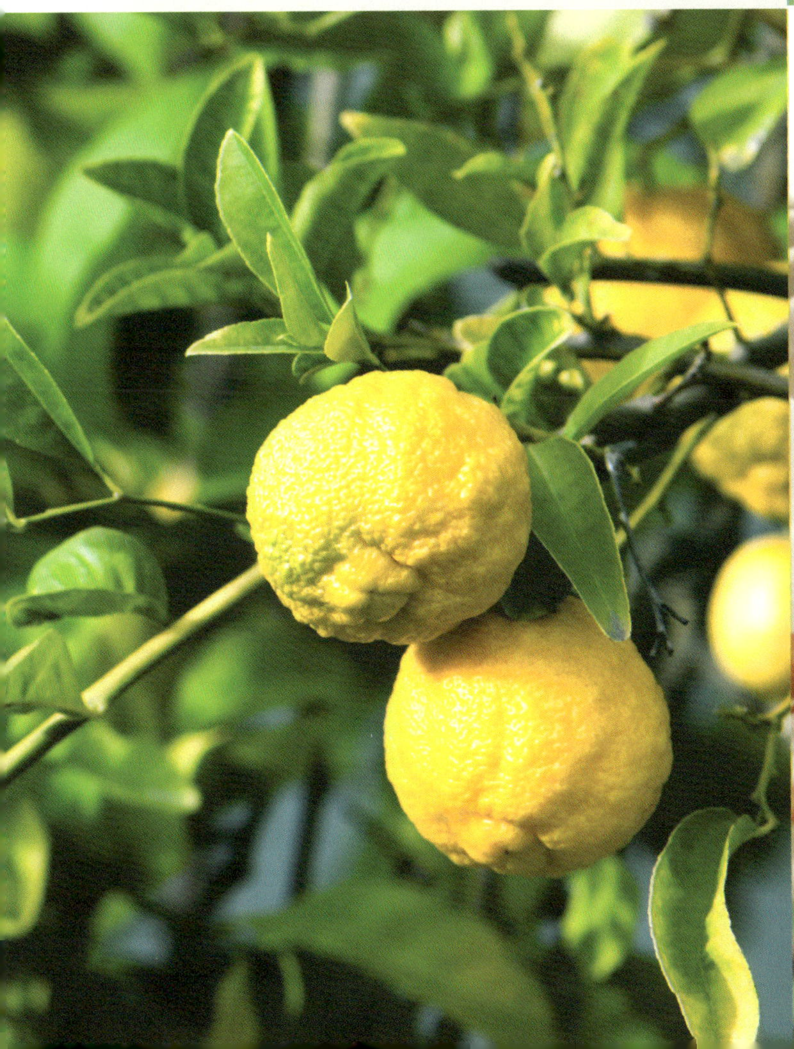
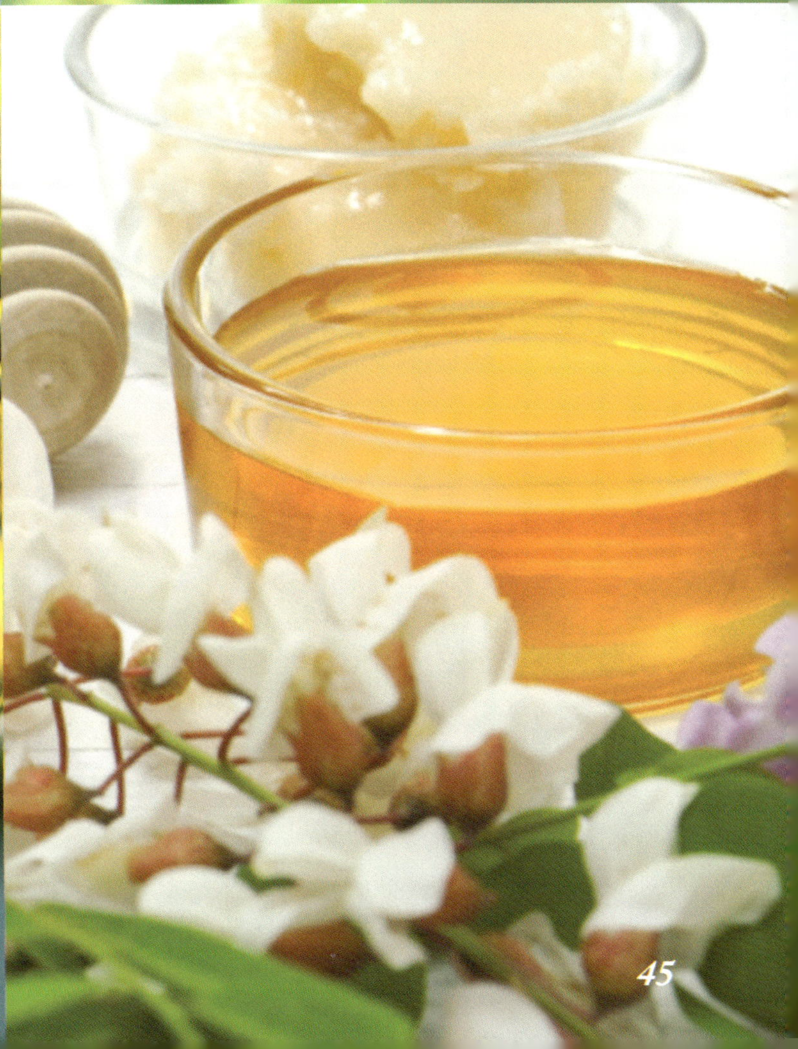

TURMERIC AND HONEY COLD REMEDY

Natural antibiotic for colds and digestion

This traditional magical potion has powerful anti-inflammatory activity, which not only destroys bad bacteria but also promotes natural defenses. Unlike synthetic antibiotics, this medicine has no negative effect on intestinal microflora. Consuming the two ingredients together improves digestion and increases the activity of beneficial flora in the gut. So don't run to the doctor at the first symptoms of a cold, instead use the golden honey mixture. Can also be used in treatment of respiratory diseases.

7 Tablespoons raw honey
2 Tablespoons ground turmeric

Mix well and place the mixture in a jar and use within 3 days. Take at the first symptoms of a cold. The mixture must stay in your mouth until it's completely dissolved.

> *Day 1 Take half a teaspoon of the mixture every hour throughout the day.*
> *Day 2 Take half a teaspoon of the mixture on every two hours.*
> *Day 3 Take half a teaspoon of the mixture three times a day.*

A great way to have it is in milk or tea.

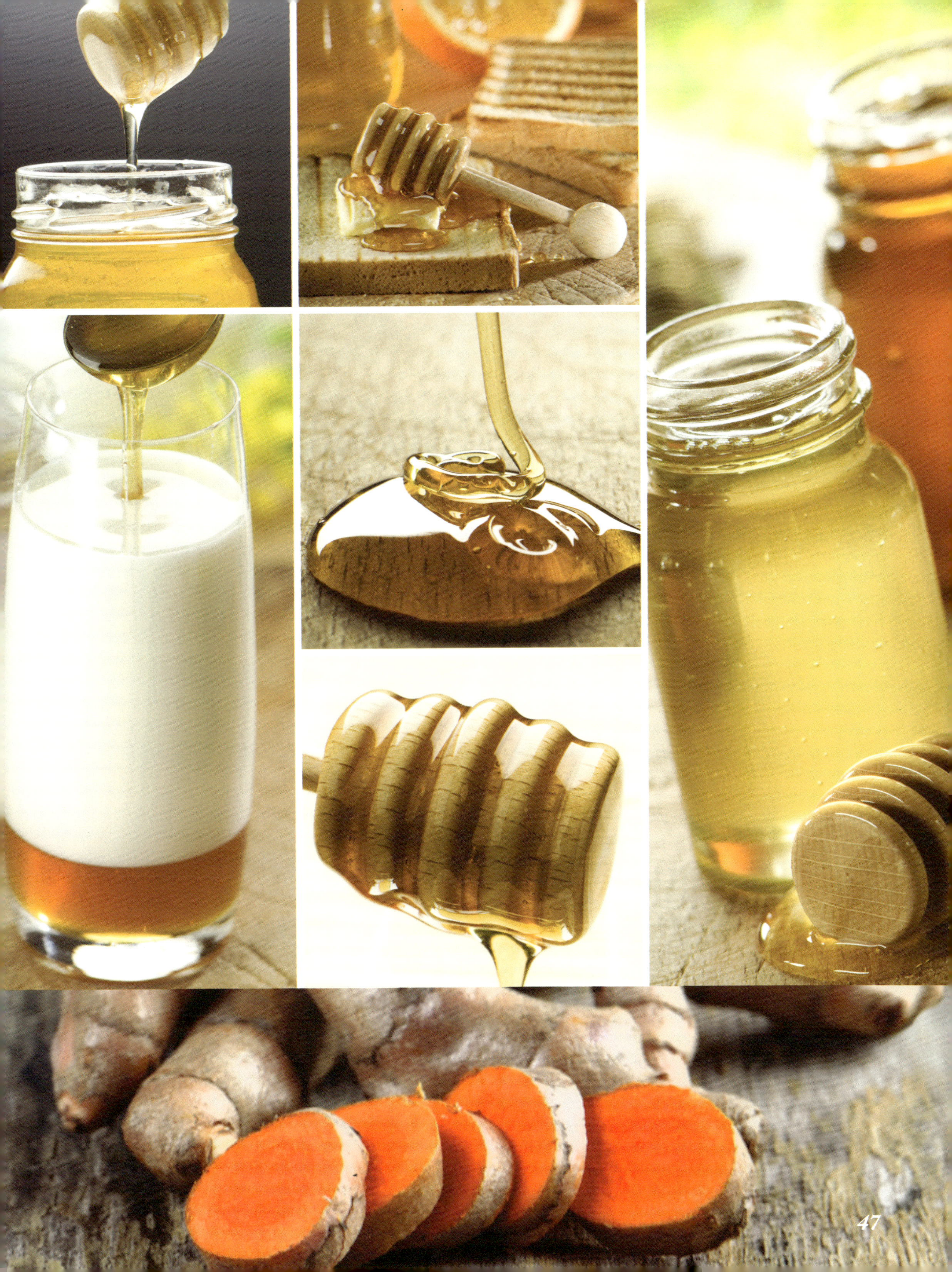

BLOOD CLOT REMEDY

7 Tablespoons Manuka honey
2 Tablespoons turmeric
4 Tablespoons coconut oil
2 Tablespoons fresh pineapple juice

Mix well and place in a jar, leave for 24 hours at room temperature. Then keep at room temp till finished.

Week One - Take half a teaspoon of the mixture every hour throughout the day.

Days 8 –12 - Take half a teaspoon of the mixture every two hours.
Day 12 – 48 - Take half a teaspoon of the mixture three times a day.

The mixture must stay in your mouth until it's completely dissolved. This is also amazing for any respiratory infection or ailment.

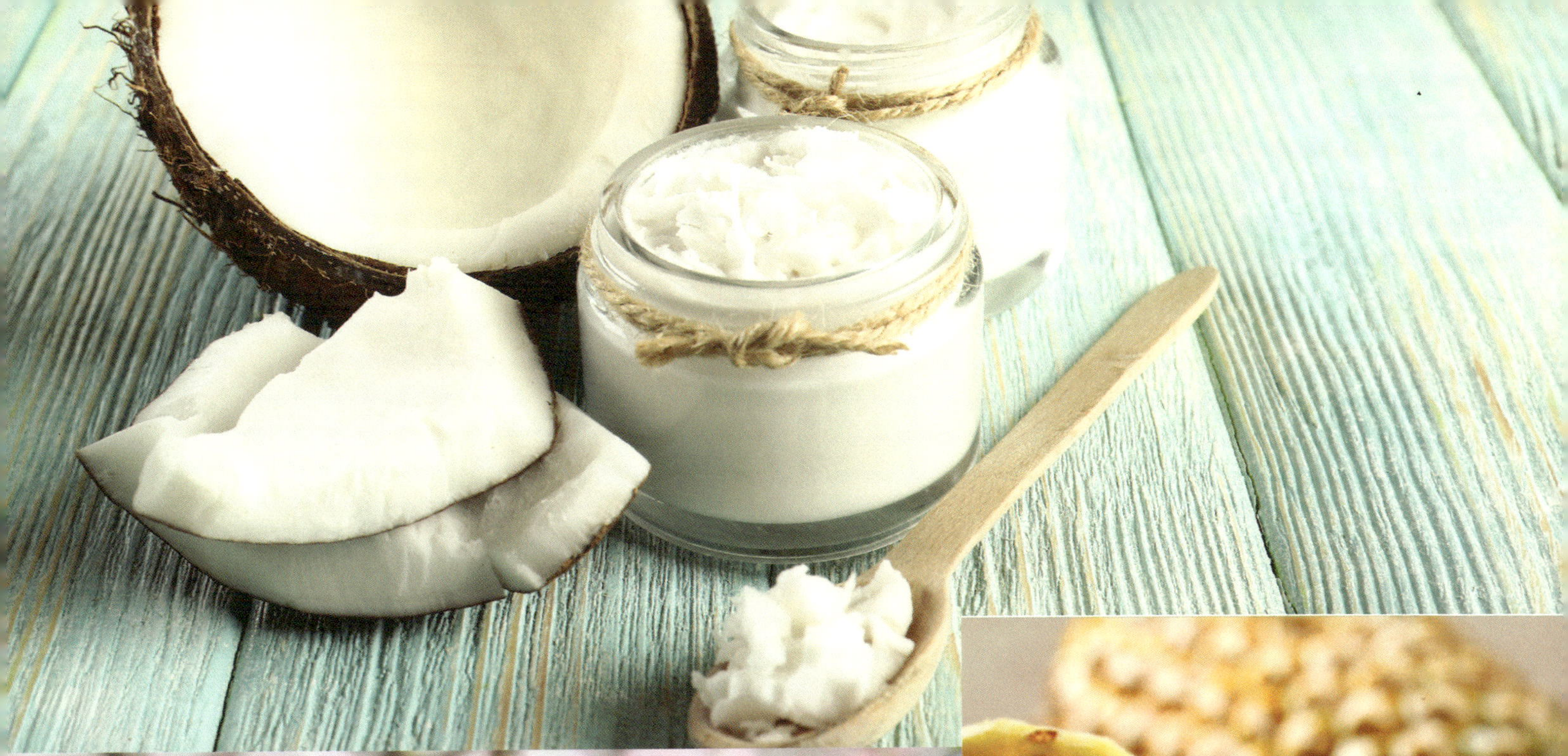
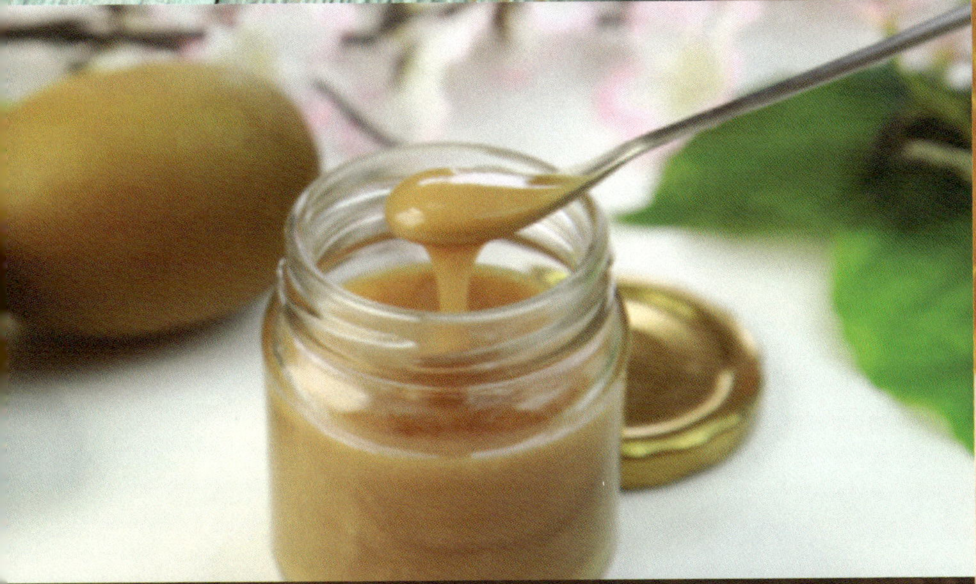
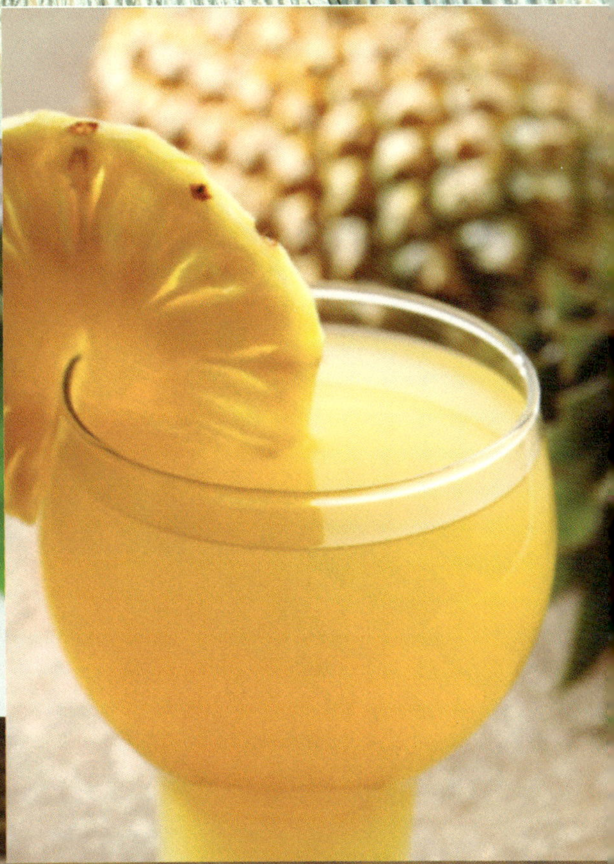
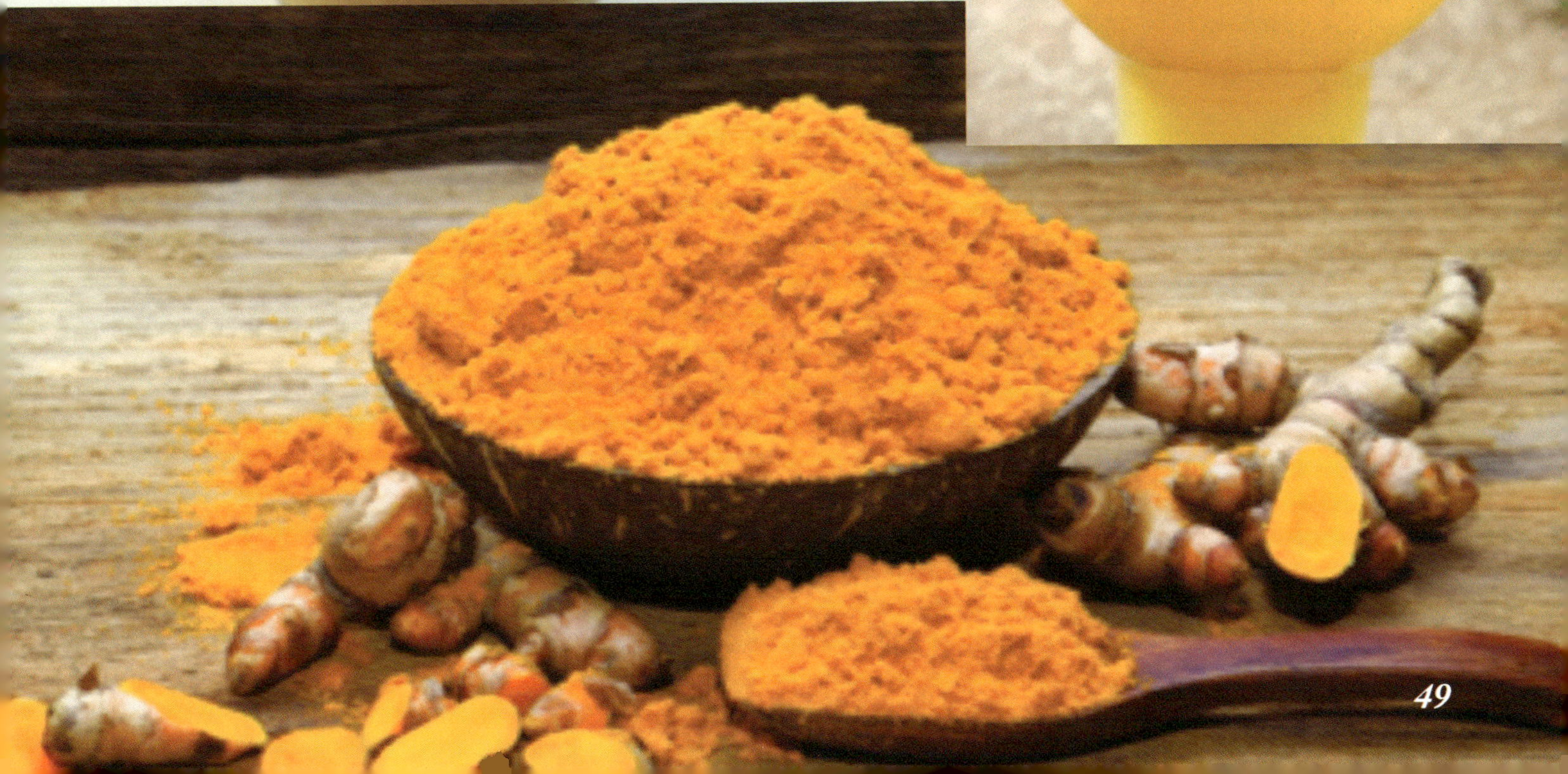

FOUNTAIN OF YOUTH HONEY ELIXIR

For Sclerosis, inflammation and kidney ailments

7 1/2 Tablespoons fresh lemon juice
15 Tablespoons raw honey
3 1/2 Tablespoons unprocessed virgin olive oil

Mix all ingredients thoroughly and pour the mixture into a glass jar. Close the lid and store in a cold and dark place. Drink the mixture every morning, on an empty stomach, just one tablespoon is enough to boost your energy and promote your overall health.

For Anti-Aging

Twice a year this elixir of youth should be consumed every day for one month. You'll feel refreshed and rejuvenated, look younger and you'll resolve many of your health problems.

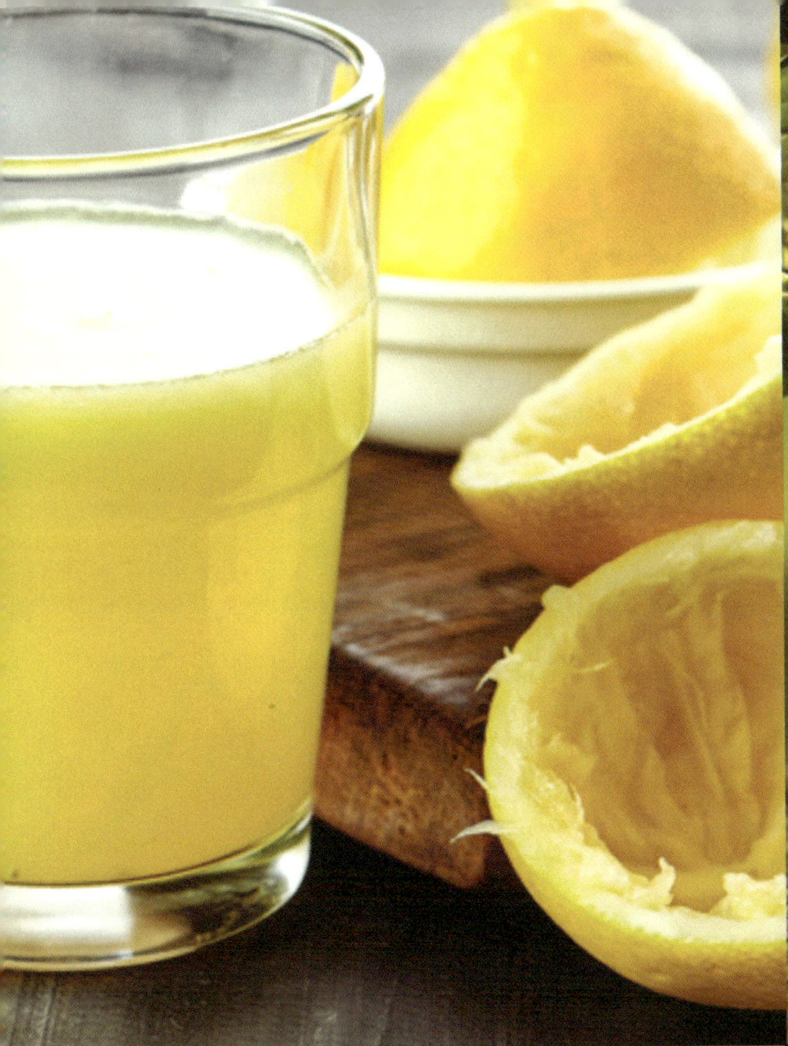
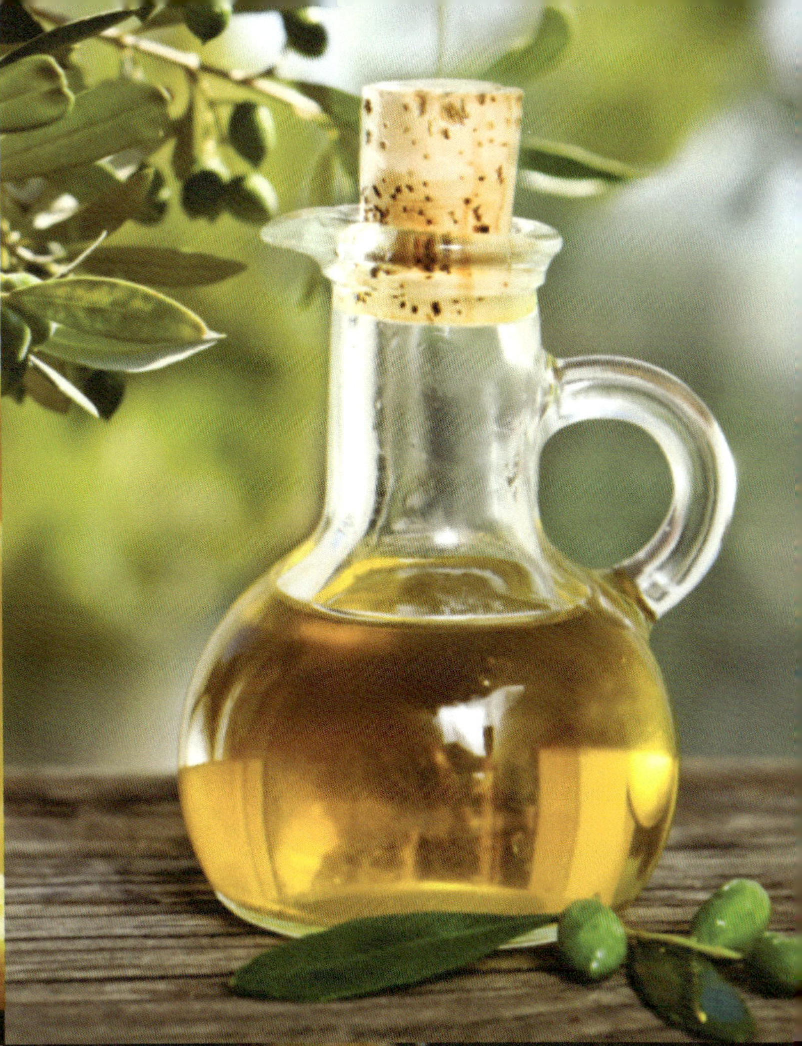
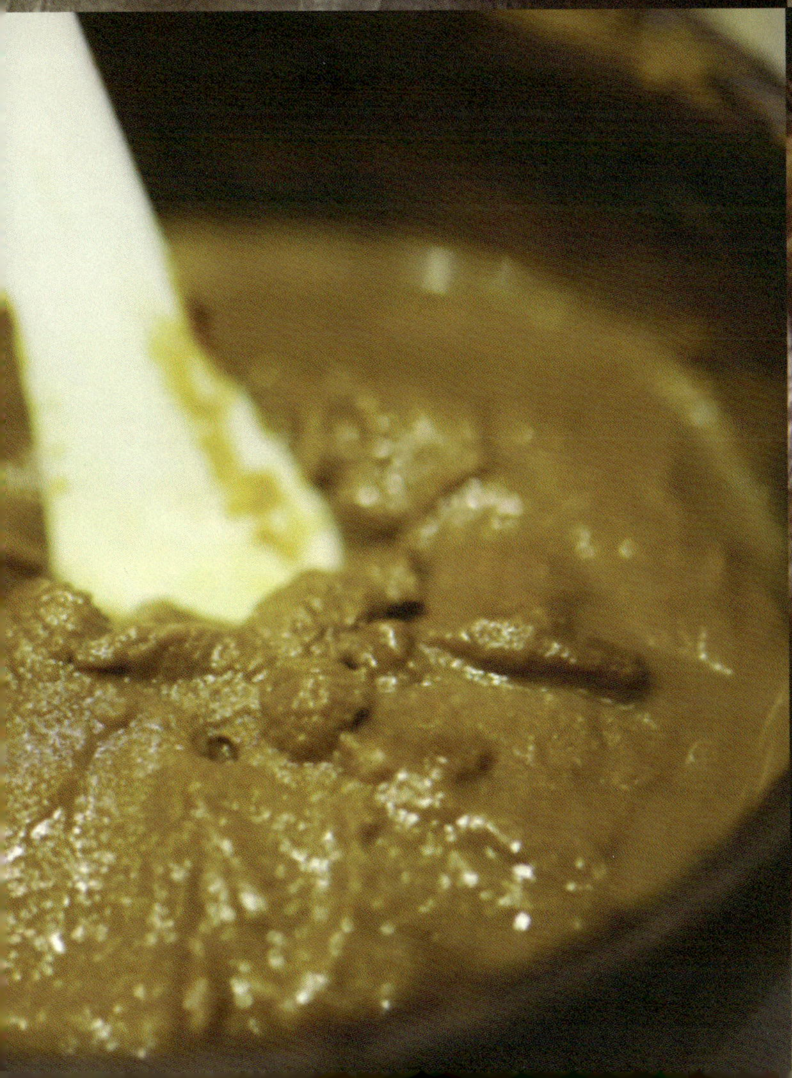
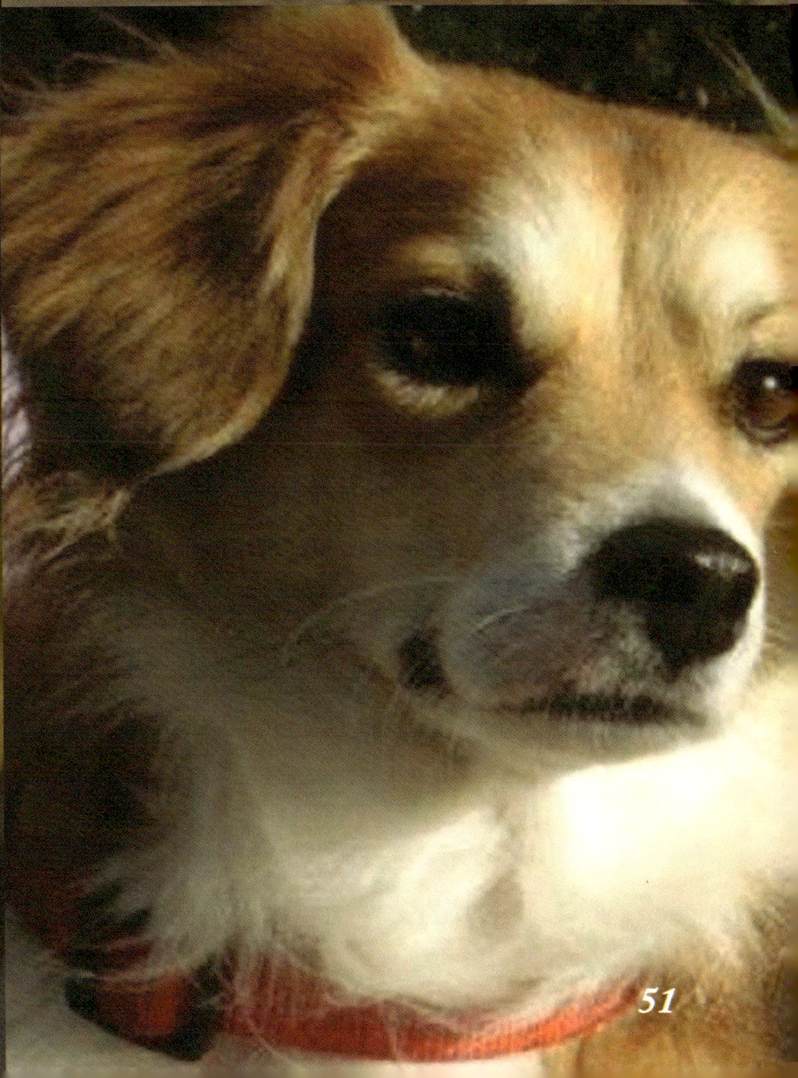

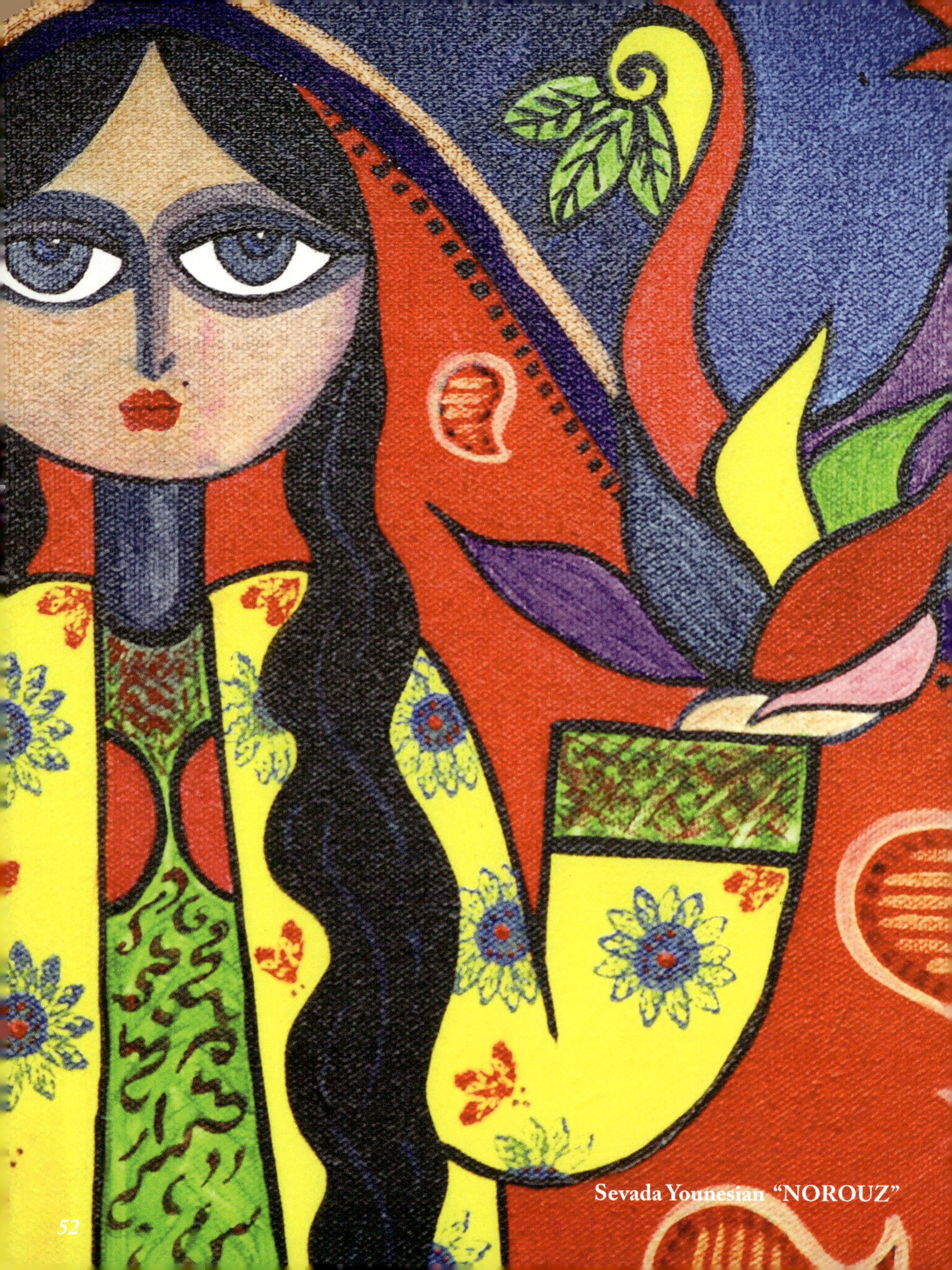

Sevada Younesian "NOROUZ"

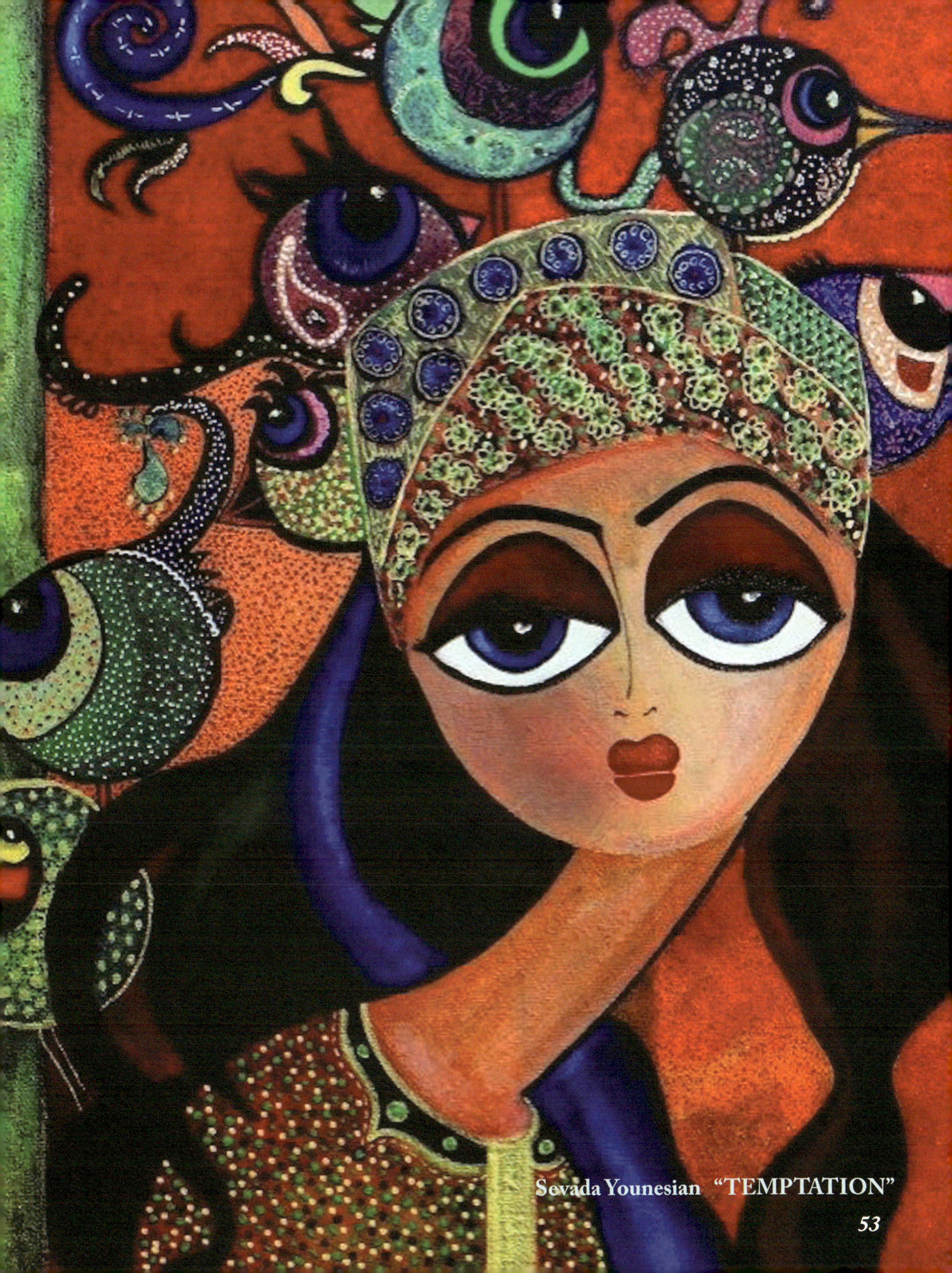

Sevada Younesian "TEMPTATION"

LEMONADE LIVER DETOX (MASTER CLEANSE)

For clear skin and more energy and health.

Juice of 5 organic lemons
1/4 Teaspoon cayenne
1 Tablespoon raw organic maple syrup
1 Gallon distilled water

Mix together and drink all day everyday for four weeks. You can also do a 7-day Liquid Detox where you only drink the lemonade. Prior to doing a fast you need to take 2 weeks to eat clean food, no alcohol.

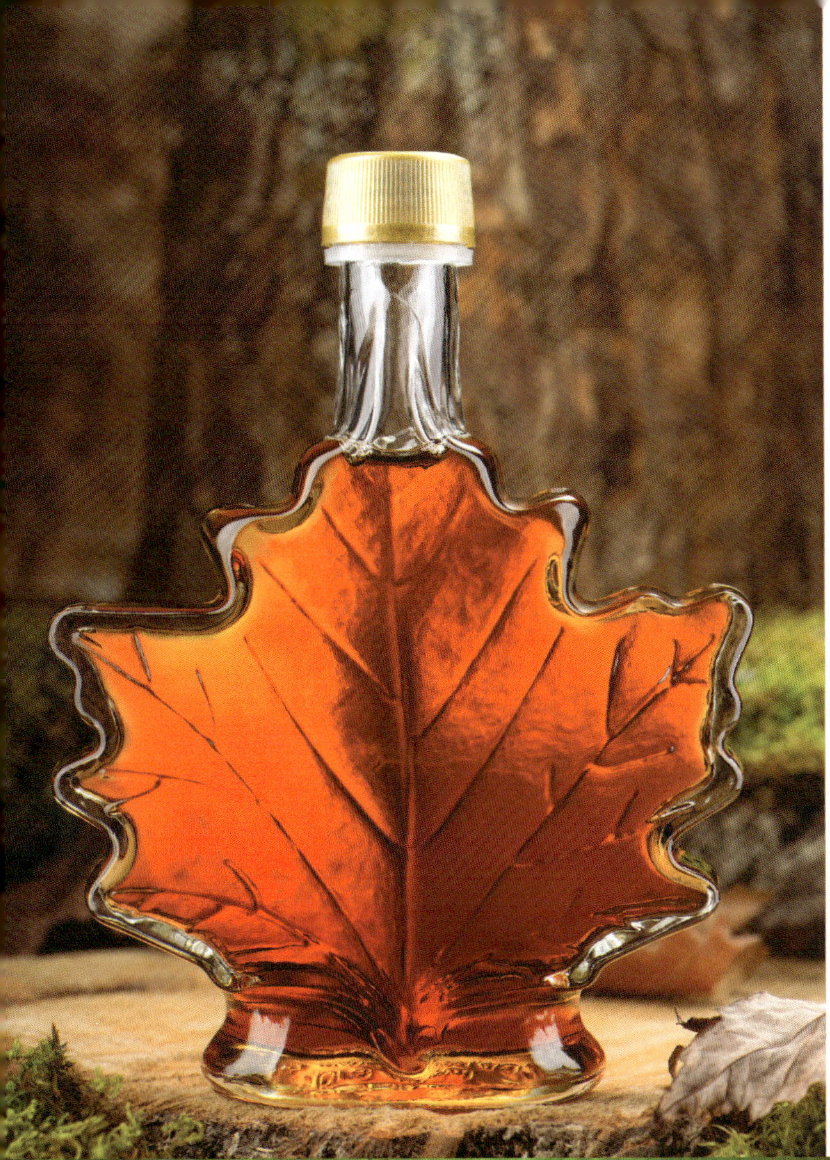

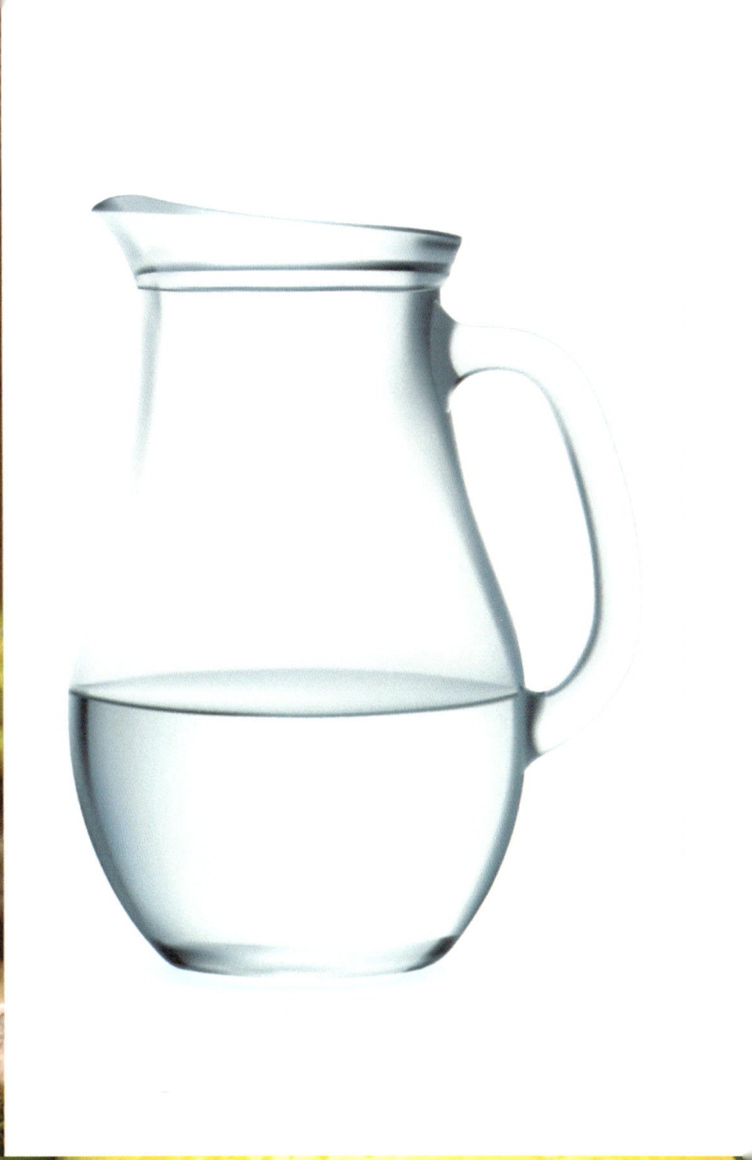

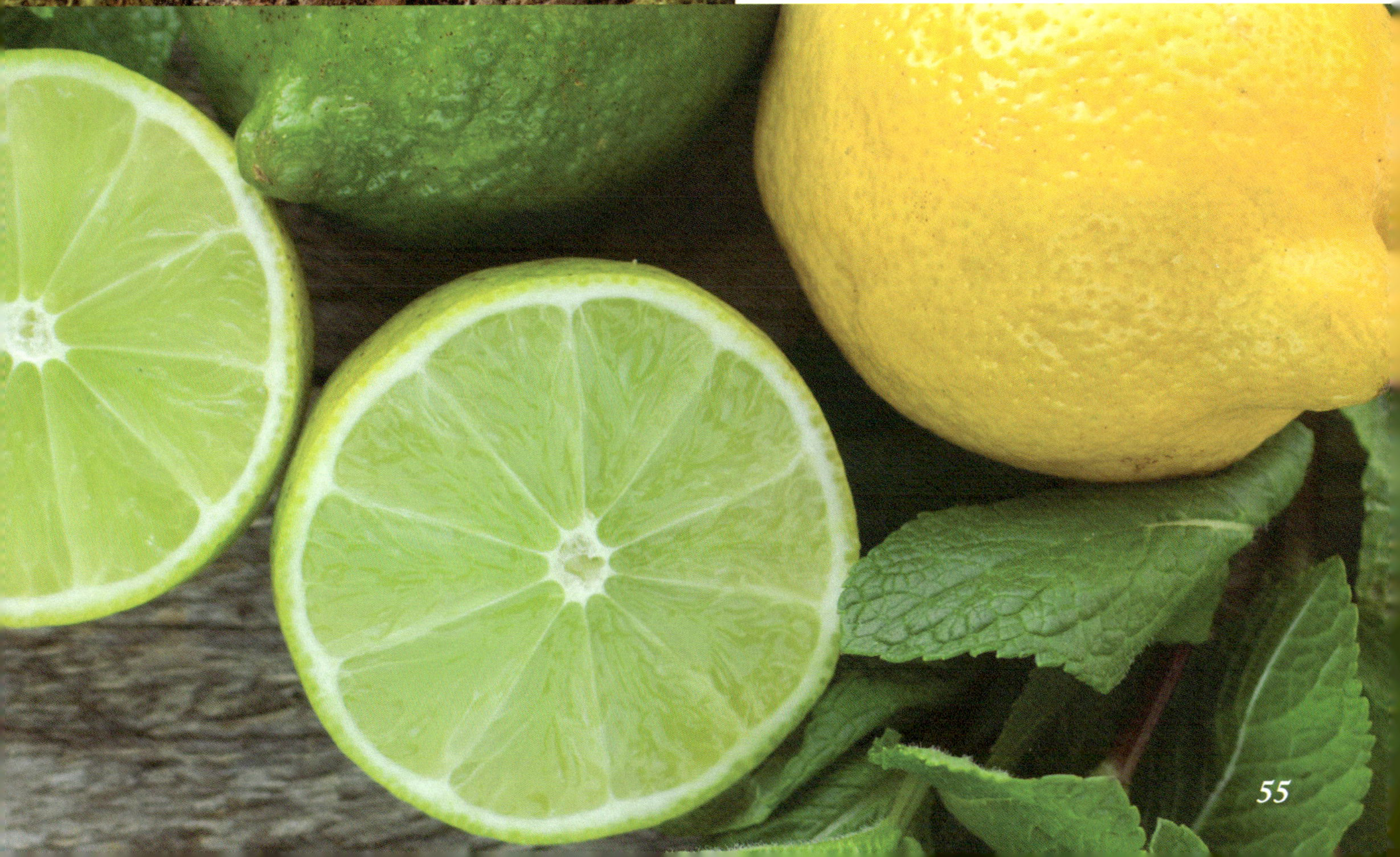

LIVER DETOX 2

A more gradual detox, do this regimen for 48 days.

½ Organic lemon
1 Tablespoon virgin olive oil
1/4 Teaspoon cayenne pepper

Mix the ingredients well and drink so the oil does not settle.

Drink once in morning, 30 minutes before breakfast and at night 30 minutes prior to sleep.

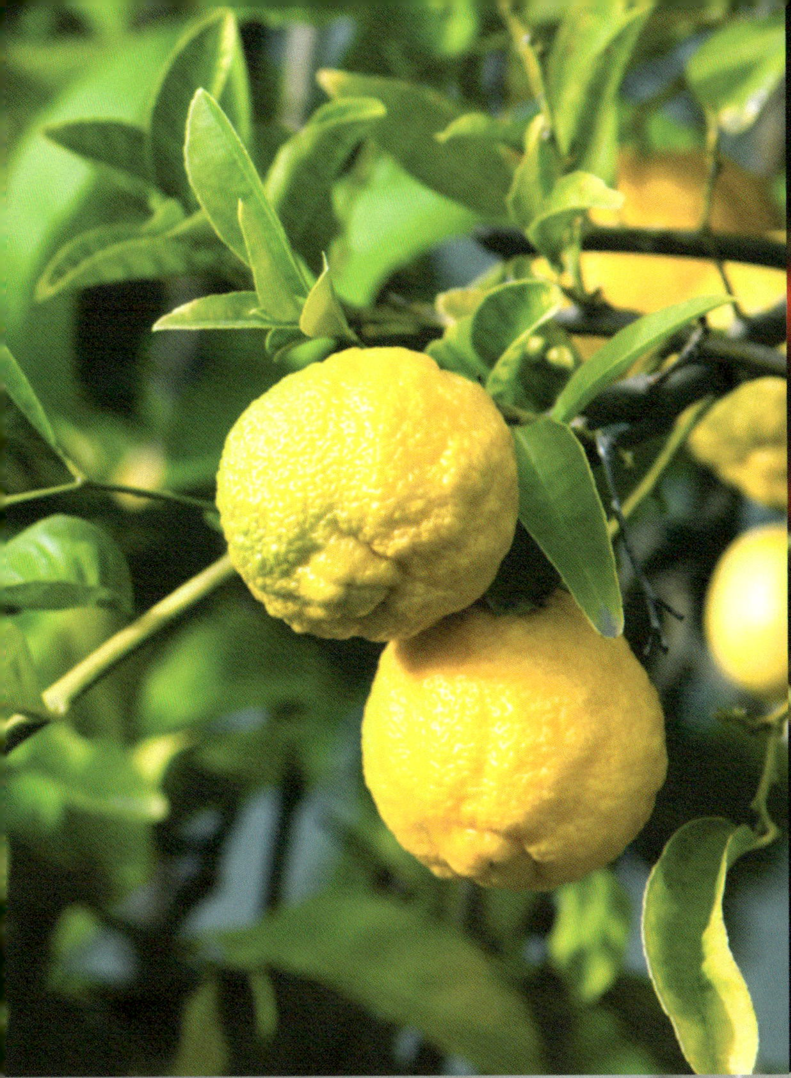
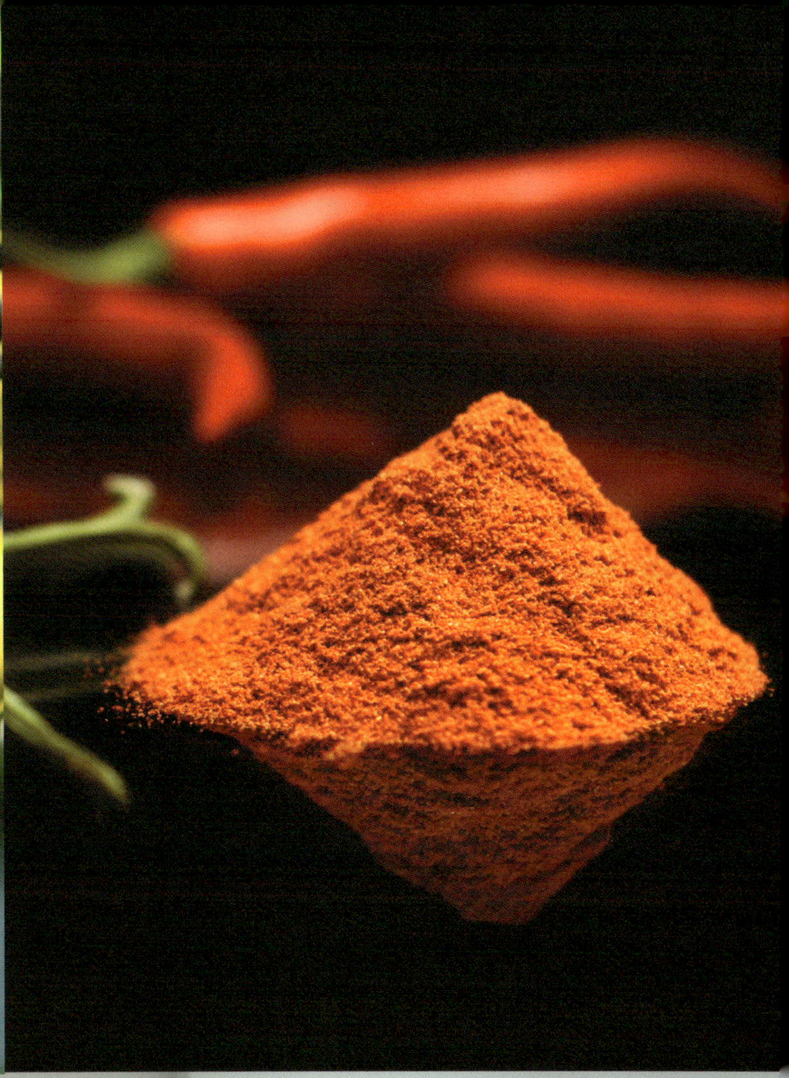
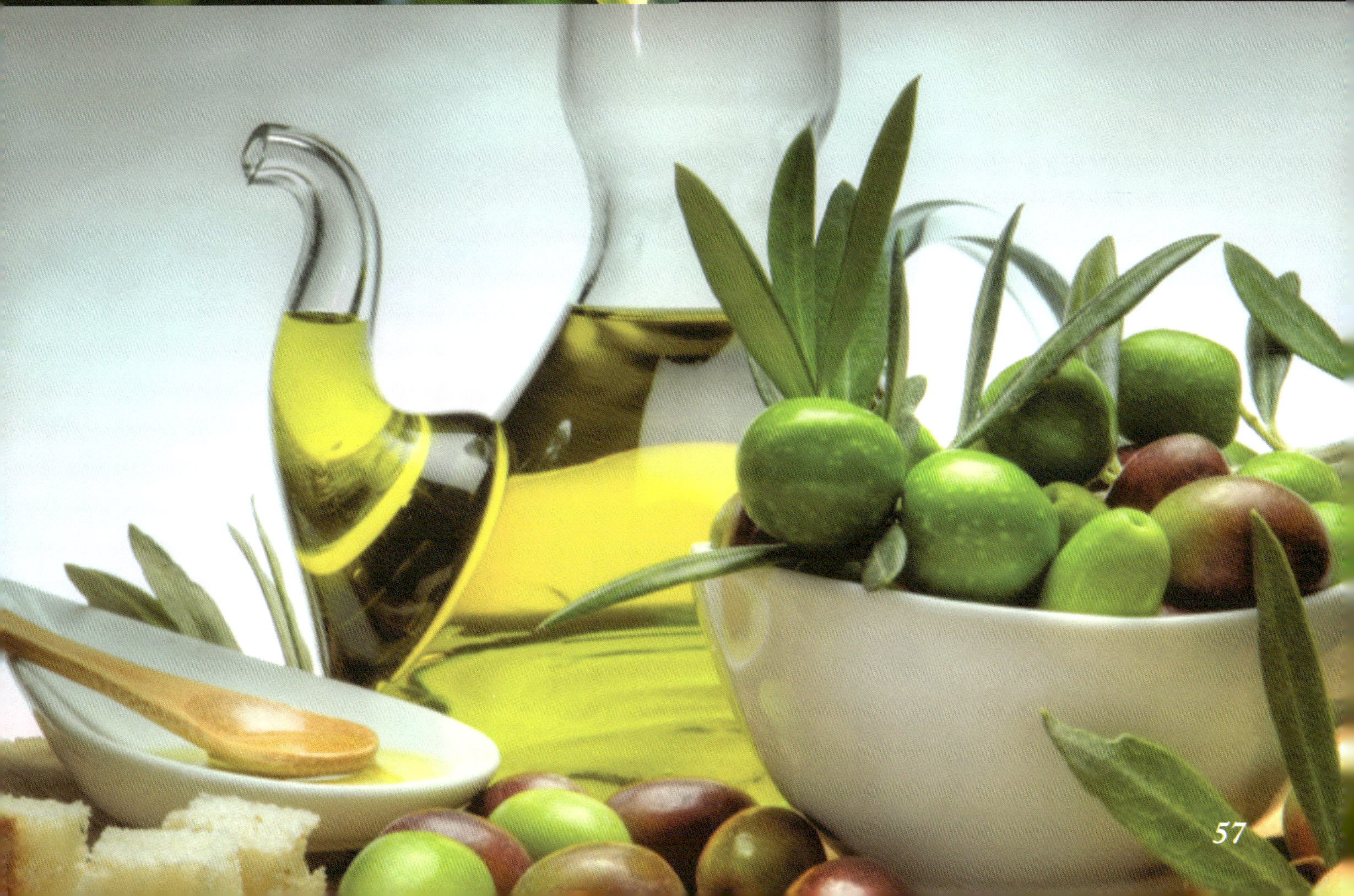

LYMPHATIC DETOX LEMONADE

3-6 days Liquid fast

Juice of 5 organic lemons
½ Teaspoon ground turmeric
12 Slices raw ginger (grated)
1 Tablespoon raw honey (or Manuka honey if you can not find organic local honey)
1 Gallon distilled water

Add the lemon juice, turmeric and ginger to a food processor or blender. Add to distilled water and pour into a glass bottle kept in the fridge. Drink a glass every morning after a glass of chilled water upon rising and proceed to drink 3 large glasses a day for 48 days. You can also do a 7-day fast where you drink only water and this lemonade.

Important note: To prepare your body for the liquid fast, prior to your lemonade fast, it is vital for 12 days , to eat mainly organic cooked vegetables with grass-fed beef and organic chickens and eggs, cutting out sugar, dairy, alcohol and coffee, and drinking half of your body weight in ounces of water. (If you weigh 100 pounds you would drink 50 ounces of filtered or spring water per day.)

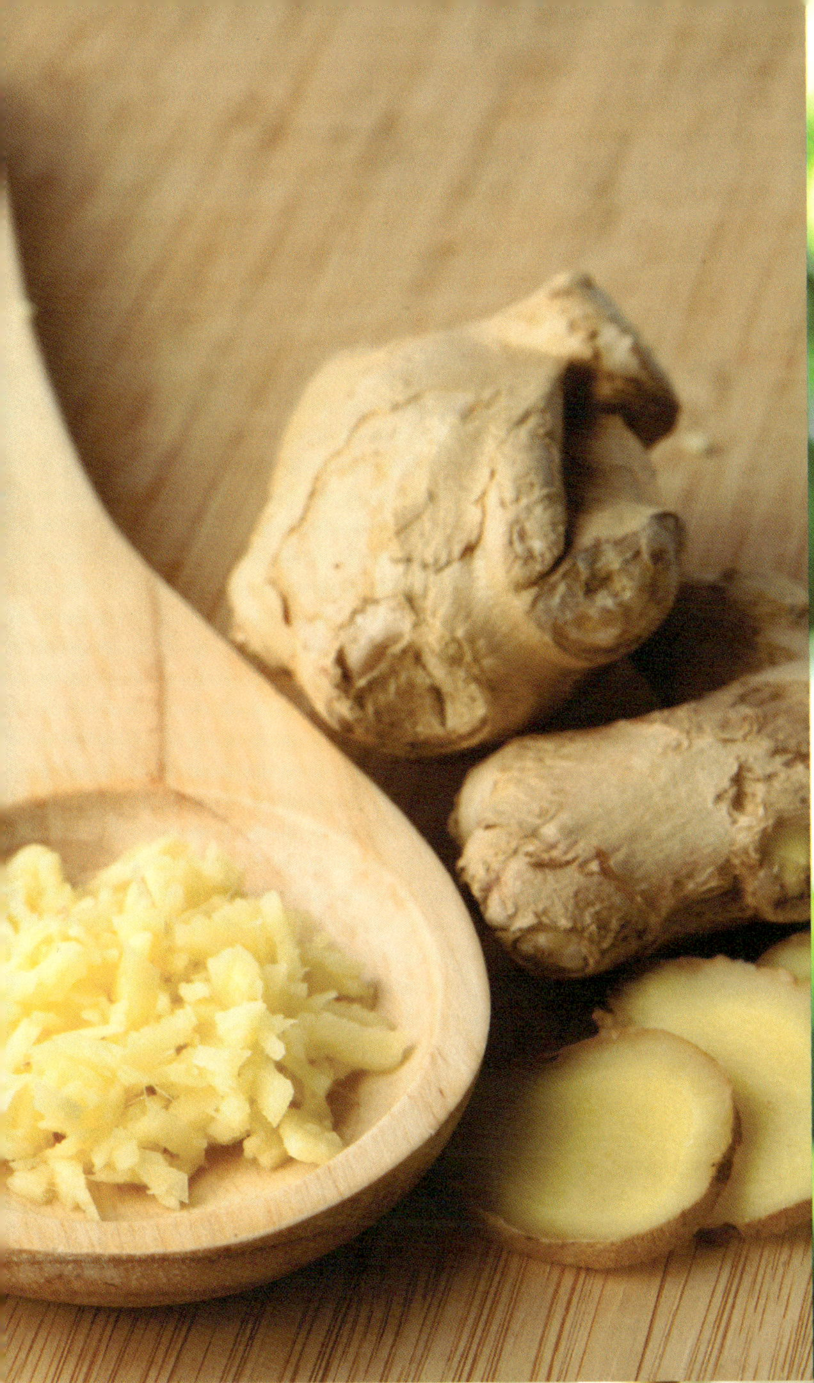
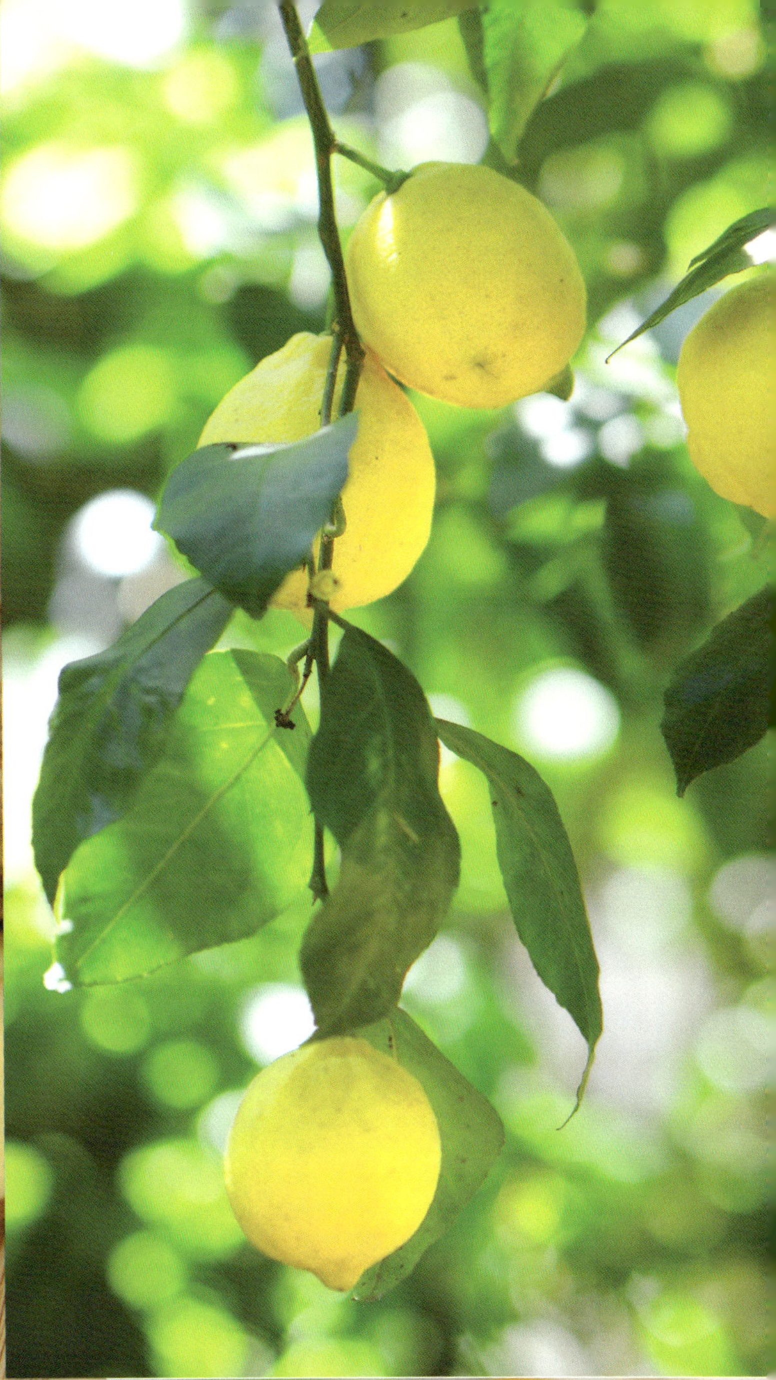
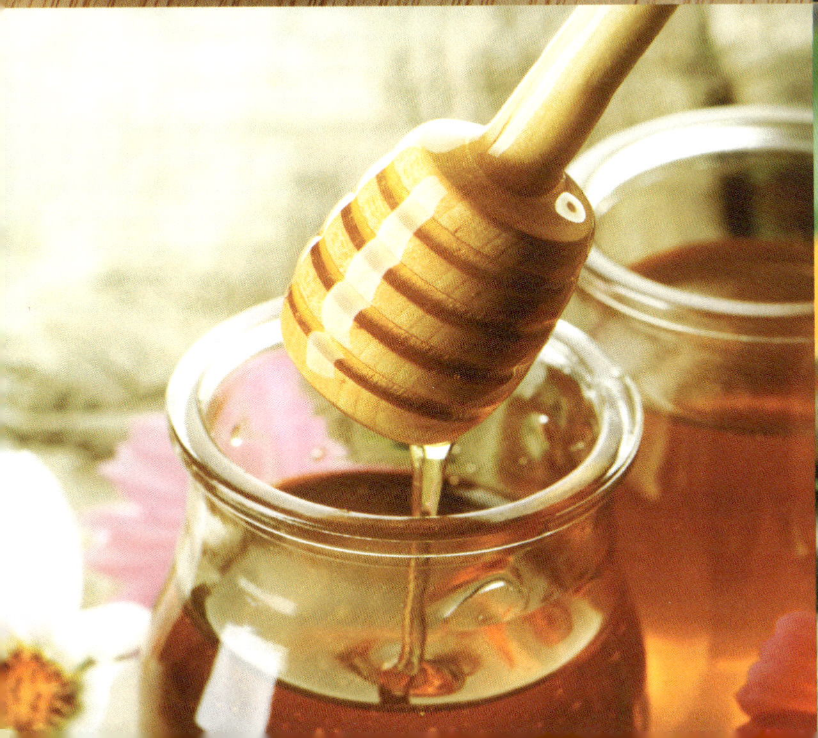
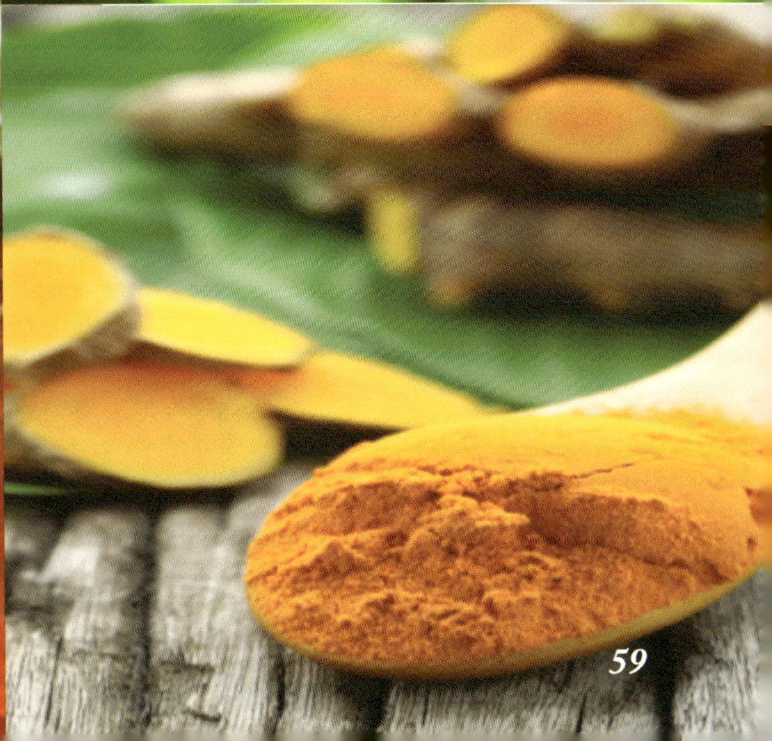

MAMANJOON'S SPECIAL REMEDIES
ULCER REMEDY

1 black beetroot (found in Chinese markets)
1 Teaspoon raw honey

Take black beet, shave out the core so that it resembles a hollow cup. Put a teaspoon of raw honey into the hollow. Leave overnight. In the morning you will see it has filled with juice. Drink that juice on an empty stomach an hour before breakfast. Continue this regimen every morning for 144 days and you will be ulcer free.

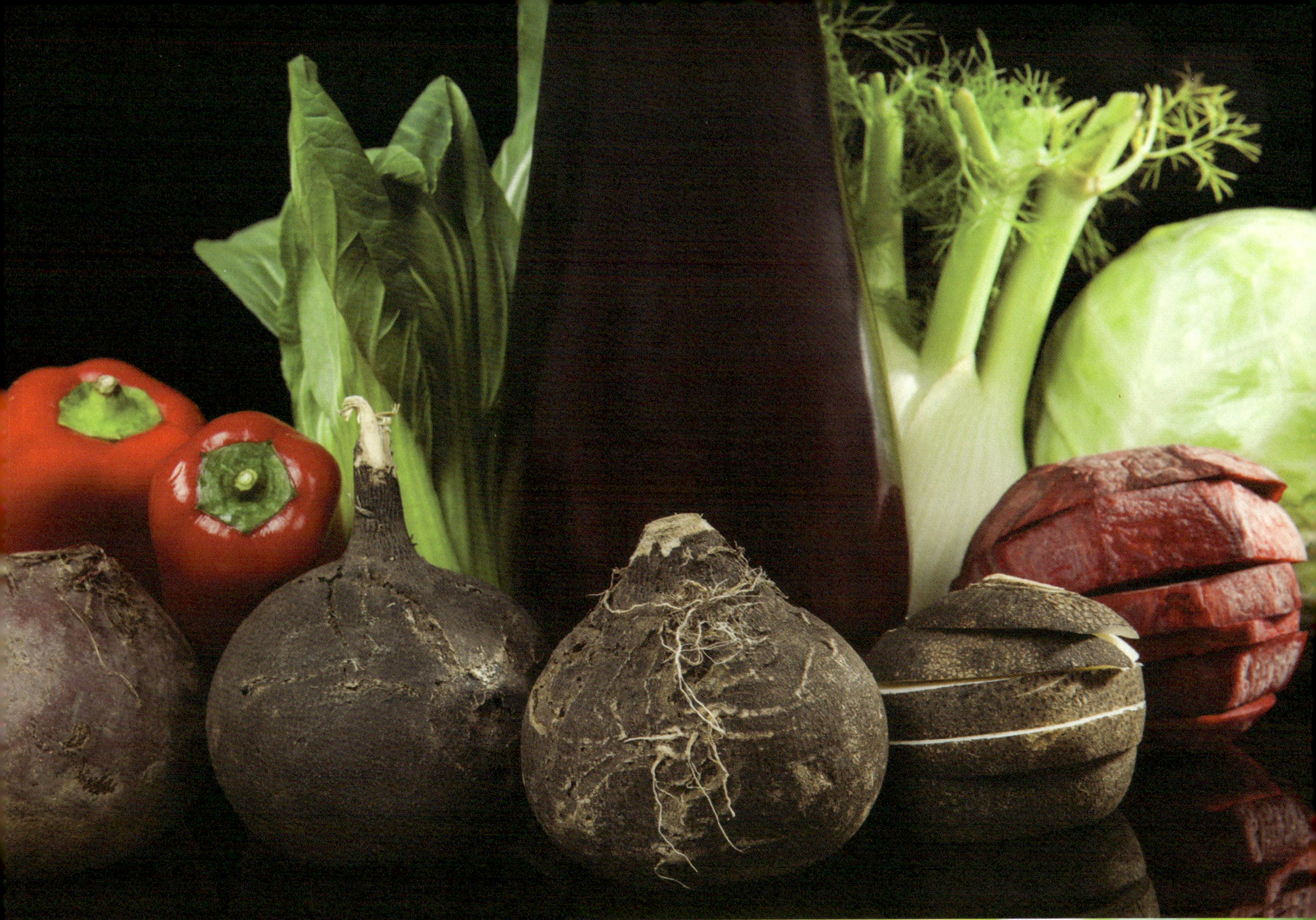

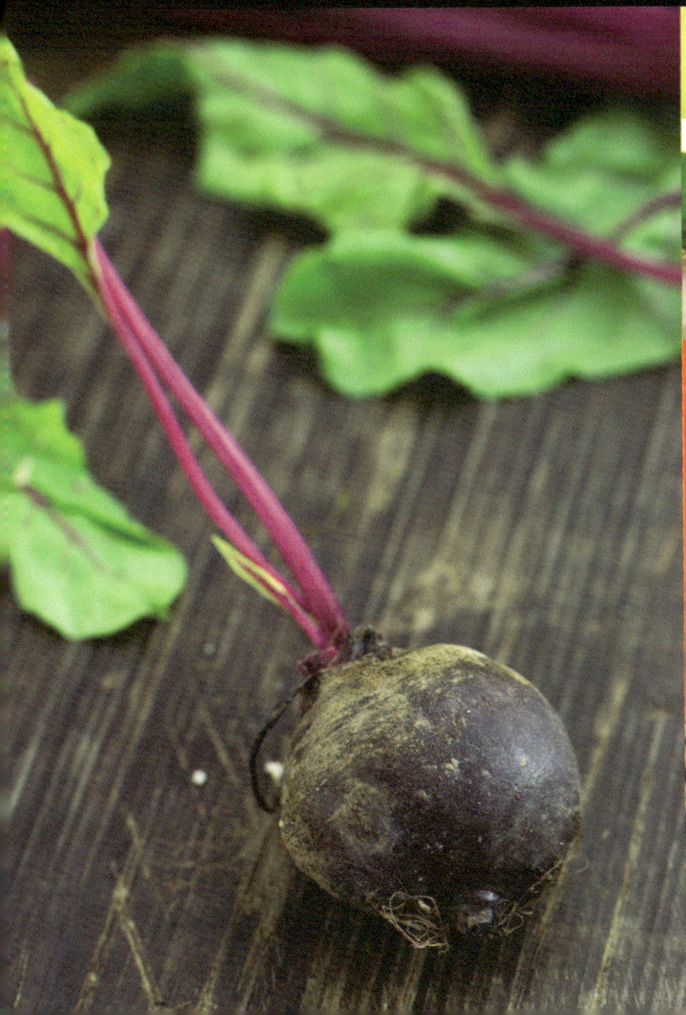

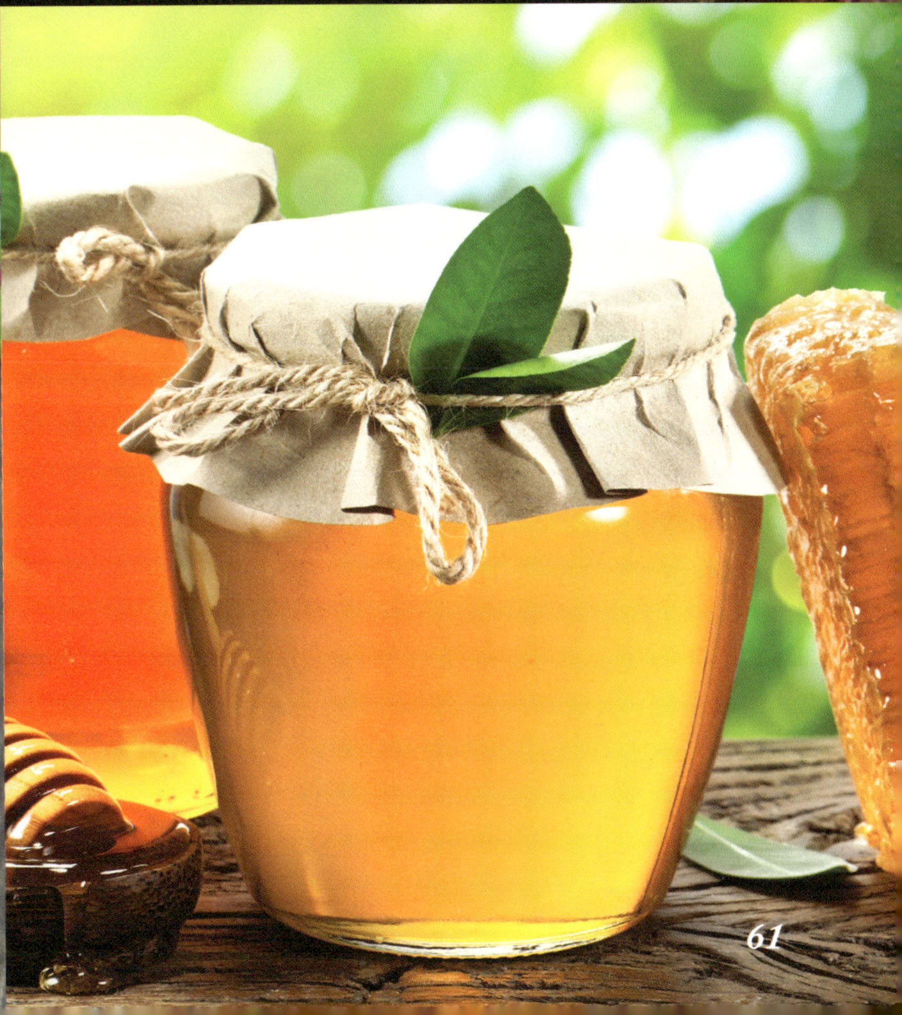

ONION JUICE EAR INFECTION CURE

1 medium red onion
Natural cotton ball
10-inch piece of muslin (from sheet)
Hot Iron

When I was a baby, the story goes, I was prone to ear infections. So when once I had a temperature of 103 and was crying hysterically, Mamanjoon did a test and determined that, indeed, I most definitely had an ear infection. In Farsi the saying goes: "She has put the roof of the house over my head," meaning she was screaming bloody murder. She told my mum to find a medium red onion, natural cotton ball, long muslin cloth and an iron. You can do exactly as she did:

MamanJoon shaved the onion with small grater to "juice" it, then put a piece of natural cotton in the juice and let it absorb well. She followed by folding the cloth in fours and putting the hot iron on it for 30 to 40 seconds until very hot. She then squeezed the wet cotton ball slightly and placed the moist ball in my ear. She placed the warm sheet of muslin on top of the ear and held it for two minutes to draw the infection out onto the cotton. After three or four repetitions the pain will subside.

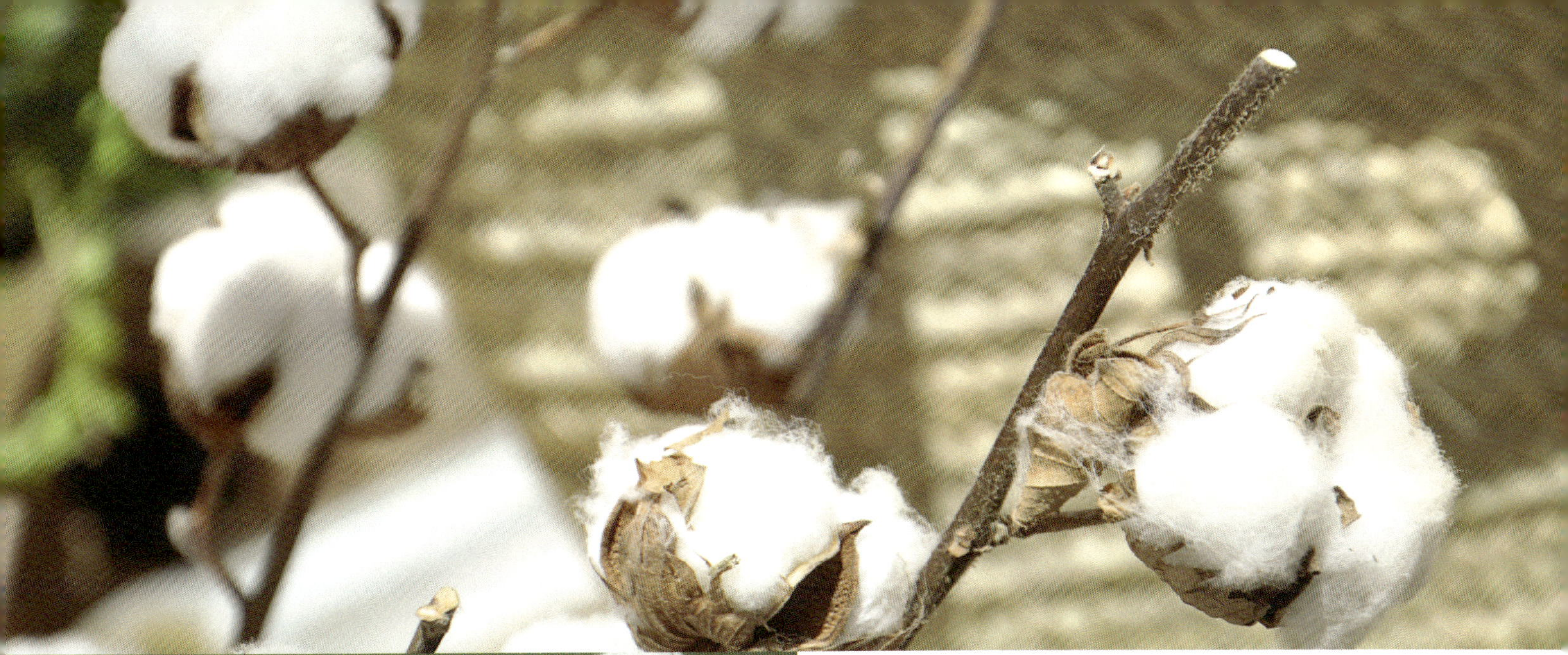
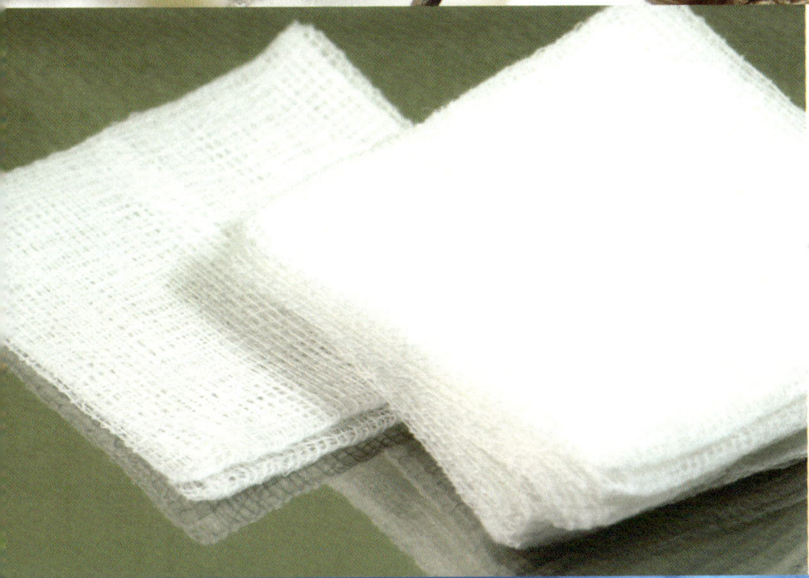
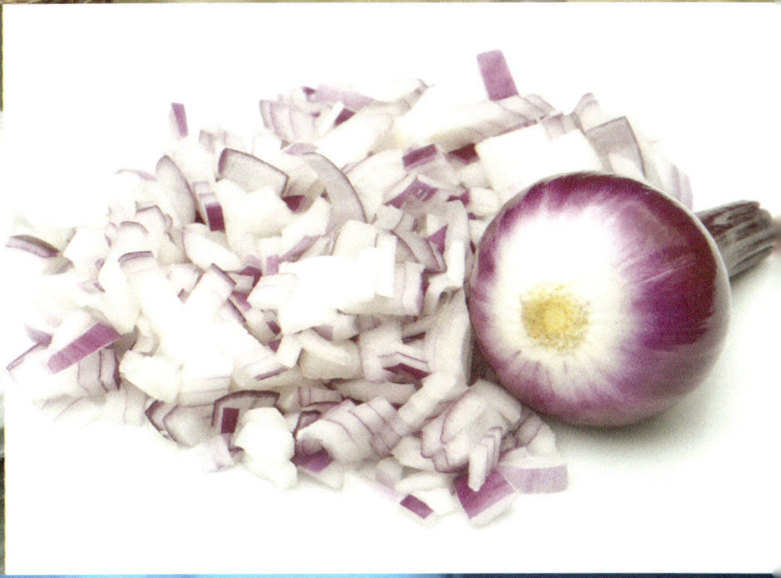
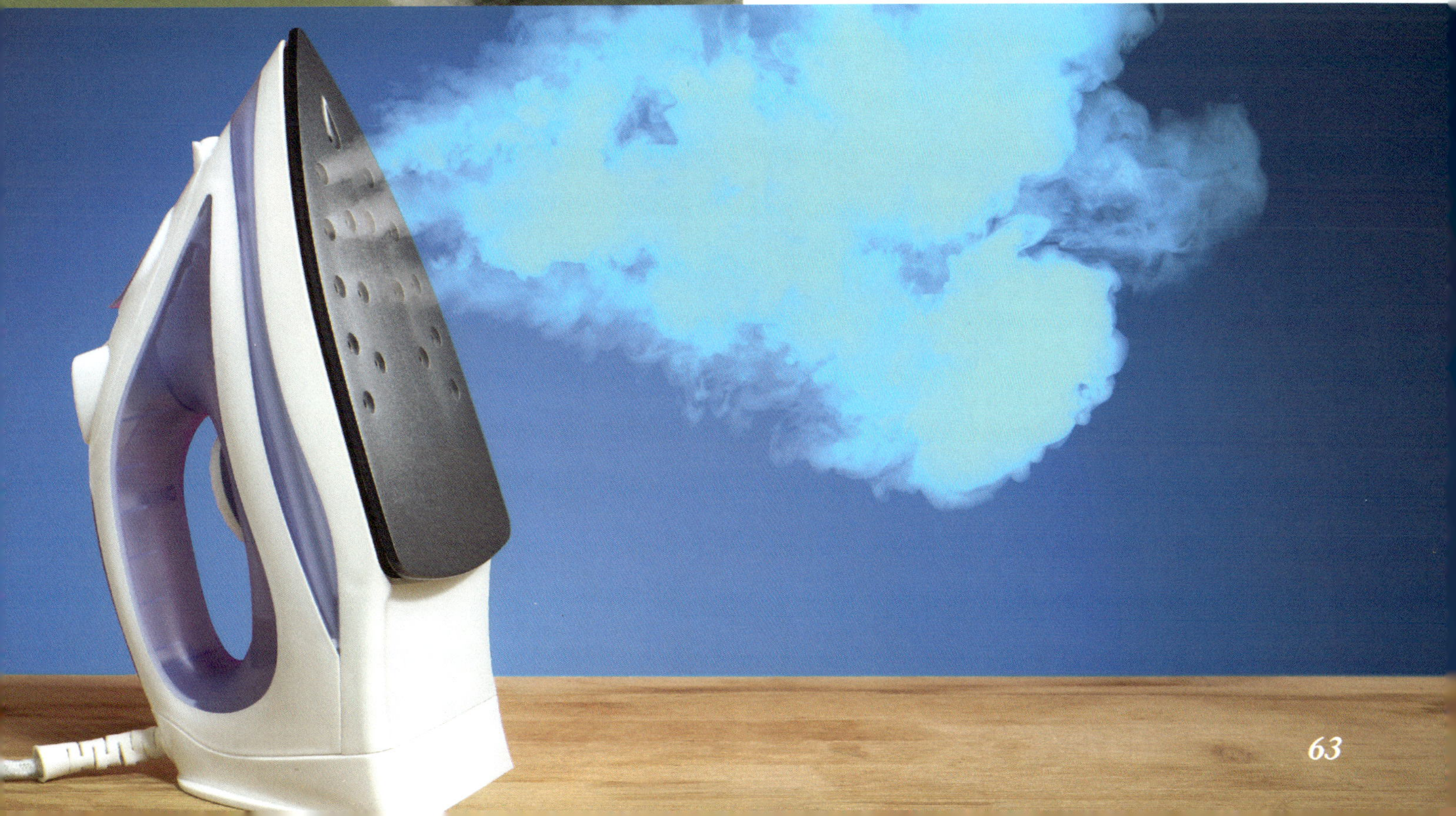

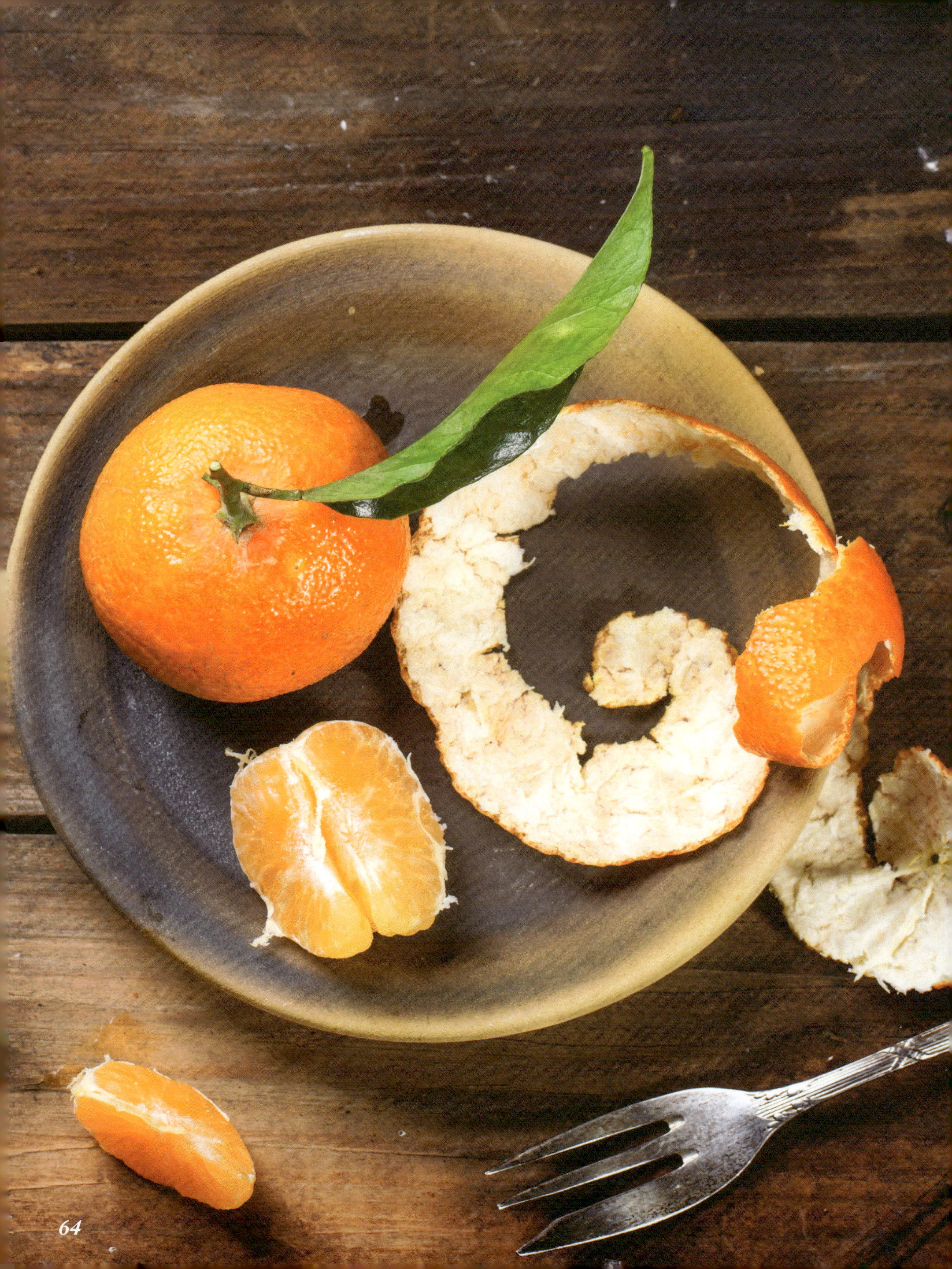

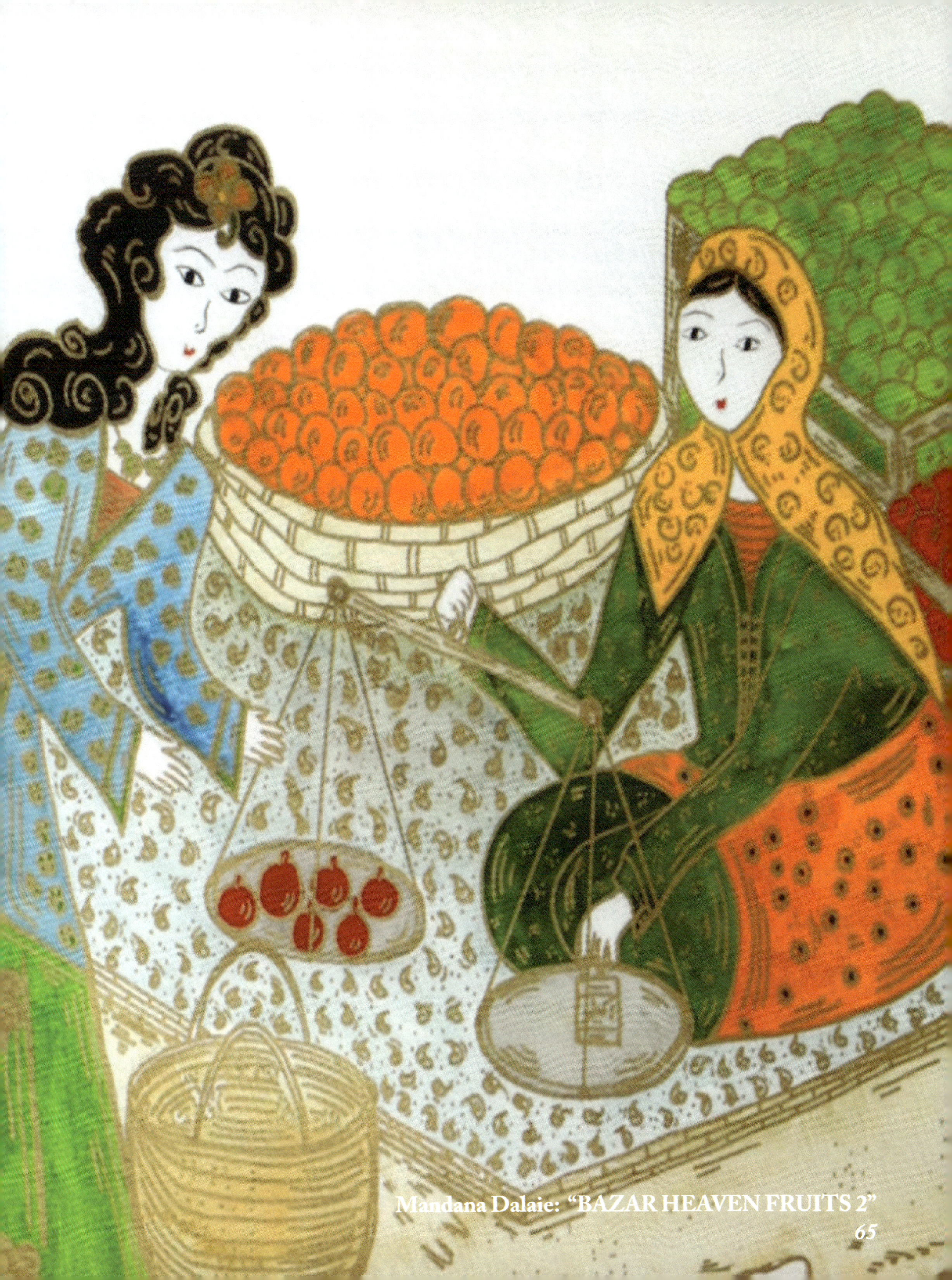

Mandana Dalaie: "BAZAR HEAVEN FRUITS 2"

ORANGE PEEL MAGIC

Natural Exfoliator

Dried orange peel beads can act as a natural exfoliator by removing dead cells and blackheads gently and naturally while also helping to remove dark spots and blemishes. Due to their cleansing, anti-inflammatory, antibacterial and antifungal properties, they work well against pimples and acne.

Dry orange peels in dehumidifier or leave in the sunlight to dry. Grind in food processor?

Air Freshener

To remove damp or musty odor in your house and fill it with beautiful fragrance, boil a few peels in water and maybe add some clove or cinnamon.

Orange Peels in Cooking

If you use organic peels in cooking the orange zest can enhance the taste and flavor of many dishes.

Dried orange peels can absorb humidity from brown sugar. Just place half a peel in the bag.

Candy made with orange peels can improve your appetite and the Vitamin-C in them protects you by boosting your immune system.

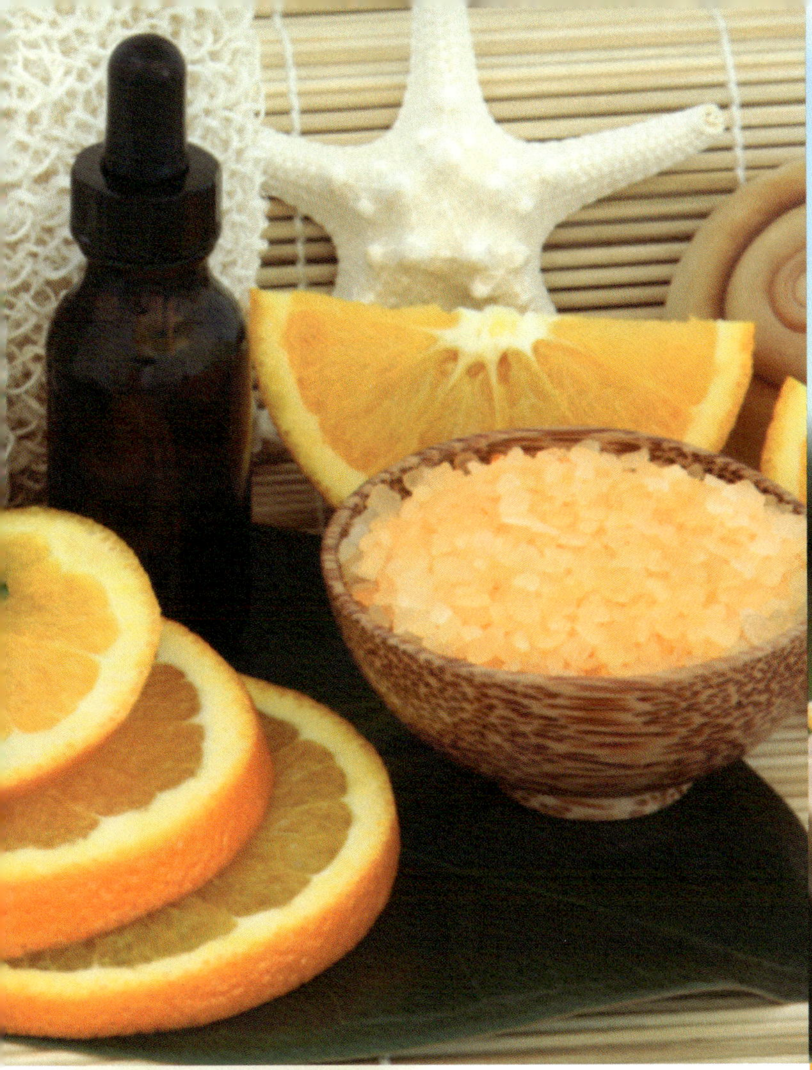
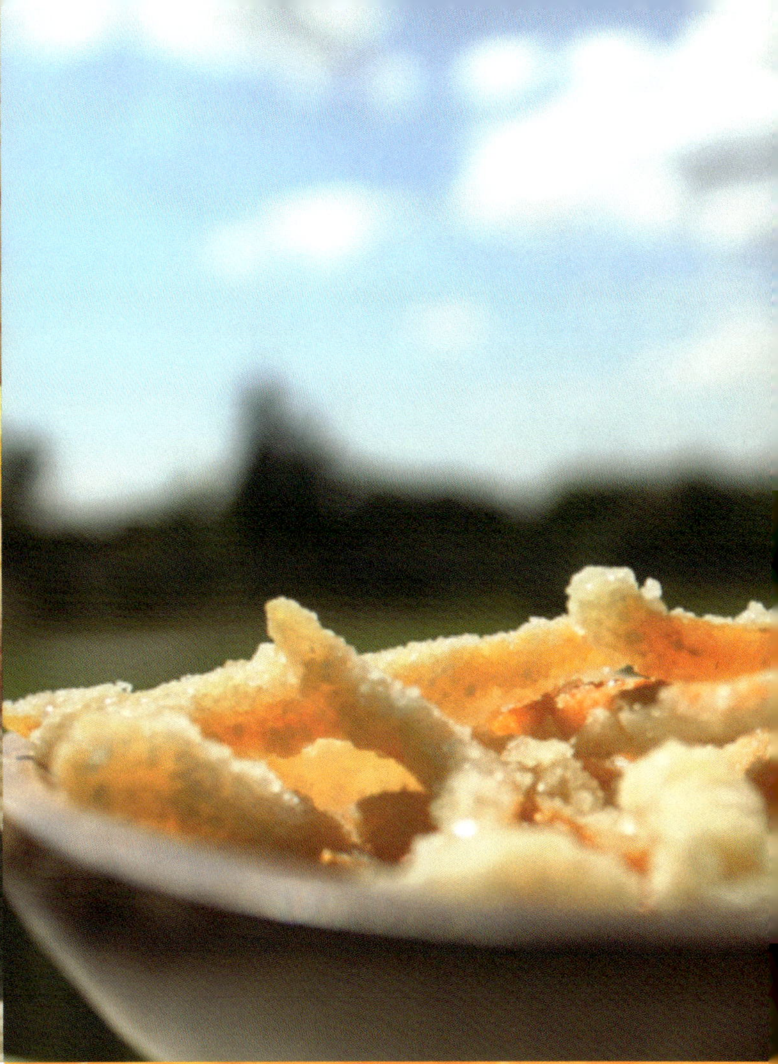
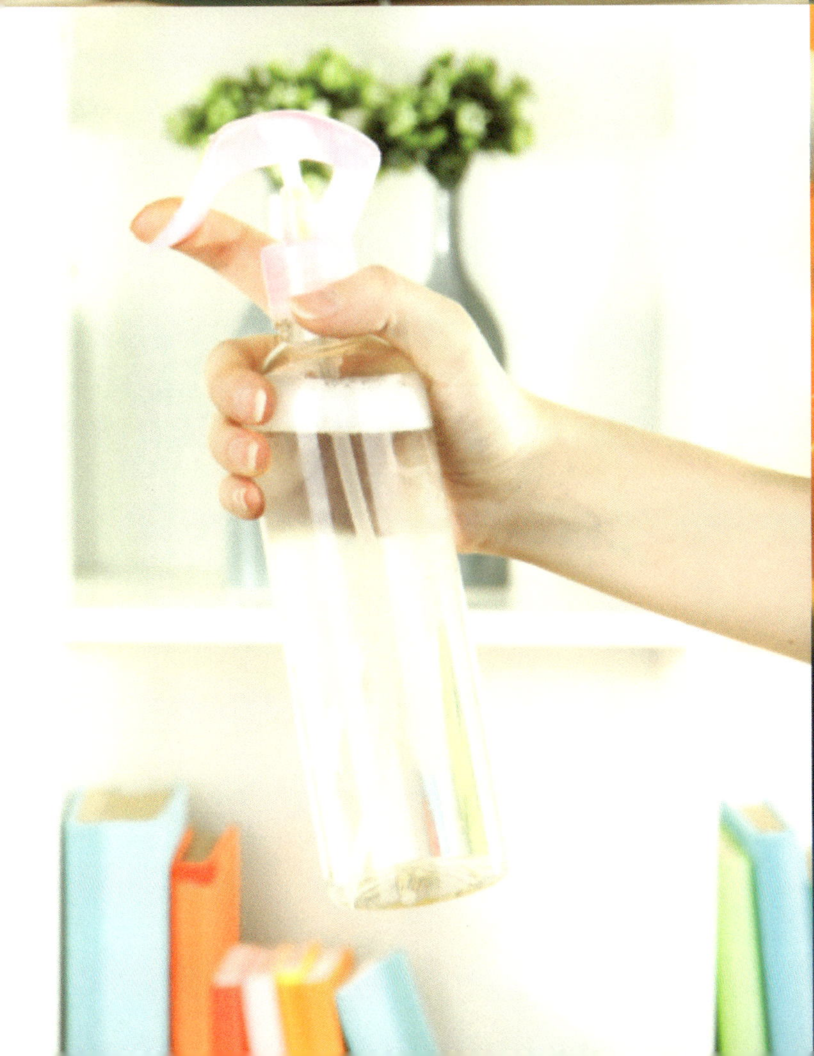
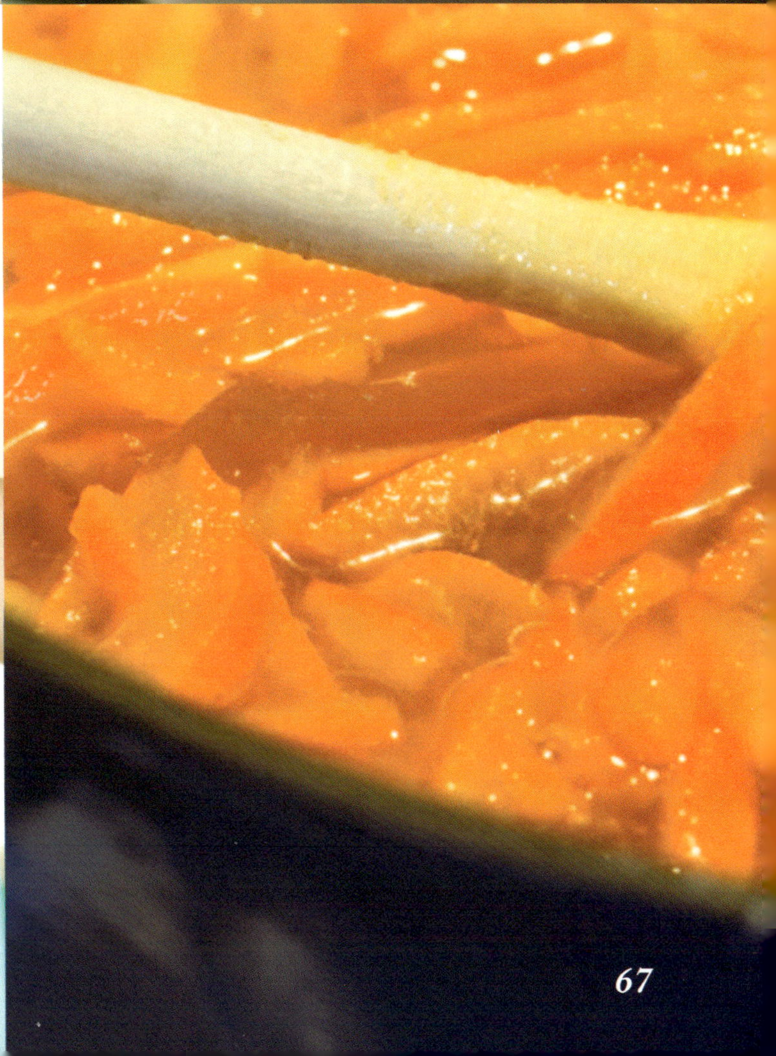

DIABETES CURE

Slows down absorption of sugar in blood stream; helps pancreas secrete insulin; helps reverse insulin resistance; improves circulation and rapid healing of the body; keeps blood sugar in balance; lowers bad cholesterol, and improves circulation.

4 oz pomegranate juice
2 Tablespoons raw coconut oil

Drink 30 minutes prior to breakfast on an empty stomach and in the evening an hour prior to sleep.

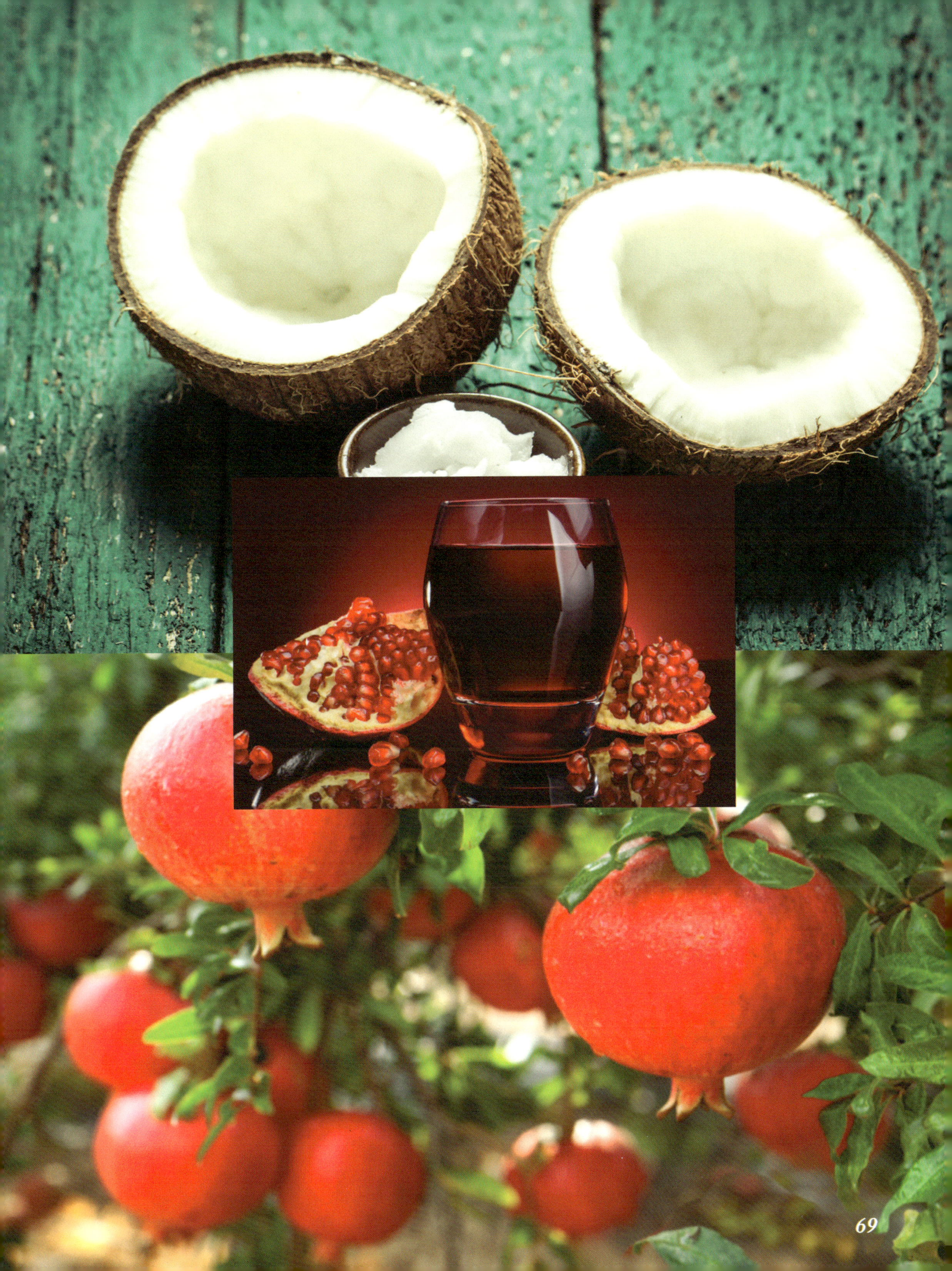

ECZEMA HEALING MASK

Many people have an issue with eczema either on certain parts of their body or all over. Eczema is related to the immune system and is often due to nerve and liver congestion.

Sedr (organic Zizyphus spina-christi) is derived from a wild fruit tree called jujube, an evergreen native to Iran, Africa and southern and western Asia. It is revered as a sacred tree. The ripe fruits are edible and the flowers are an important source of honey. The leaves are dried and made into a green powder. Sedr is filled with antioxidants and many more attributes. Sedr powder has also been used in Iran for hundreds of years to cleanse and condition hair, adding thickness and protecting hair from the elements. Some recent studies even indicate the promotion of hair growth with the use of sedr.

1 Teaspoon sedr powder
1 Tablespoon filtered water
1 Tablespoon coconut water

Mix Into a paste and brush on evenly with a kabuki or fan brush. Cover the troubled area and leave it for an hour, then rinse off with cool water. For people with severe afflictions paint the affected areas in the shower and wash off in an hour. Perform this regimen at least 3 times a week.

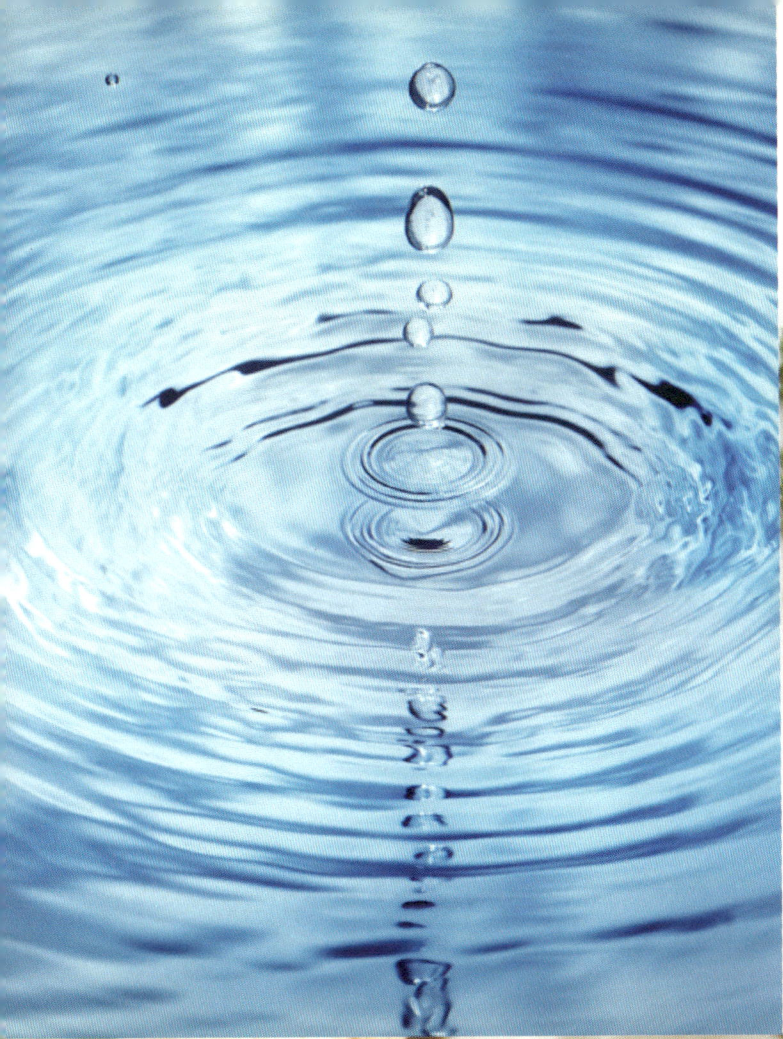
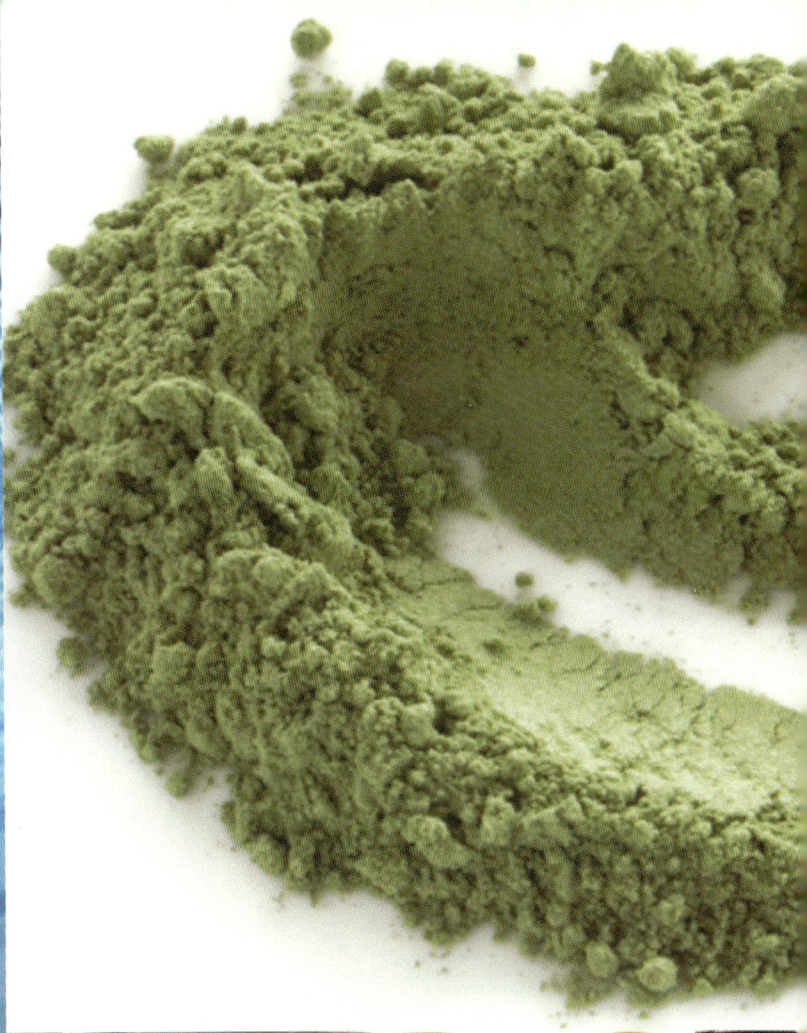
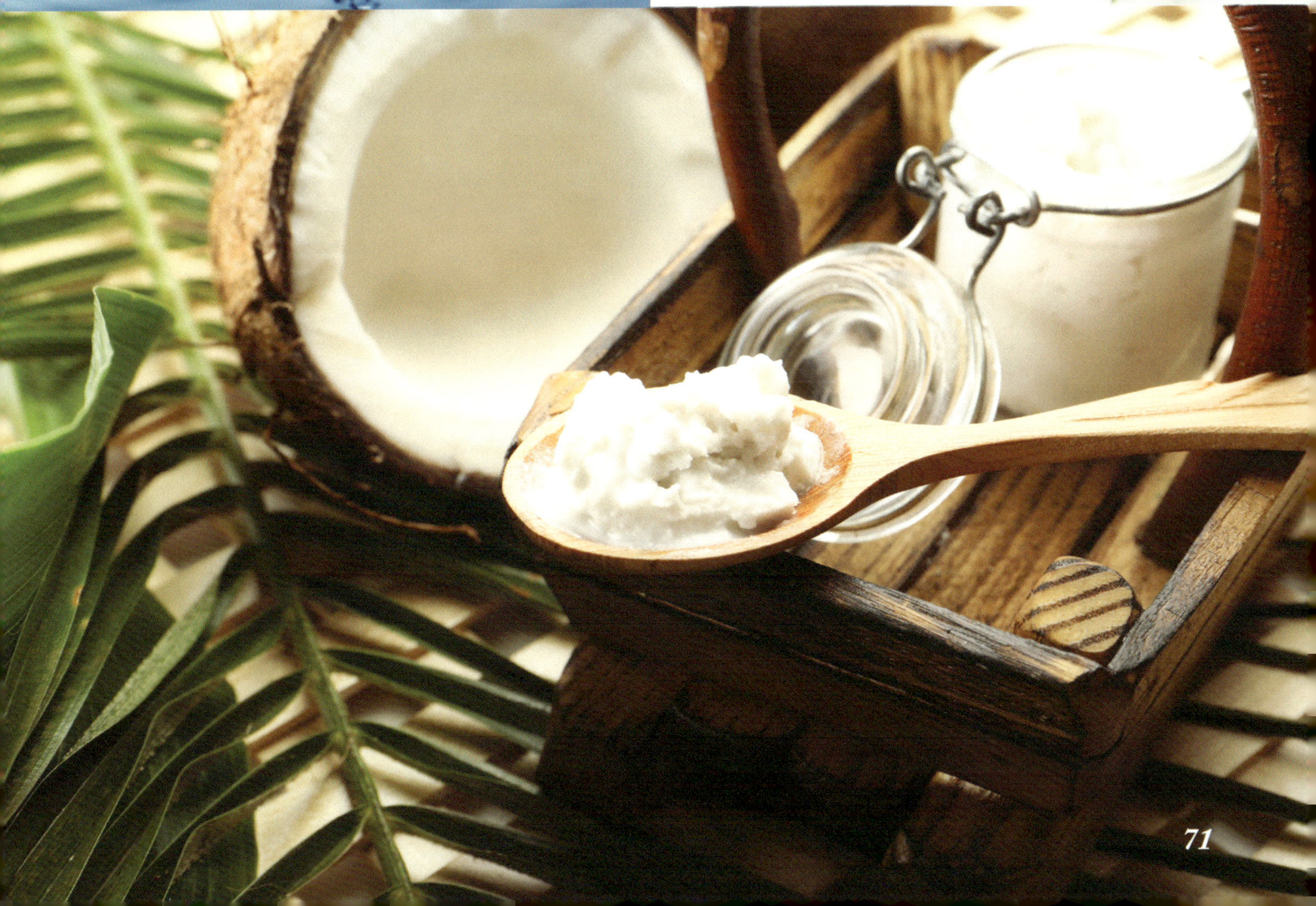

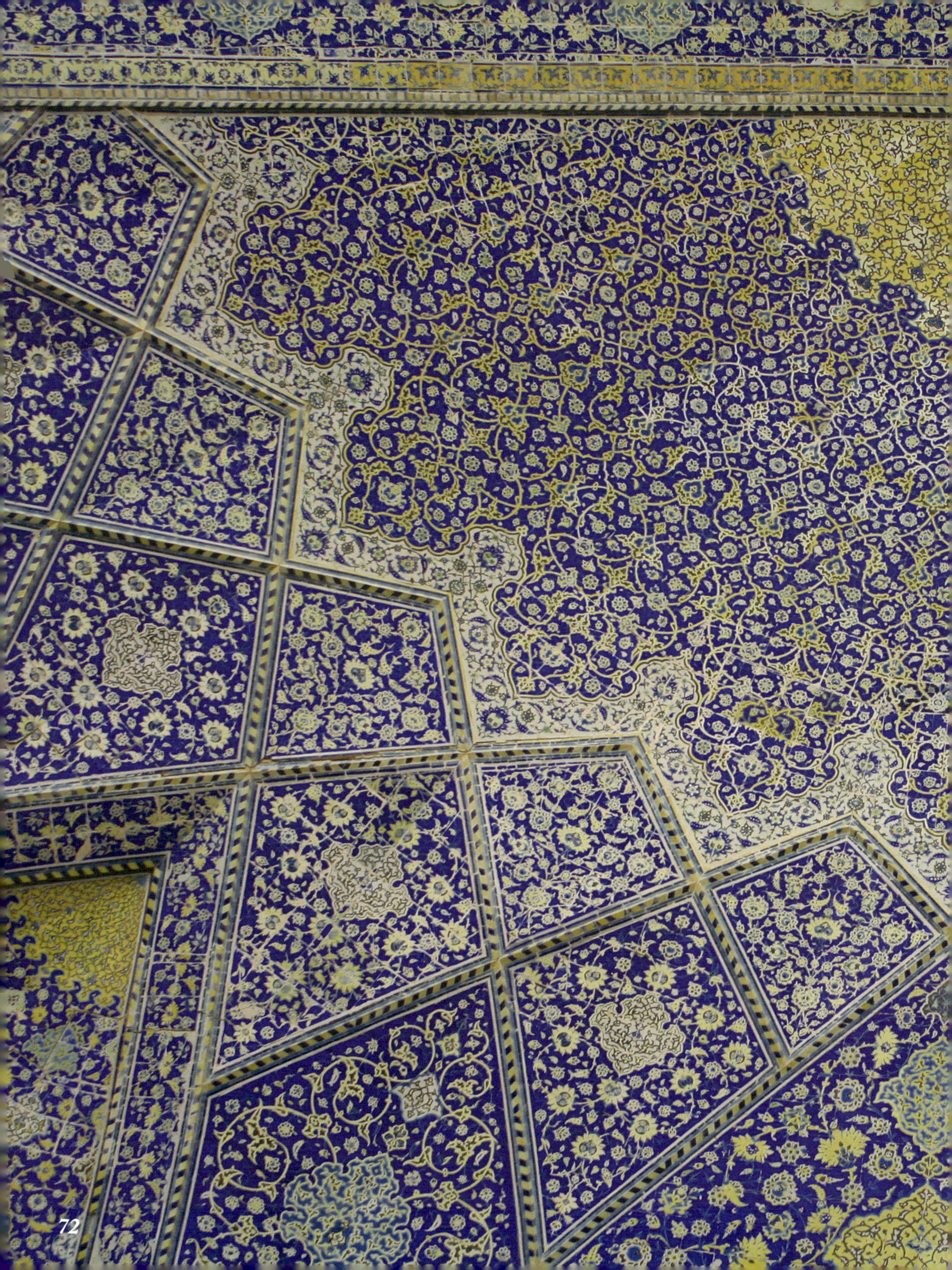

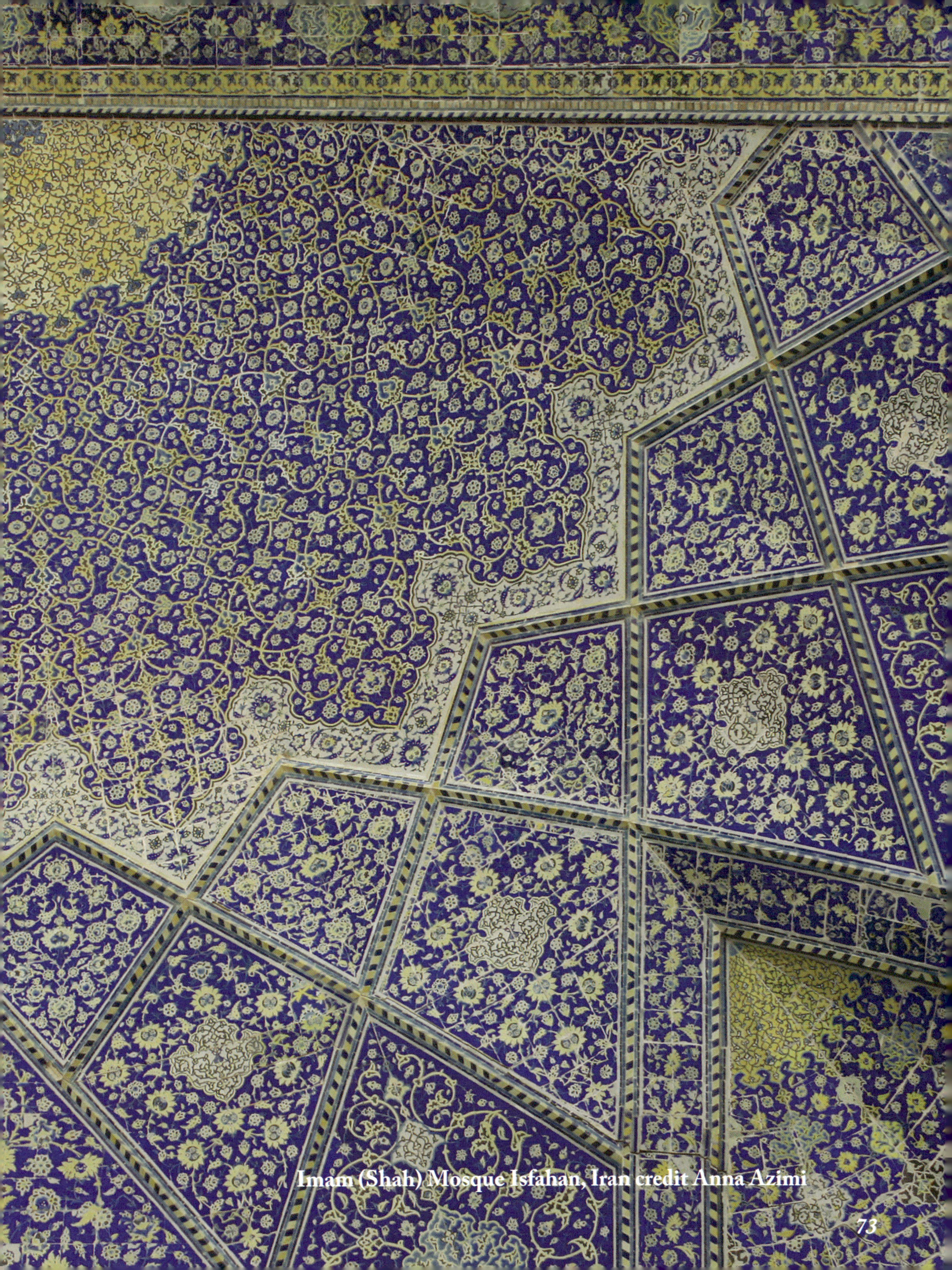

Imam (Shah) Mosque Isfahan, Iran credit Anna Azimi

THE BANANA PEEL CURE-ALL

Banana peels are full of antioxidants, minerals, and vitamins, so they can naturally cure many ailments and aid cell regeneration. (As with orange peel, make sure you use organic banana peels to reduce your exposure to pesticide levels and you might even want to try the wash described on page 86.)

Bug Bites

Just rub a banana peel on a bug bite to soothe the skin and reduce the itch.

Bruises

With regenerative properties, banana peel can speed up the healing of bruises.

Teeth Whitening

Rub the inside of a banana peel on your teeth for a couple of minutes every other day and your teeth will be noticeably whiter in a few weeks. The amazing minerals in the peel like potassium, magnesium and manganese absorb into your teeth and whiten them.

Warts

Banana peels help eliminate warts and prevent their return. Tape or somehow strap a piece of banana peel to the wart overnight for about a week or rub the banana peel on the affected area daily. This can also work for plantar warts. A potato skin has been known to be able to do the same thing.

Scrapes and Scratches

Rub a banana peel on small cuts or scratches to promote healing.

Splinters

The enzymes help dislodge the splinter and can help kick-start the healing process if you tape a piece of the peel over a splinter for a couple hours.

Acne

A banana peel can soothe the inflammation and irritation of acne. It also helps to prevent future outbreaks. Rub a peel over the acne every night. You should see a positive change within a few days.

Psoriasis

Once or twice a day rub a banana peel on a psoriasis-affected area. Bananas have properties to reduce itchiness, moisturize and heal psoriasis.

Rashes and Itches

Banana peel is good for relieving itch and promotes healing of such conditions as poison ivy, mild rashes, dry skin, irritated skin and sunburn. Rub the peel over affected area twice daily until it is gone.

Headaches

Simply take the banana peel and spread it out across your forehead and relax while the nutrients such as potassium, magnesium, calcium and sulfur are absorbed into your skin.

Wrinkles

Regularly applying banana peel to your forehead, face or cheeks can tighten the skin, shrink pores and reduce wrinkles.

Household

Banana peels are great for polishing. After removing the stringy parts from the peel, rub away tarnish on silver and to shine your shoes.

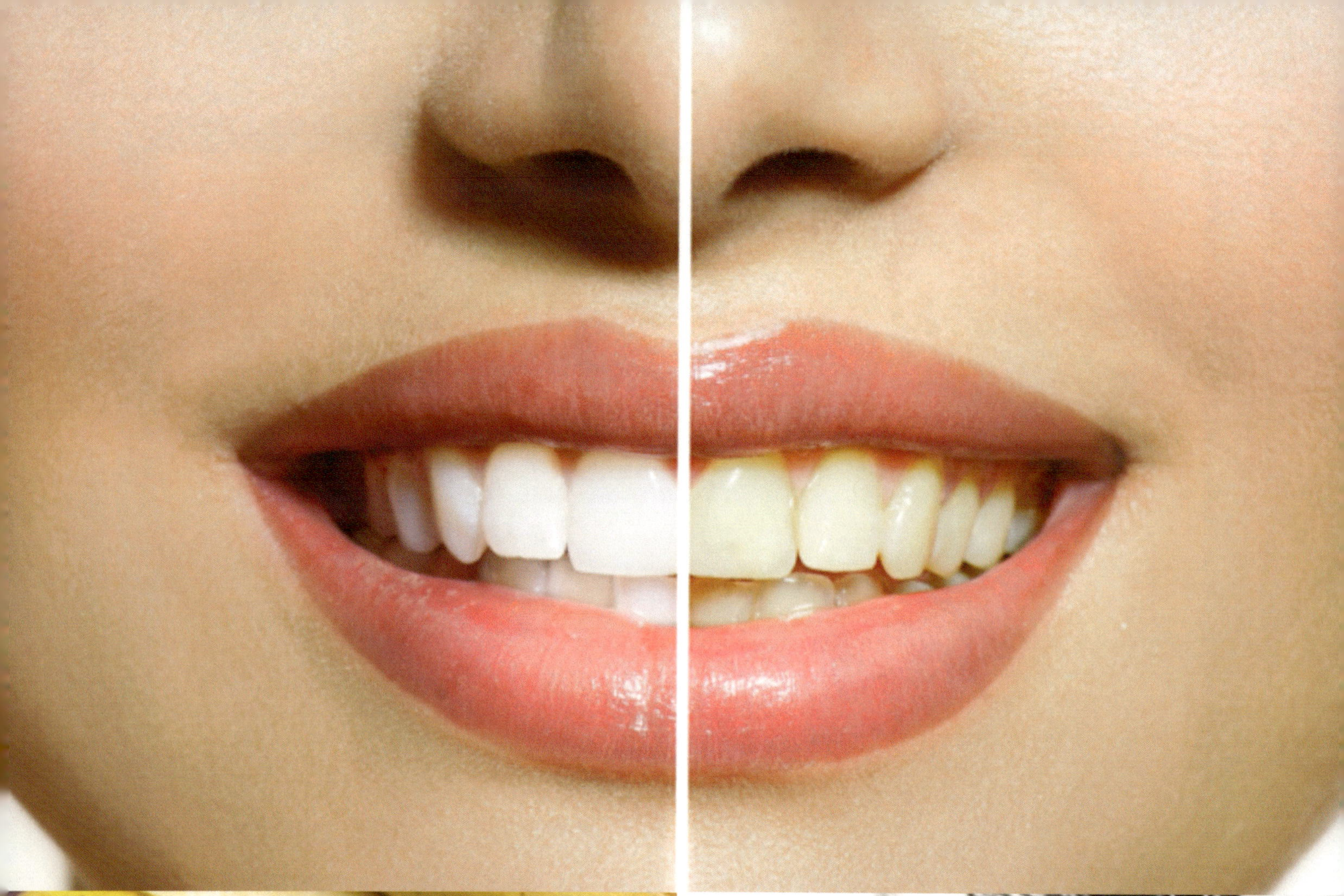
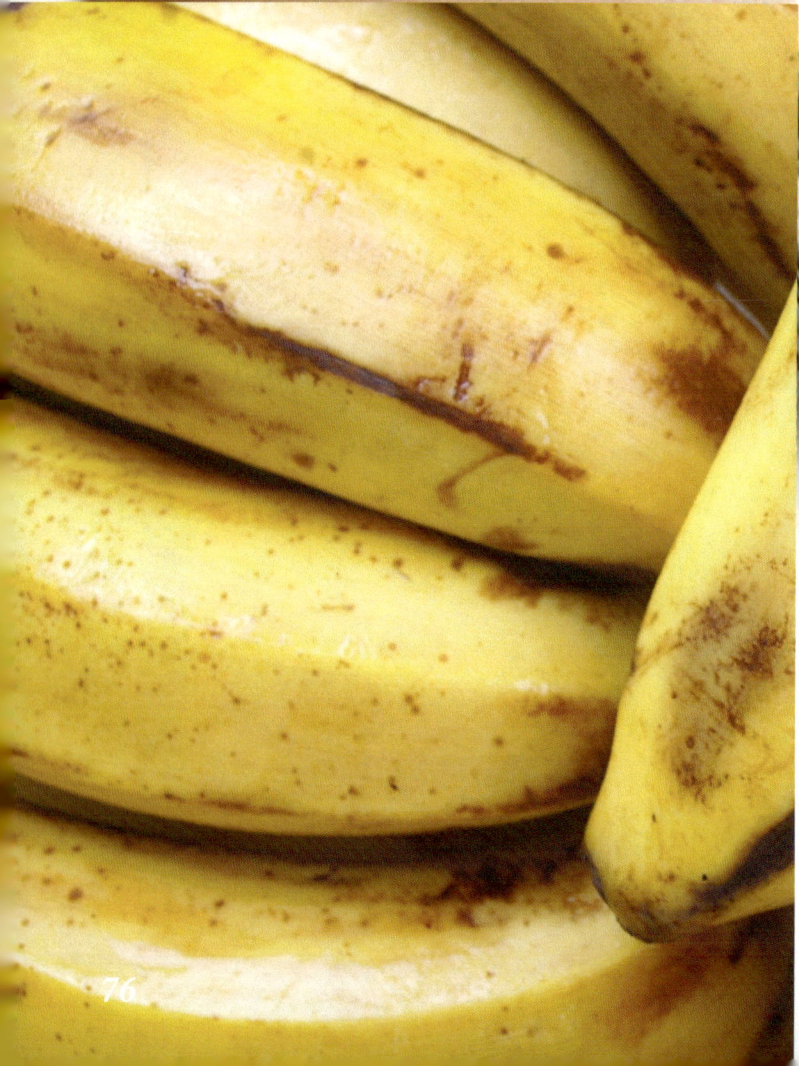
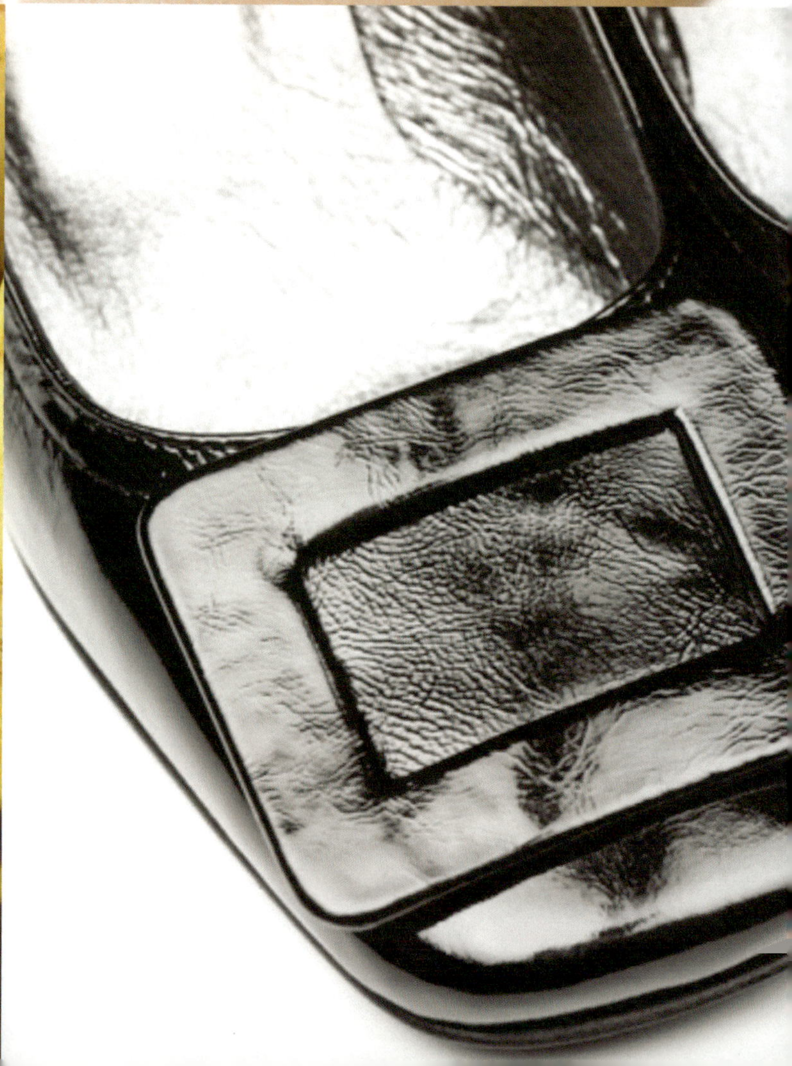

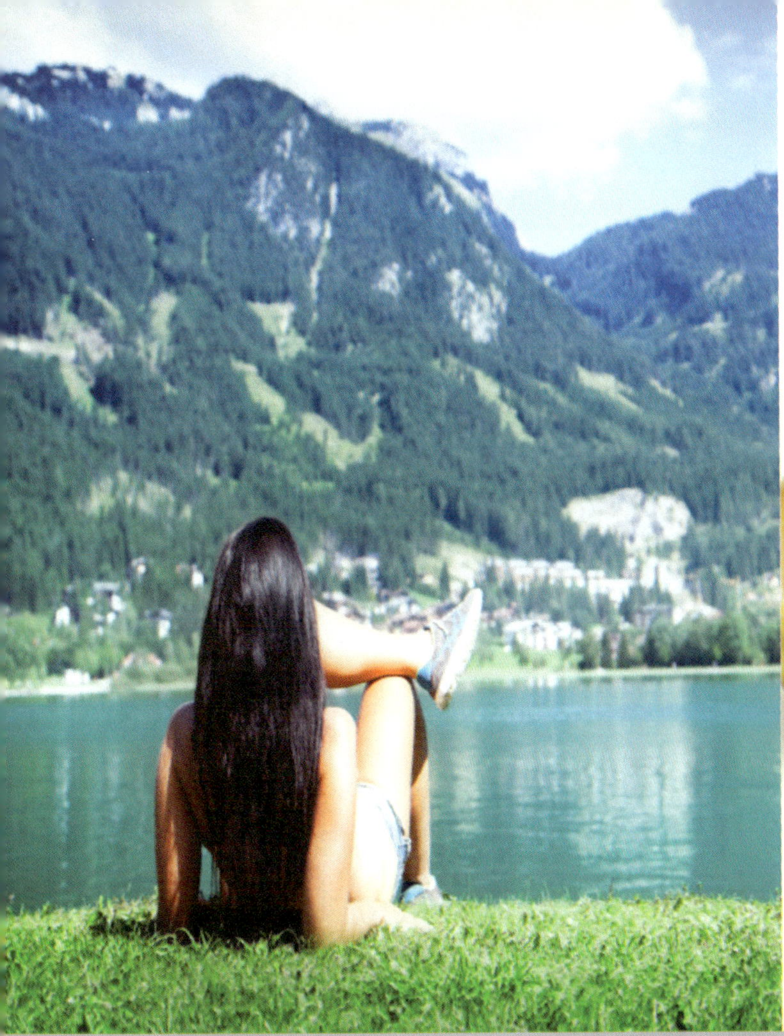
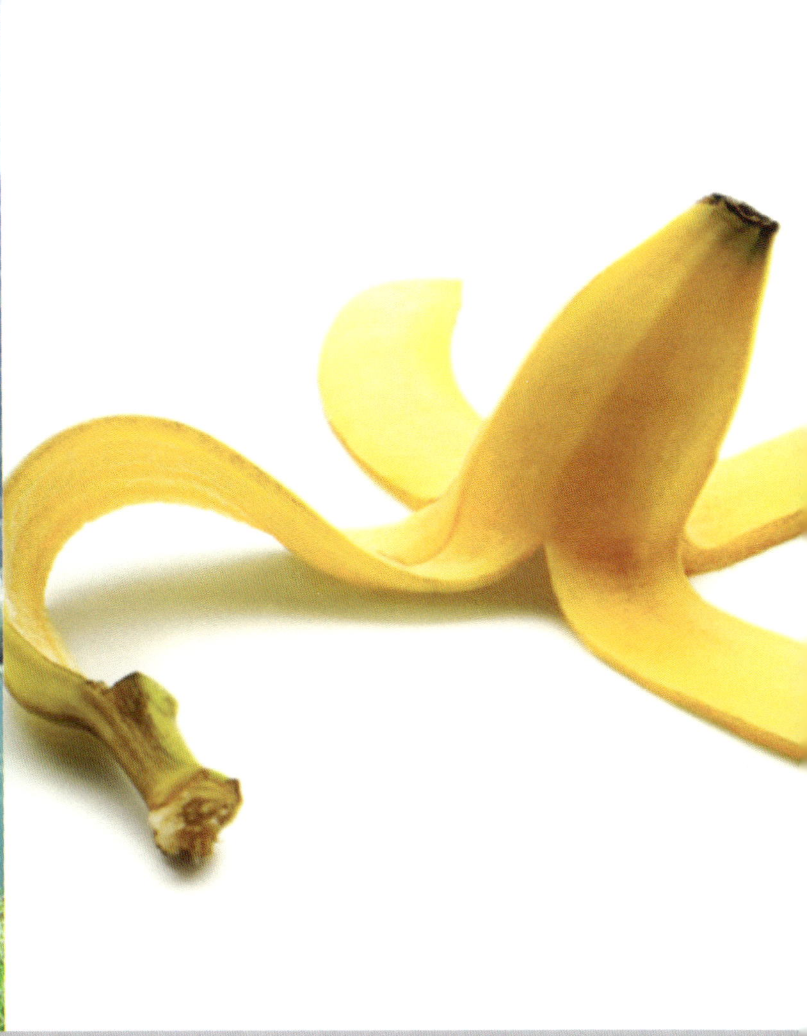
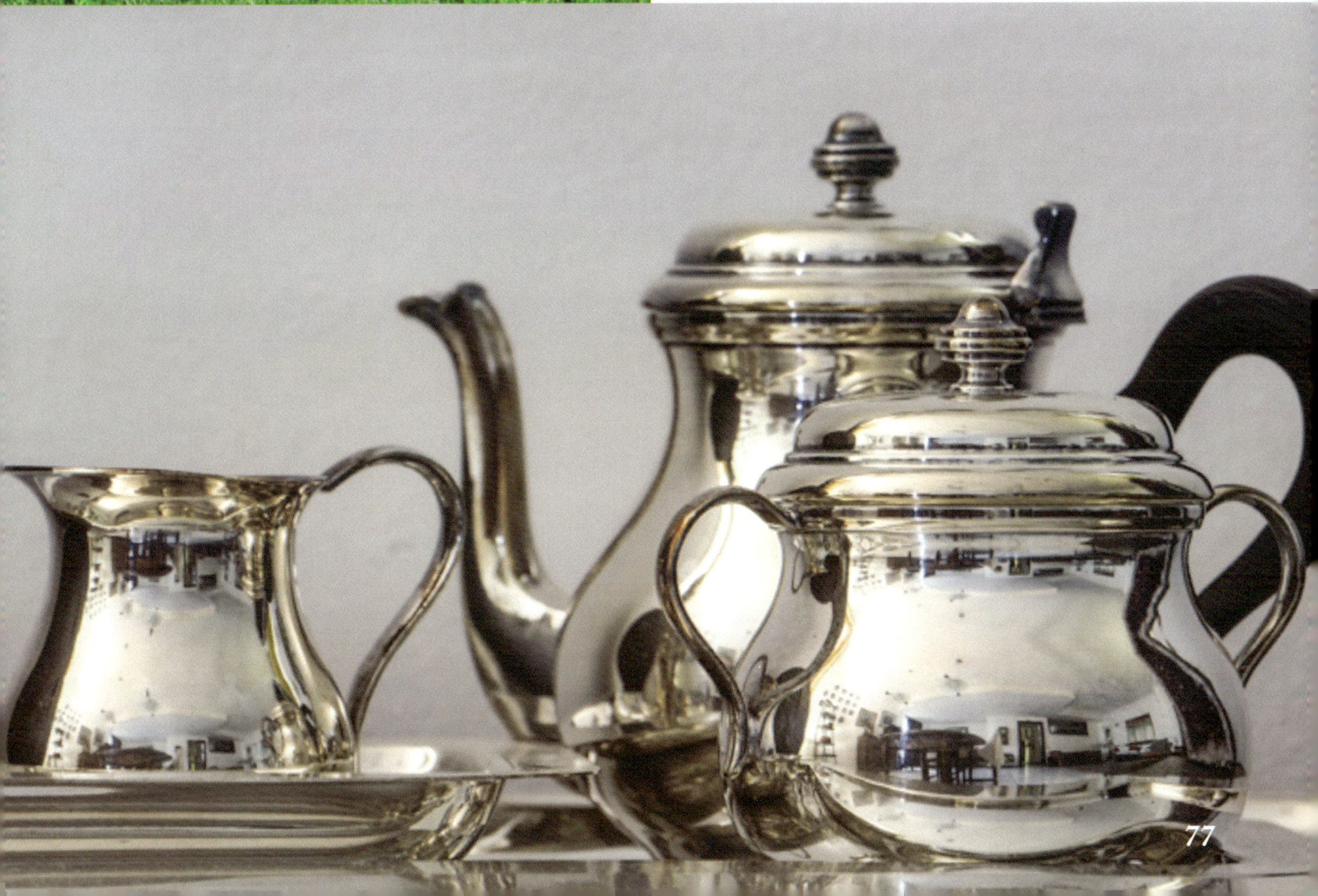

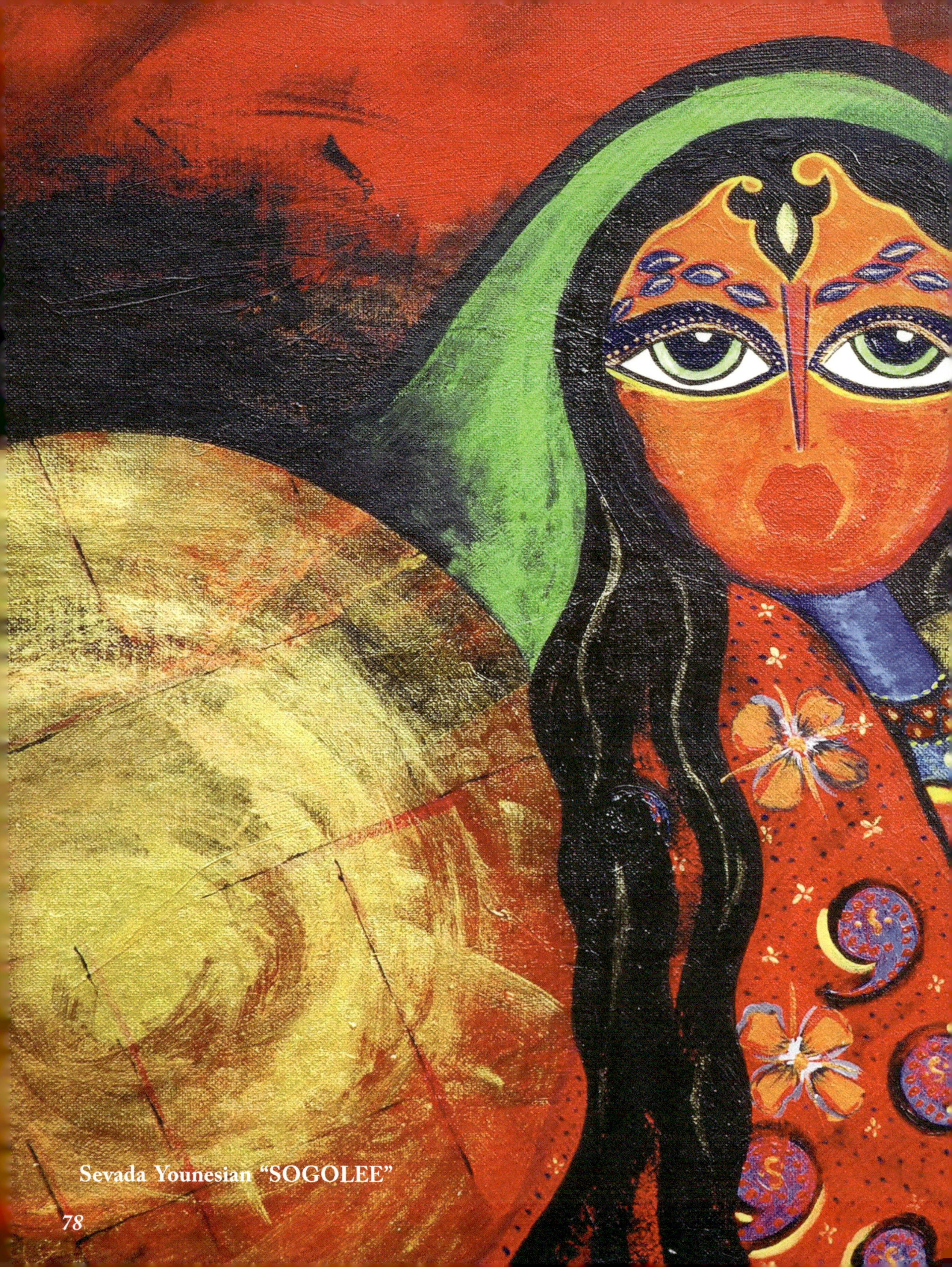

Sevada Younesian "SOGOLEE"

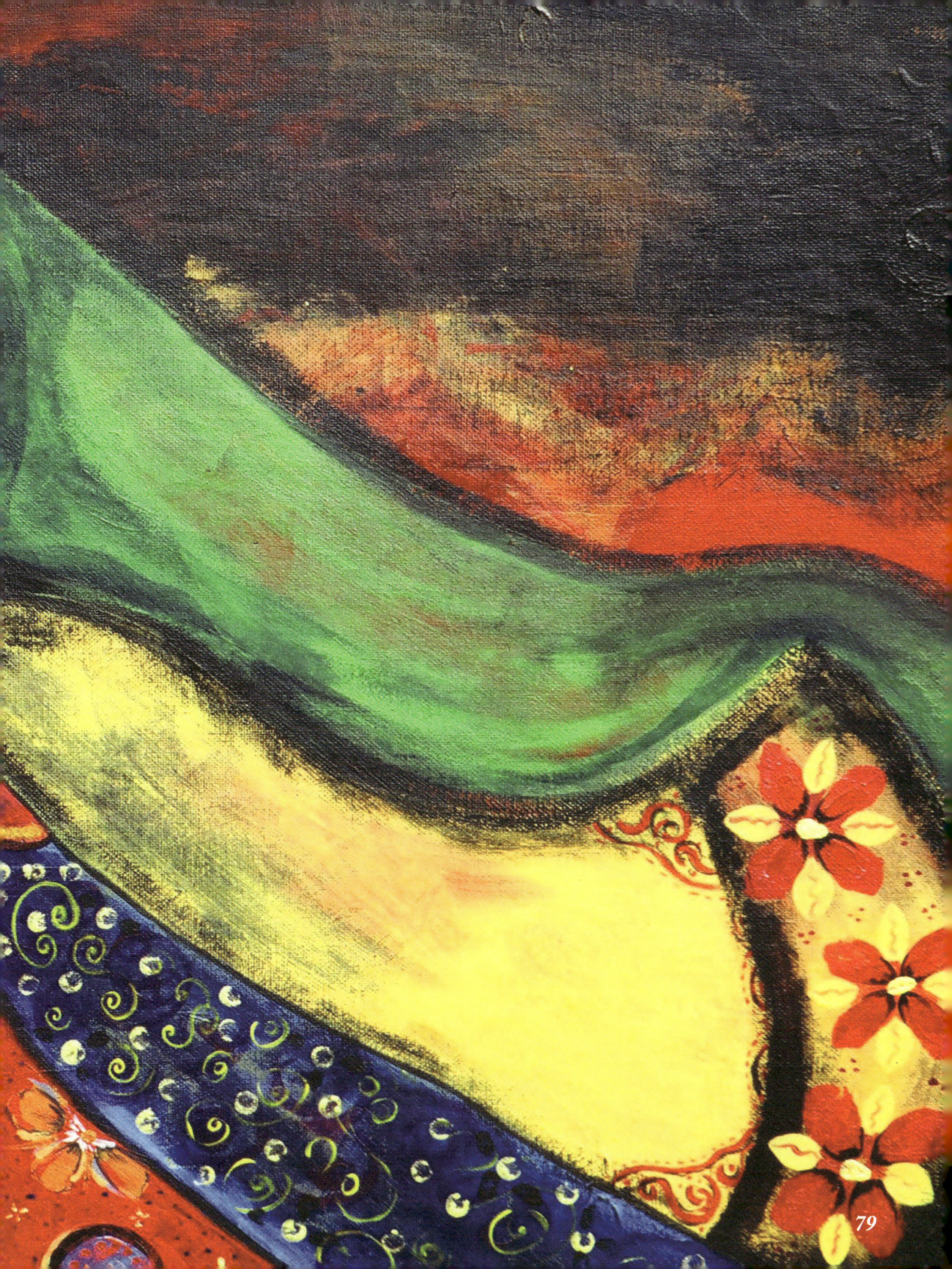

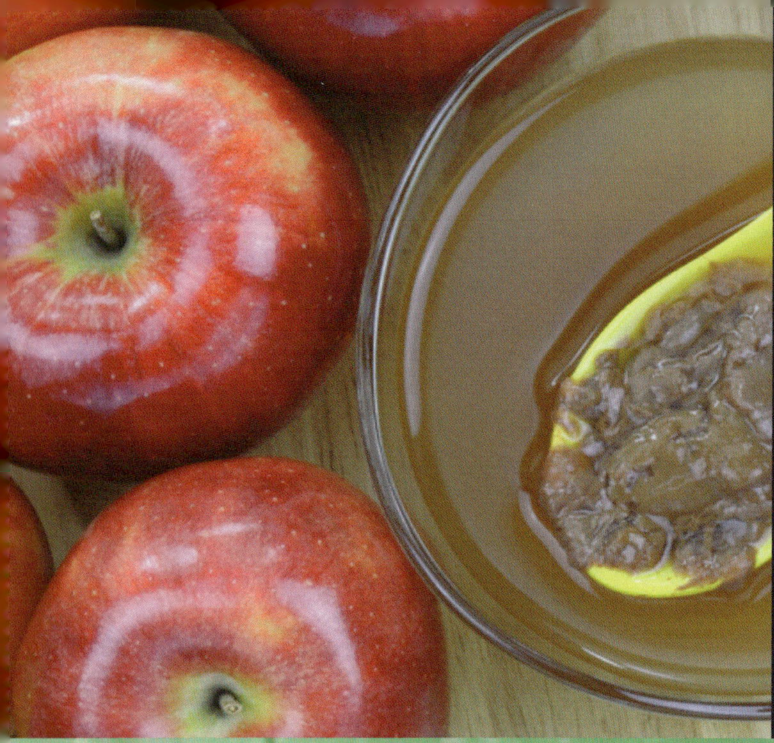

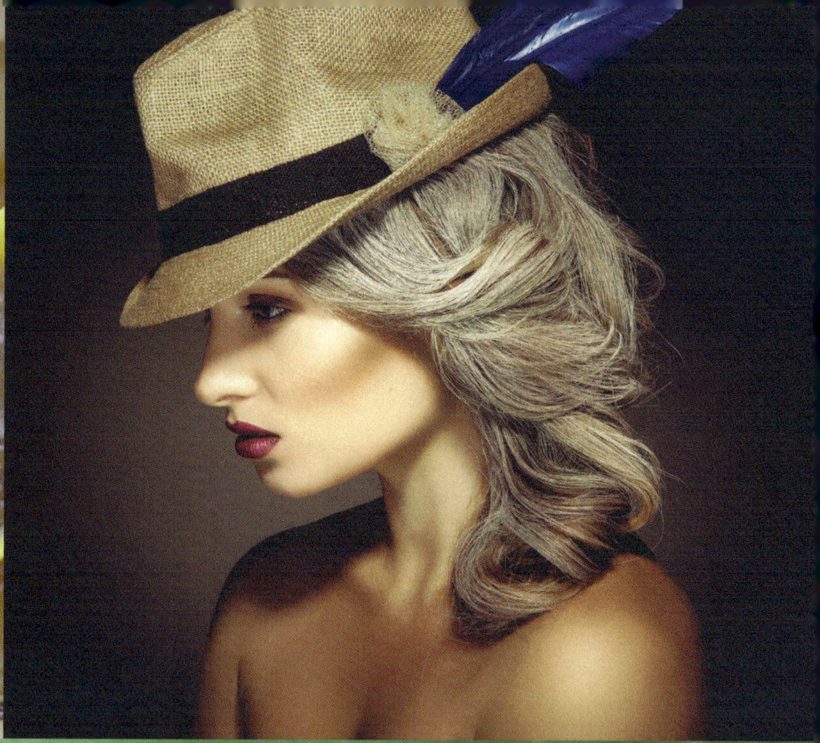

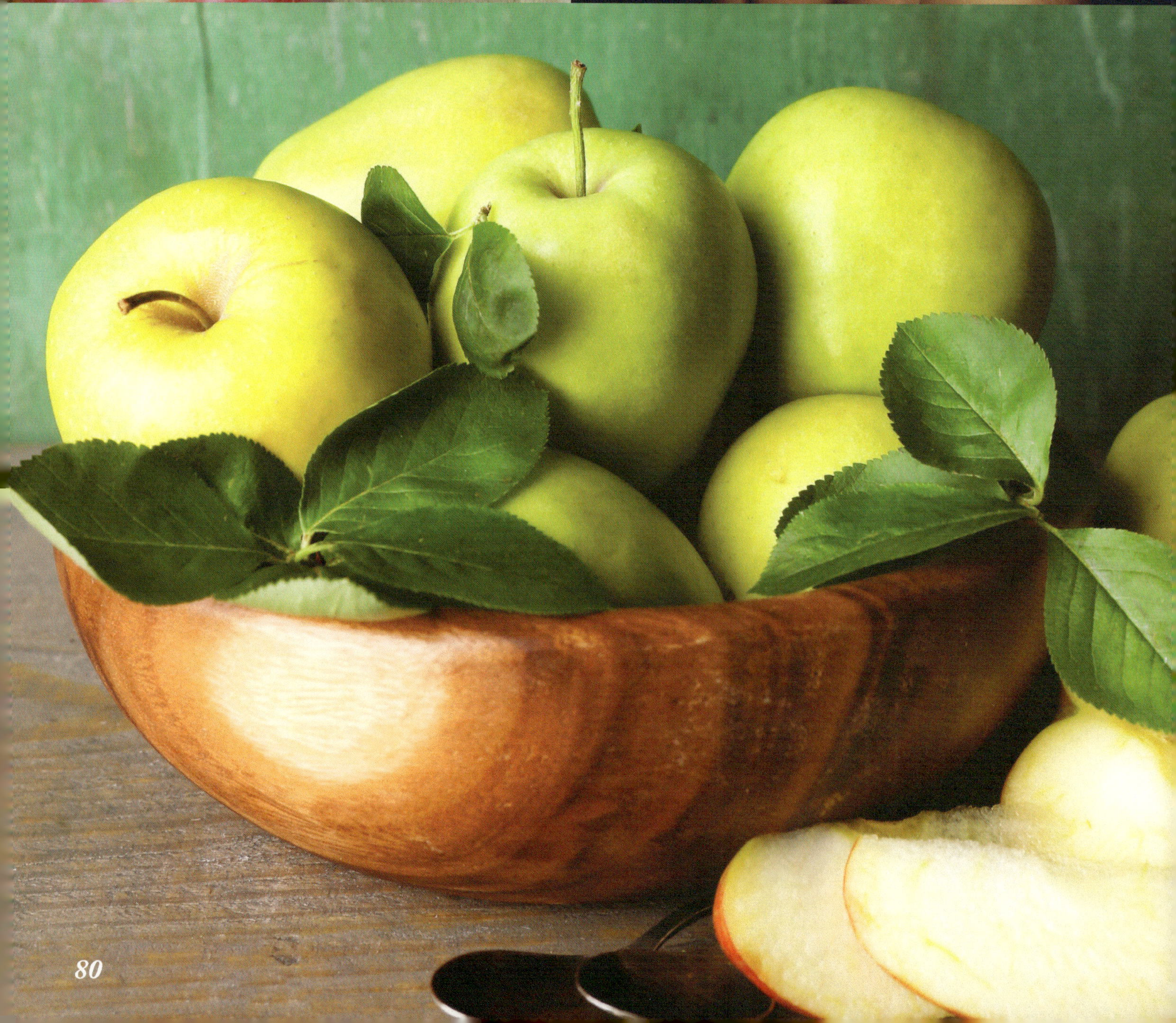

HAIR

Wash away grey

1 Organic Apple
2 Tablespoons apple cider vinegar

Juice apple with seeds and skin, then mix with apple cider vinegar. Mix well and apply generously to the root of your hair and grey areas. Wear shower cap and leave in for a few hours or overnight. Wash out in the morning.

AVOCADO MASK

For hair loss and strong growth

1/2 Avocado
1 Tablespoon organic coconut oil
1 Egg yolk
*1 Tablespoon of cow or sheep brain**

Mix together and apply to scalp and hair. Leave overnight with shower cap or for at least one hour, shampoo.

**This was the original recipe, instead of brain you can substitute natural protein powder.*

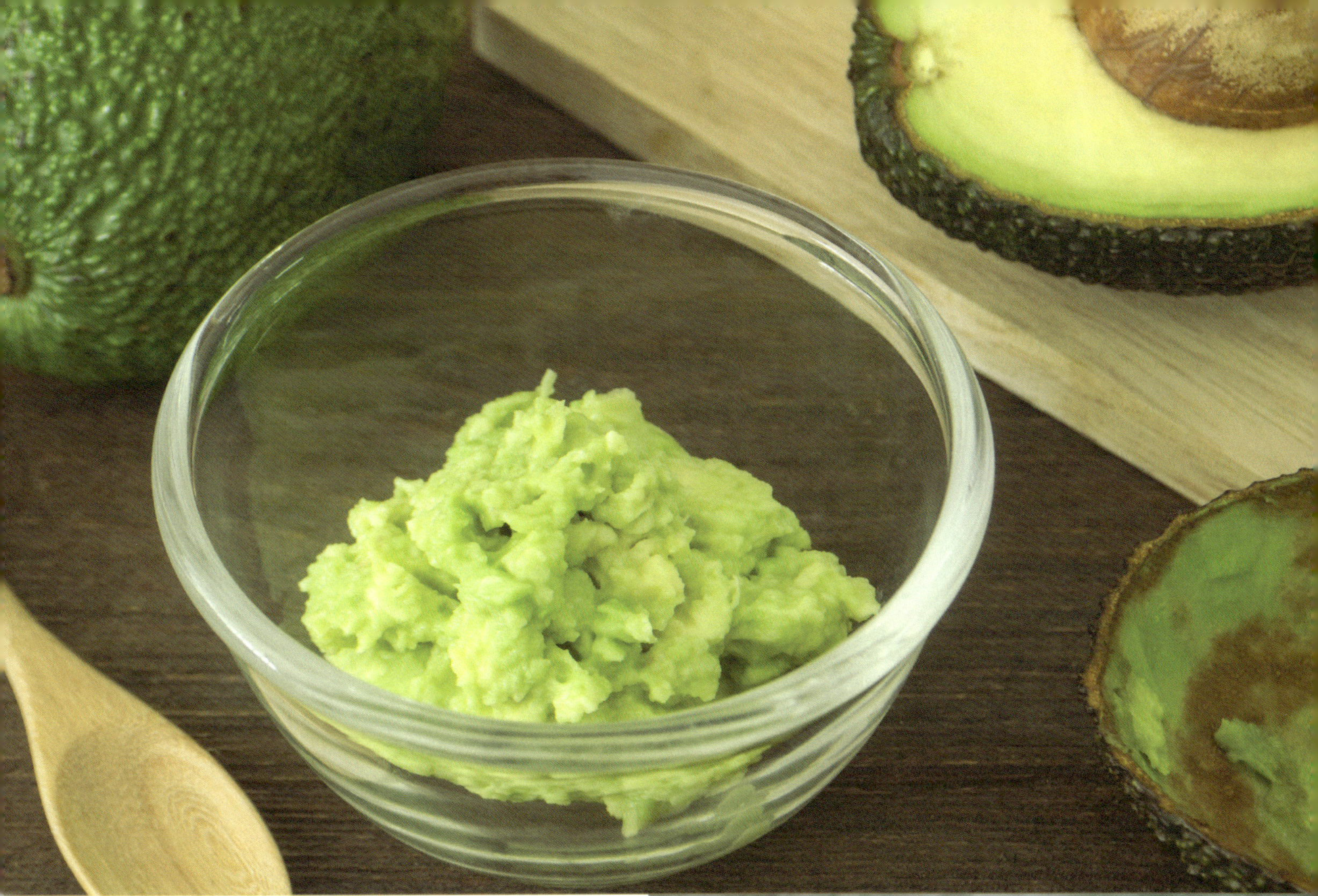

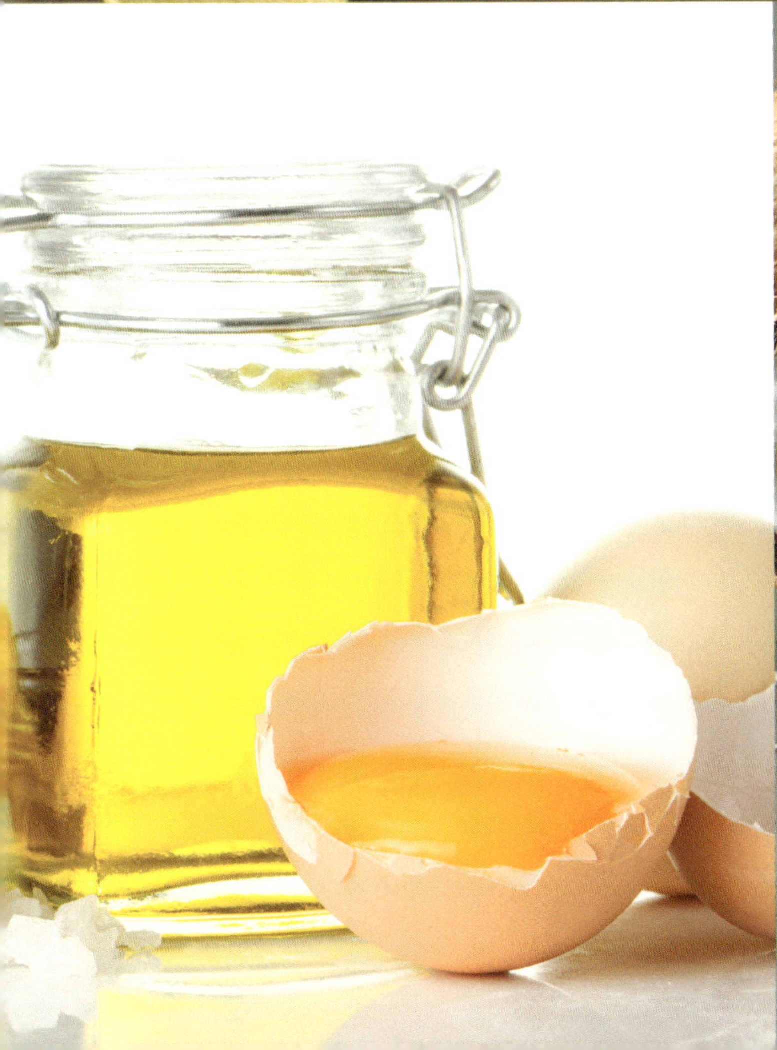

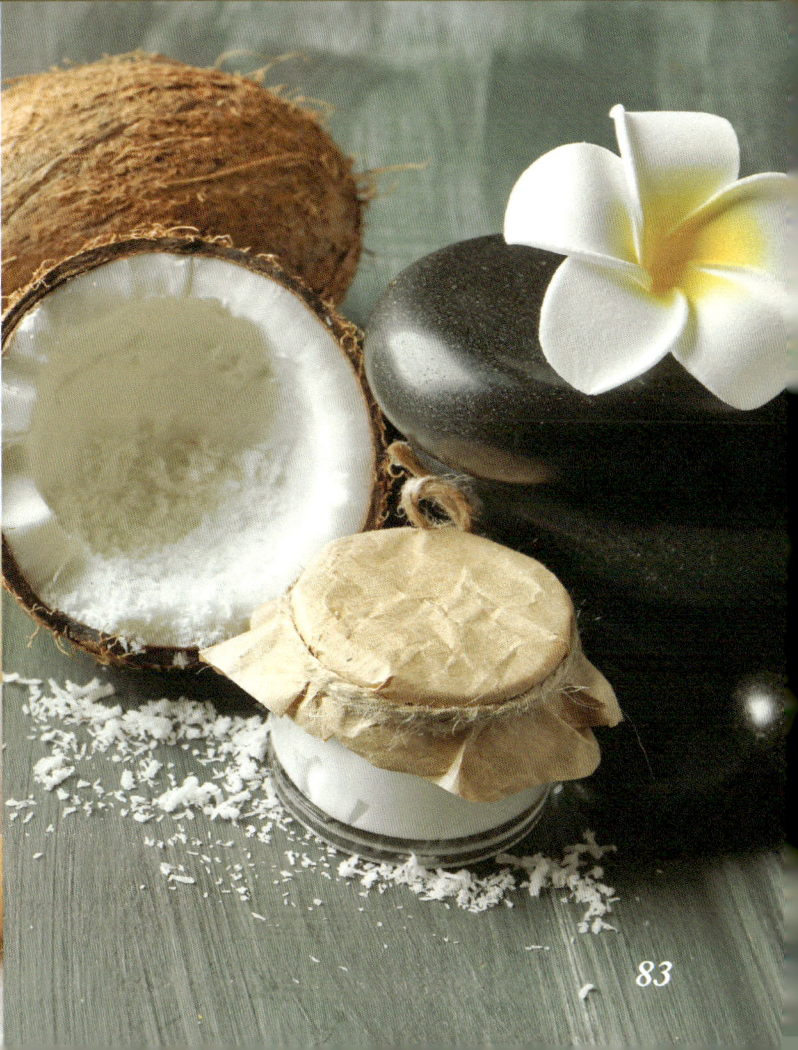

THICKENING HAIR MASK

3 Organic carrots
2 Teaspoons castor oil (from health food store, not drug store)

Juice 3 medium carrots and mix with castor oil. Apply to head and hair and leave overnight with shower cap or for at least two hours, shampoo.

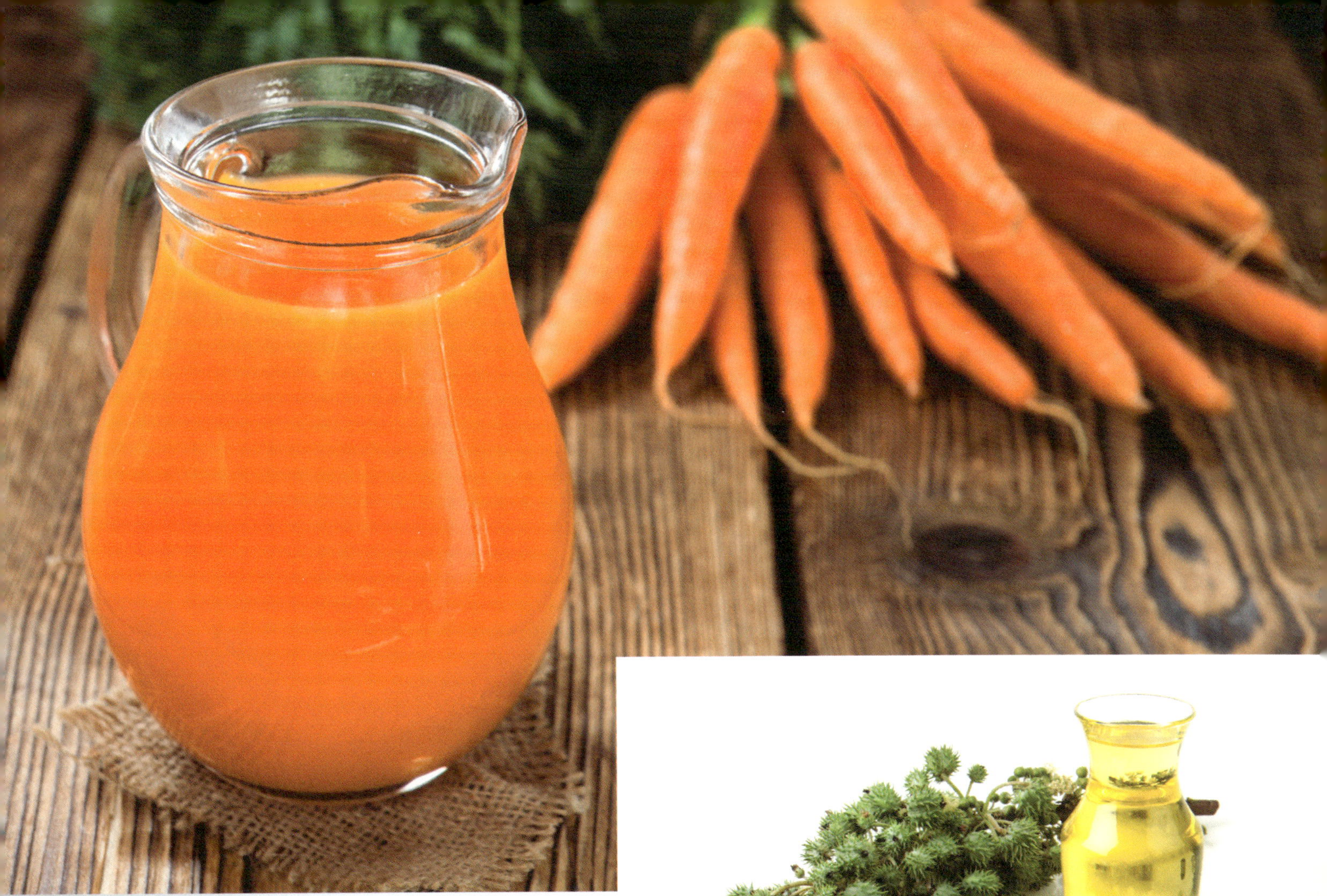
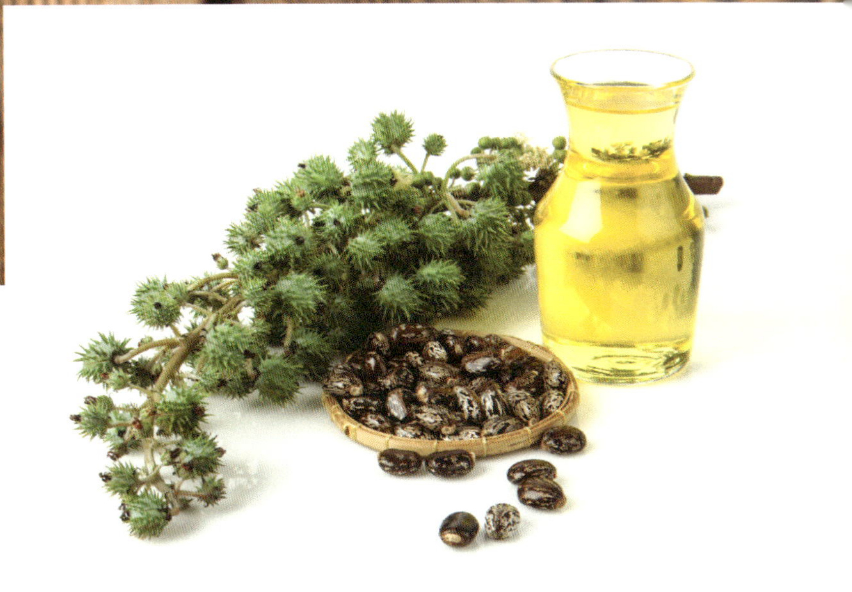
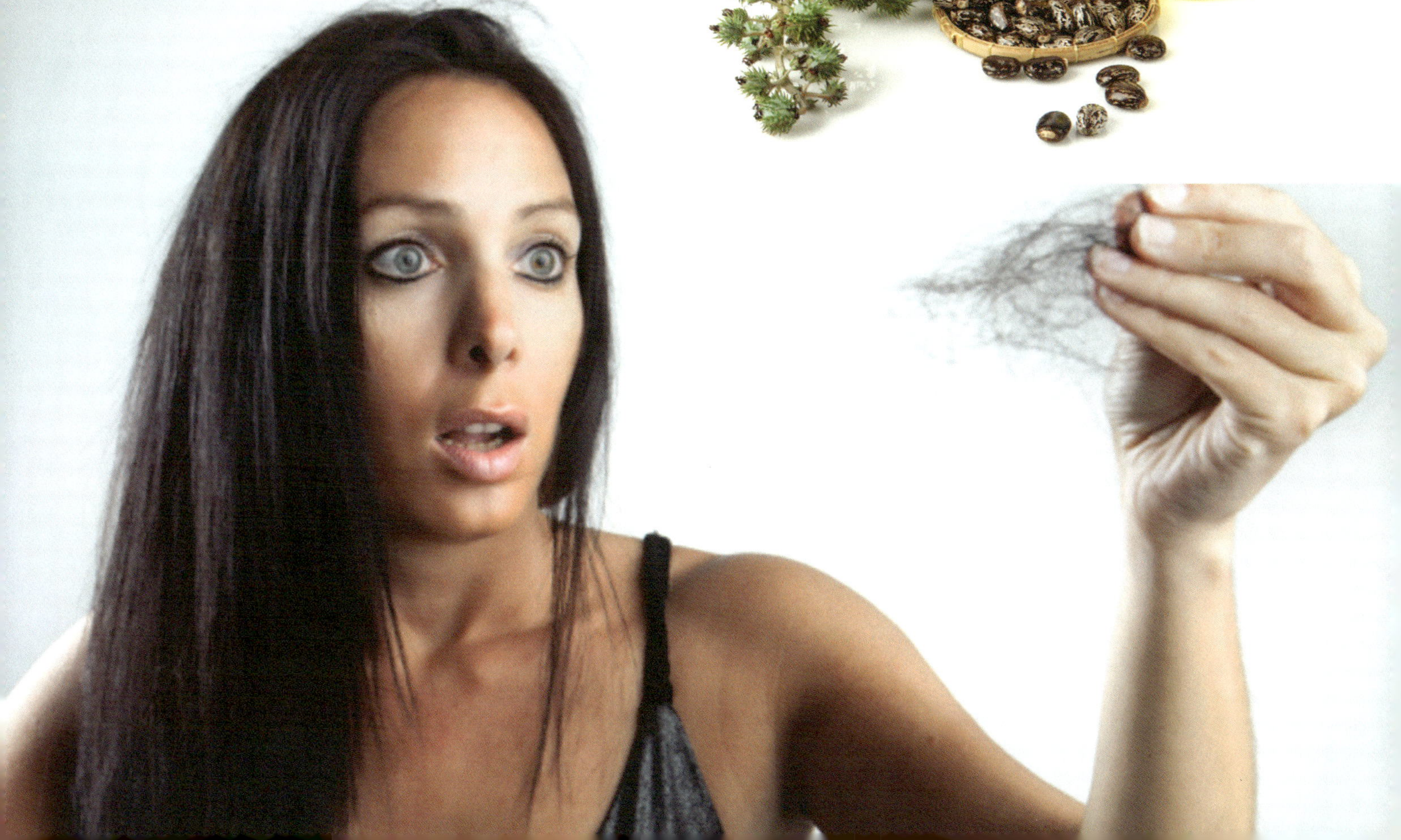

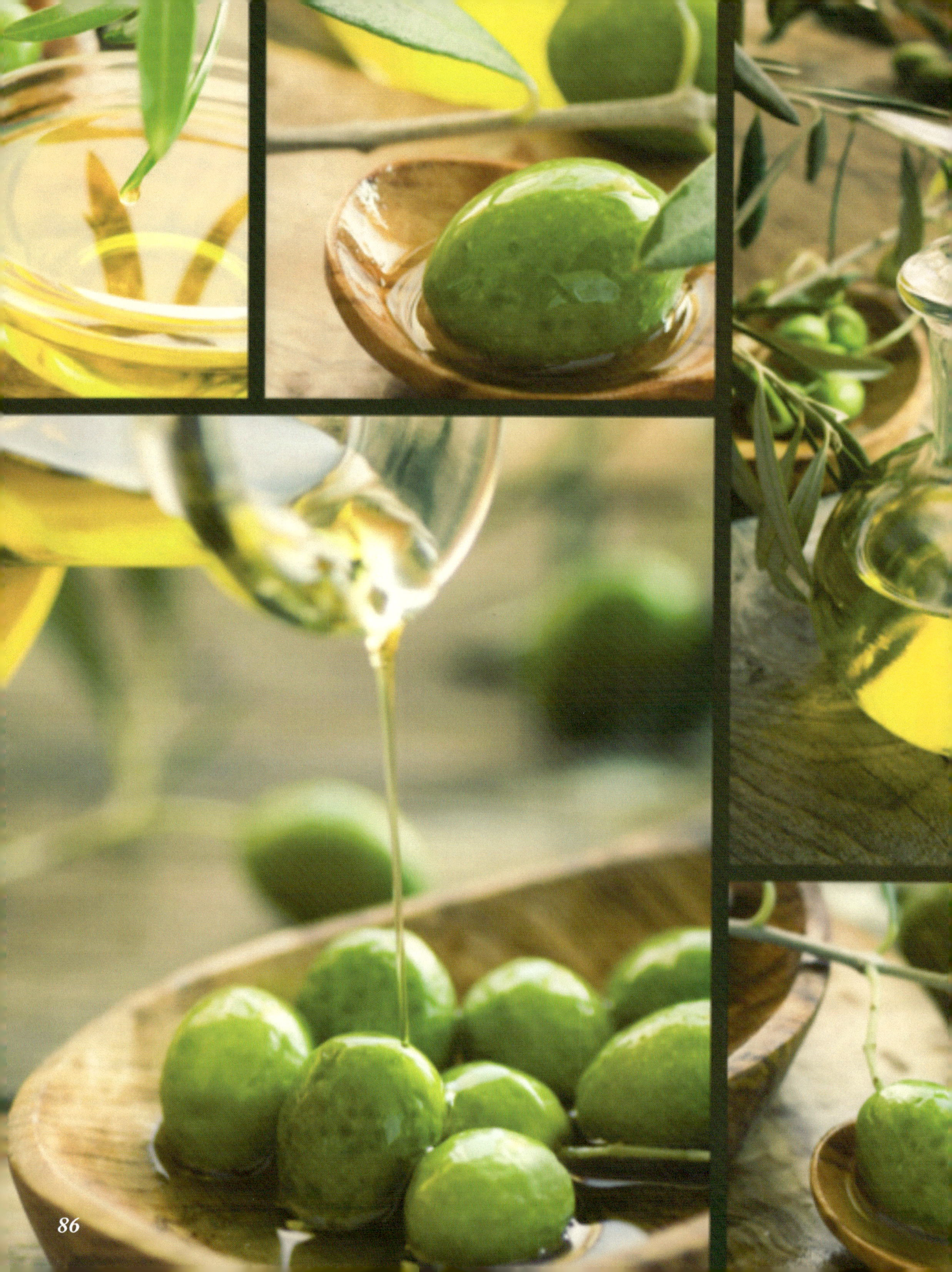

GLOWING HAIR MASK

For bright and shiny hair

3 Organic carrots
2 Tablespoons virgin cold pressed olive oil

Mix well and rub in the root of hair and leave in for a few hours or overnight with a shower cap. Wash in the morning. Leaves your hair glowing.

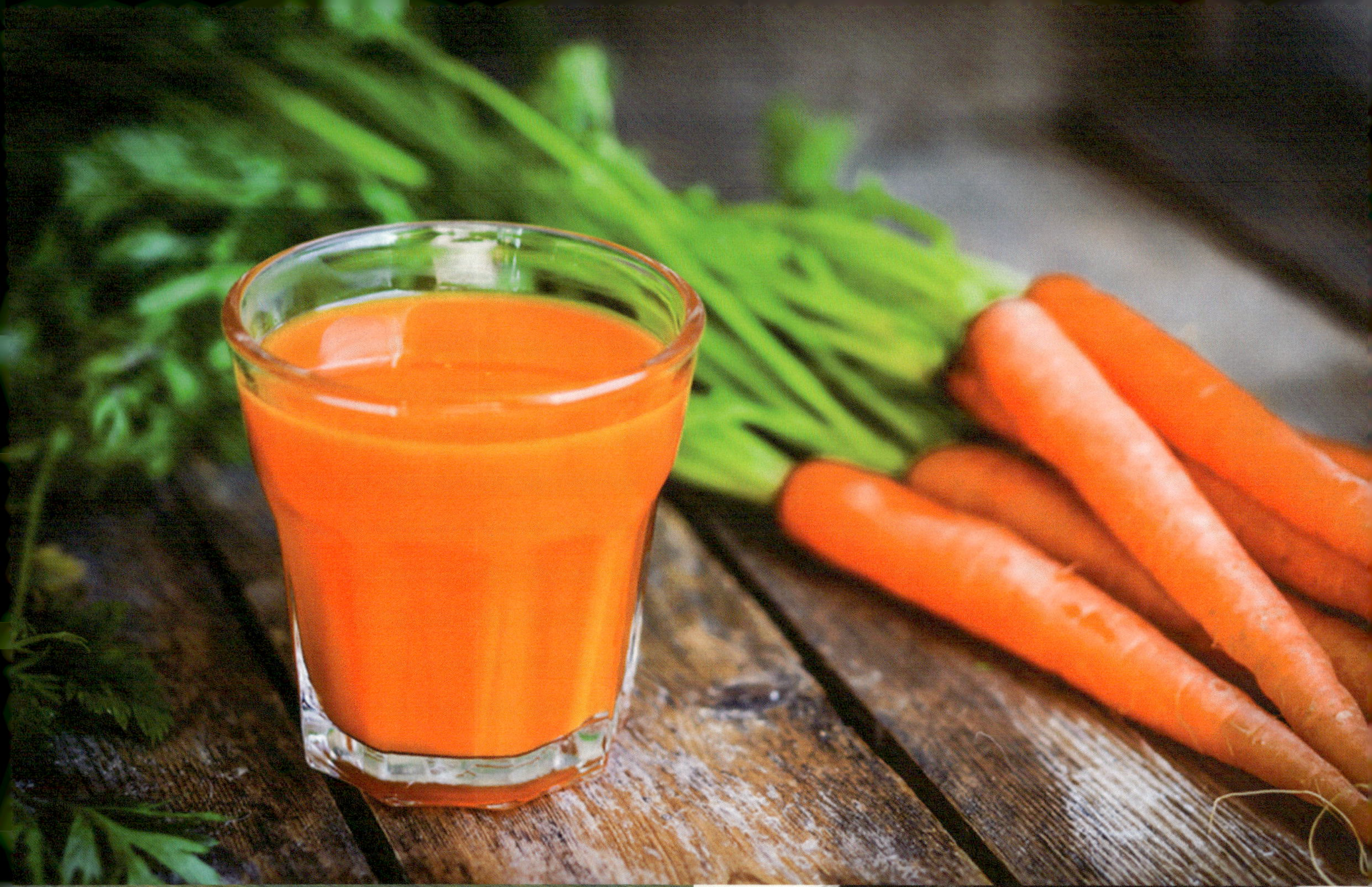

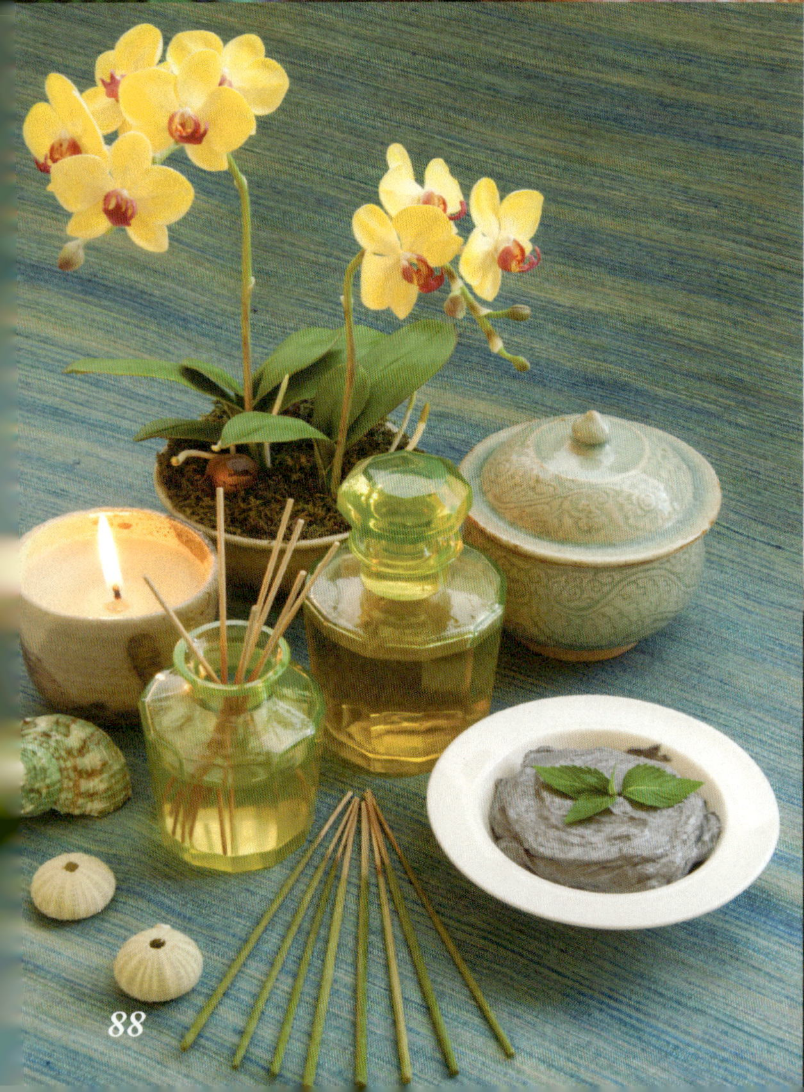

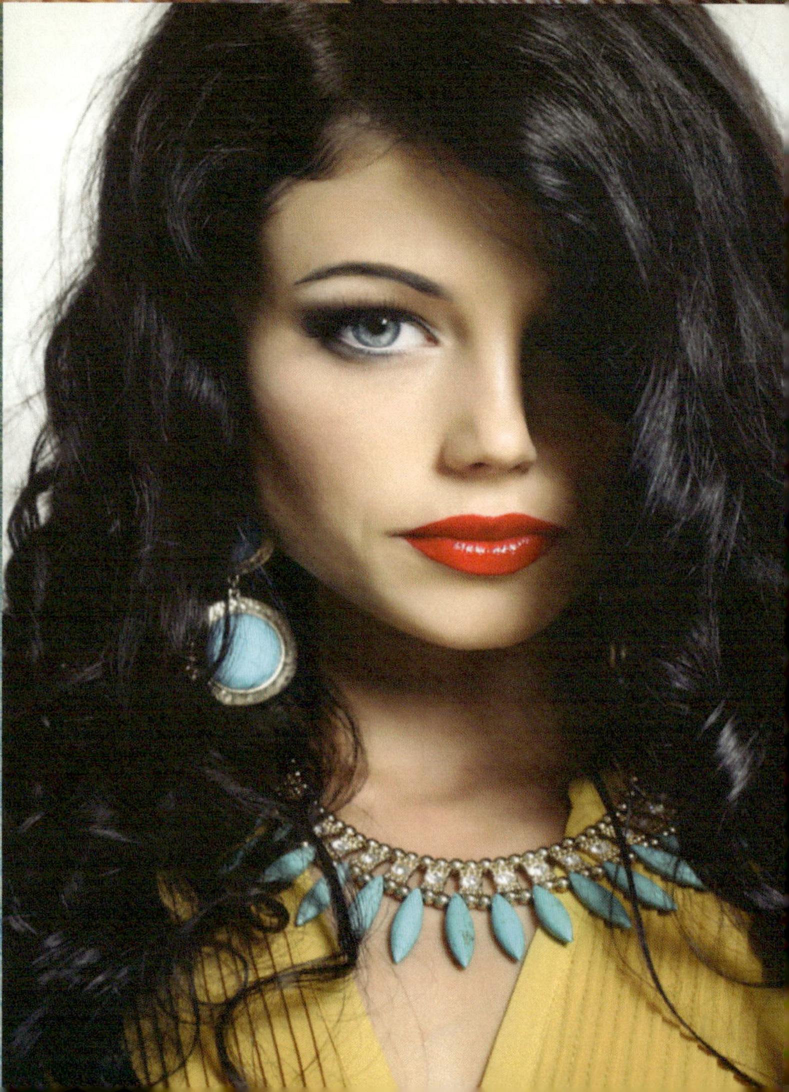

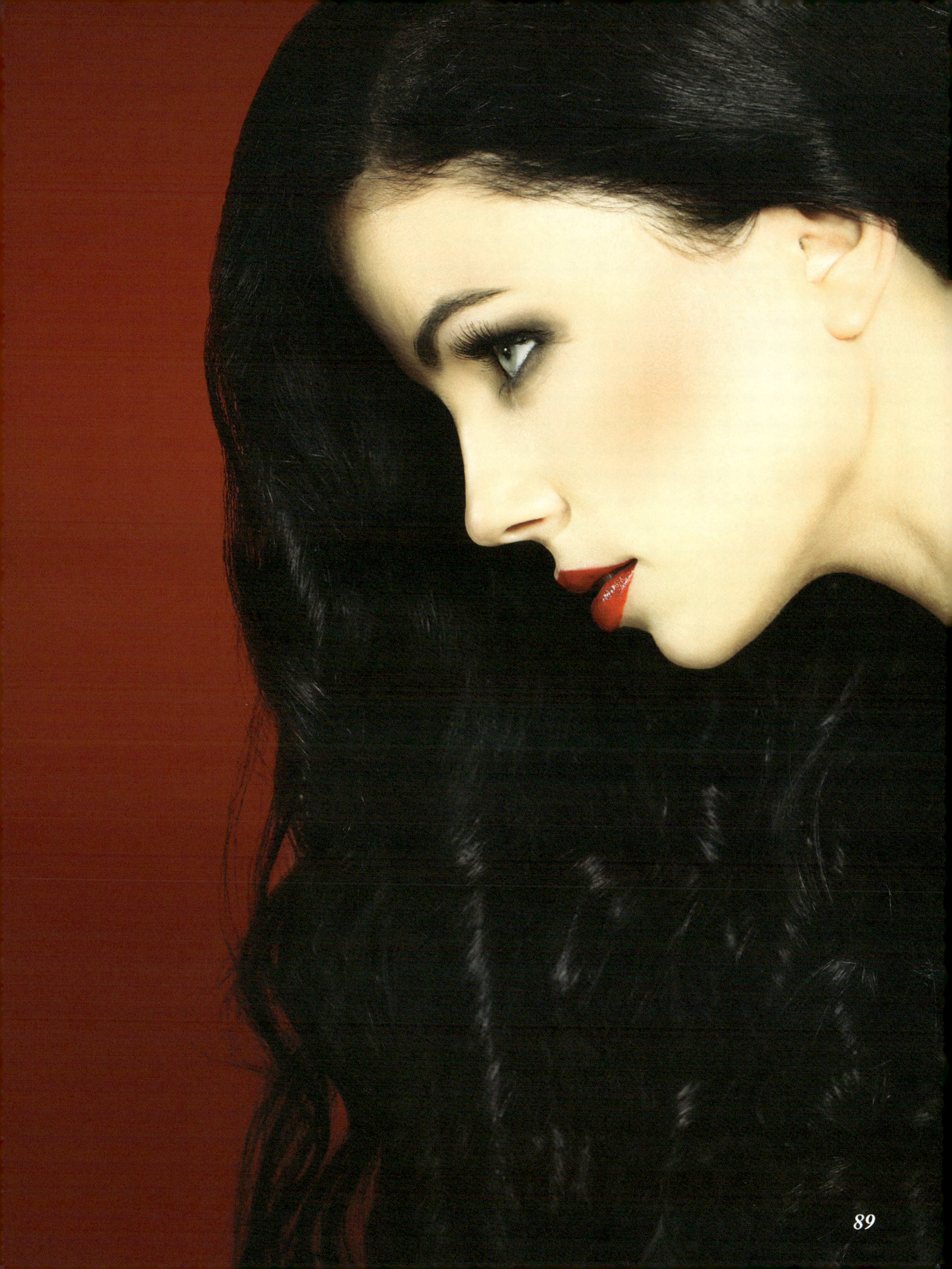

HAIR ALCHEMY

To thicken hair and make it luminous

(Amla is a sour-sweet gooseberry grown in Iran and India) Amla powder is available for purchase on Organic merchant company website.

2 Tablespoons Amla powder or 1 medium Amla
3 Tablespoons castor oil
3 Tablespoons coconut oil
1 Medium red onion
4 cloves red garlic (a little spicier than white)

Chop ingredients then place in a blender to mix well. Simmer on very low flame for about 15 minutes. Cool and strain. Part your hair in sections and massage the oil into your scalp. Leave on for 3 hours or more, preferably with a shower cap. Shampoo. For optimum results repeat twice a week.

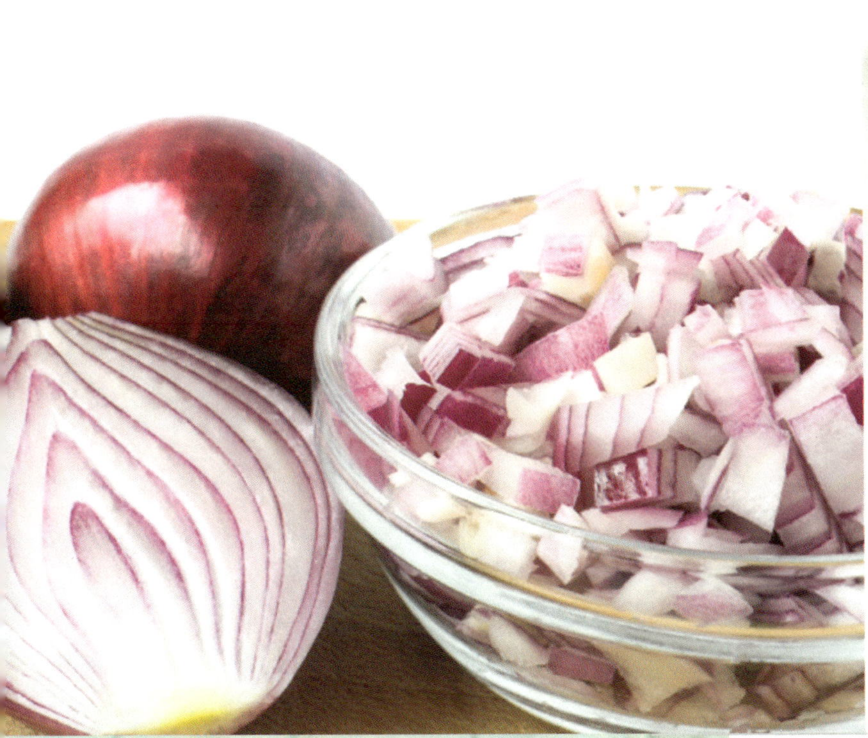
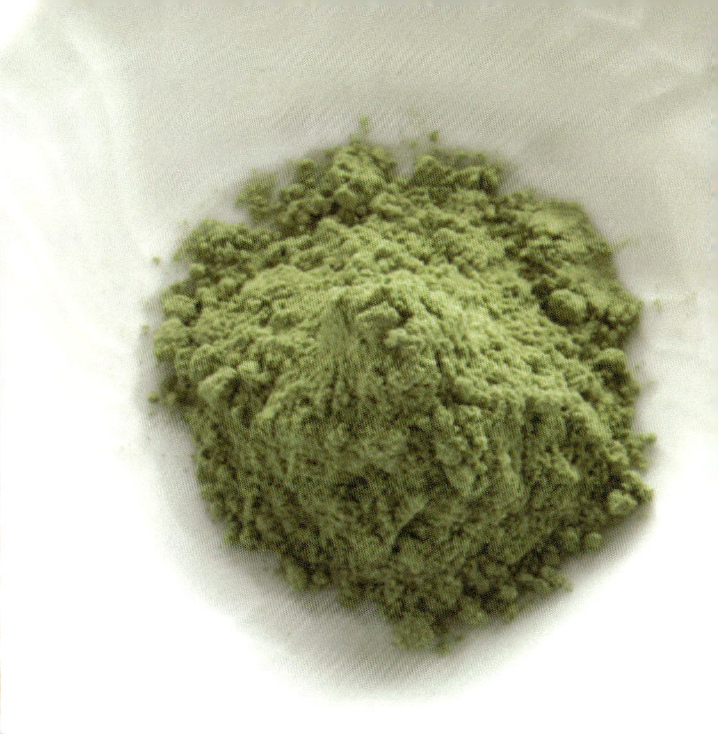
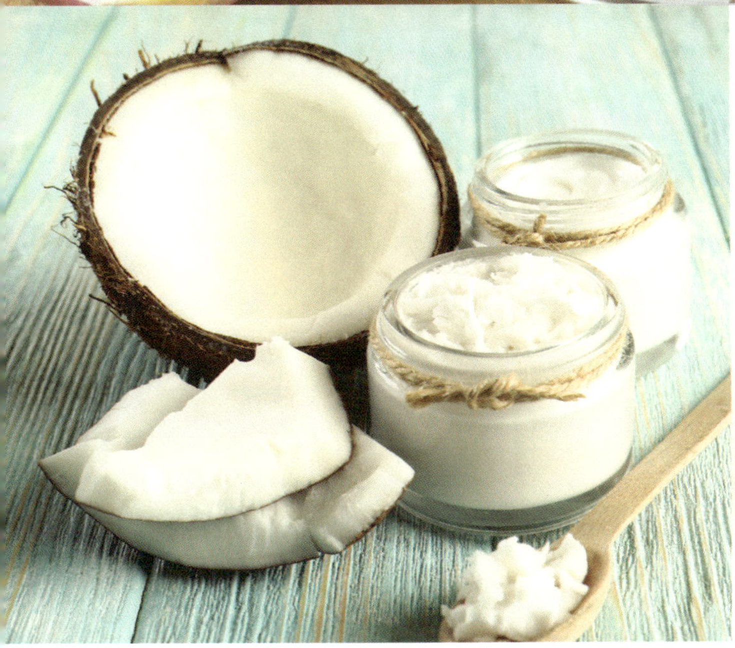
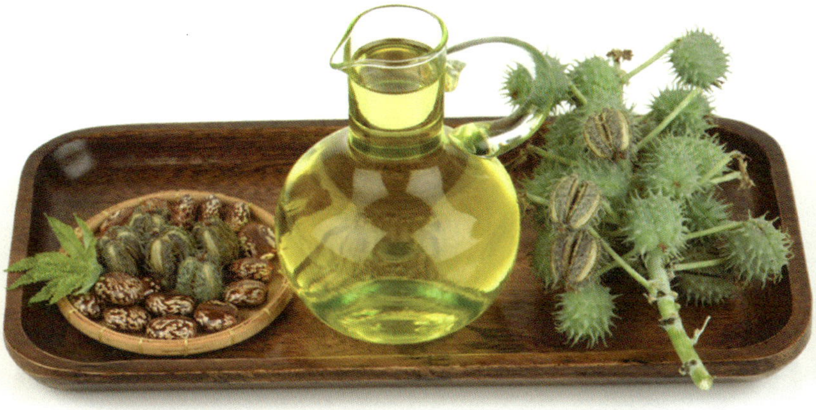
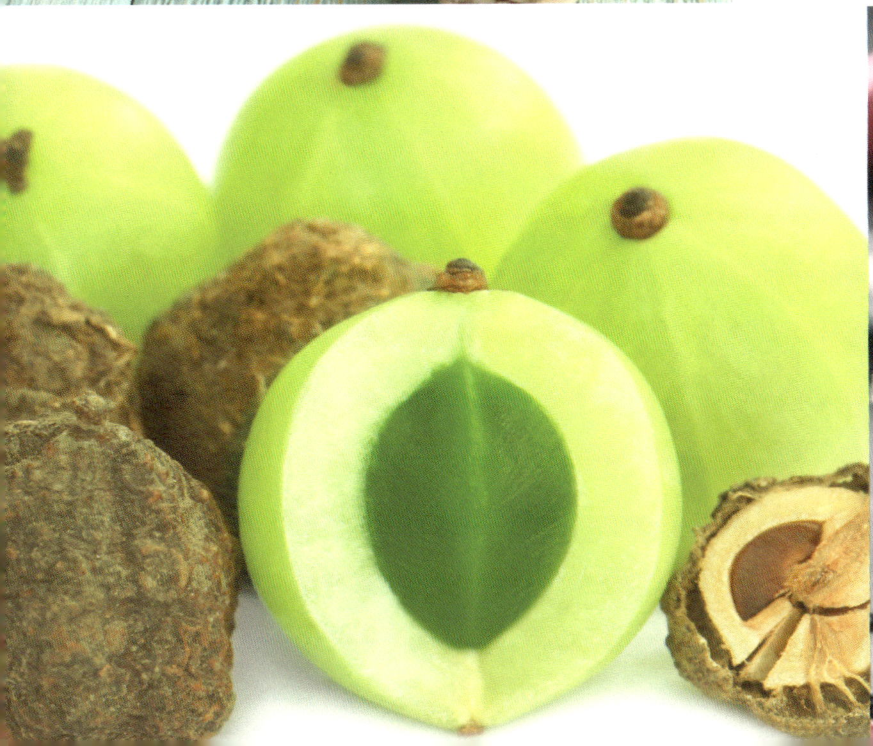
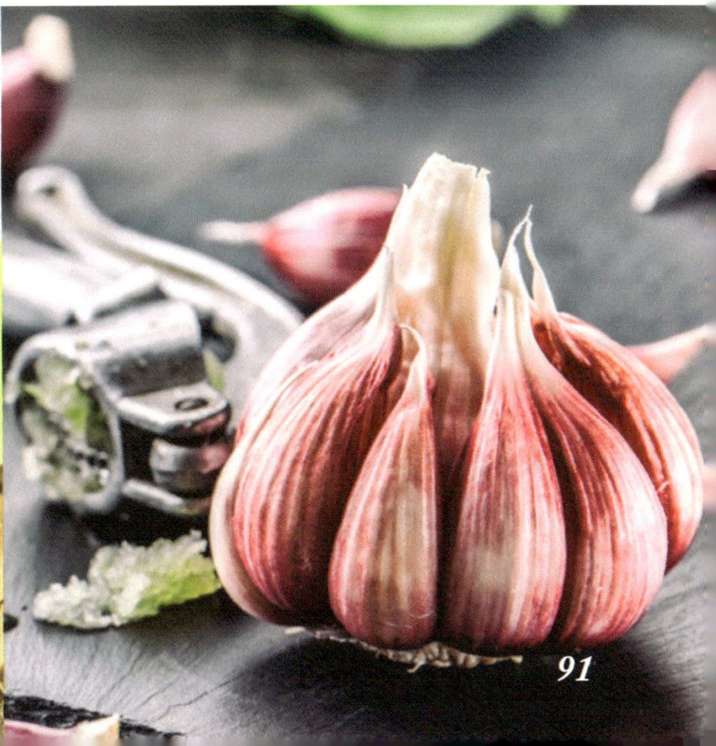

SEDR MASK
For dandruff (eczema of hair)

Sedr (organic Zizyphus spina-christi) is derived from a wild fruit tree called jujube, an evergreen native to Iran, Africa and southern and western Asia. It is revered as a sacred tree. The ripe fruits are edible and the flowers are an important source of honey. The leaves are dried and made into a green powder. Sedr is filled with antioxidants and many more attributes. Sedr powder has also been used for hundreds of years in Iran to cleanse and condition hair, adding thickness and protecting hair from the elements.

Some recent studies indicate the promotion of hair growth with the use of sedr.

1 Tablespoon sedr
1 Egg yolk (organic)
1 Tablespoon coconut oil

Mix to a paste and leave at room temperature for an hour, then apply to the hairline and comb through hair. Put a shower cap on and sleep with it if you can or leave in for 3 hours, then wash it out.

Sedr is also considered as a natural shampoo. You can purchase sedr powder at Sadaf Company, Sehat or Henna Sooq.

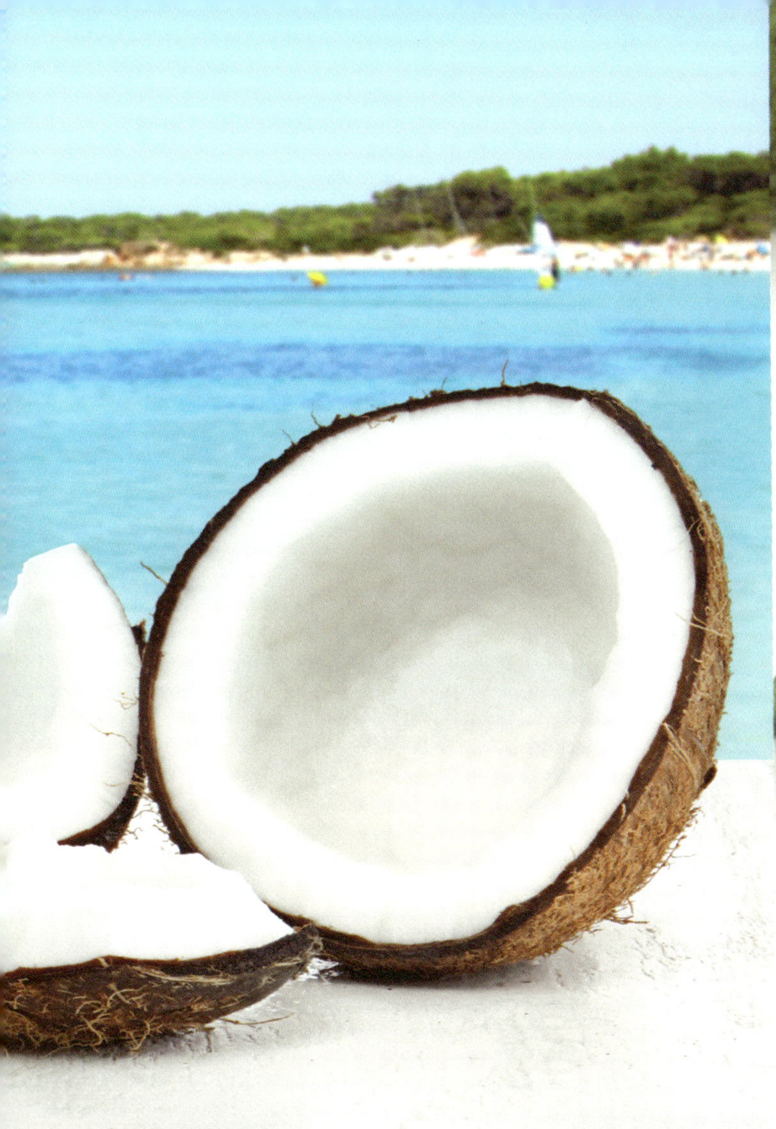

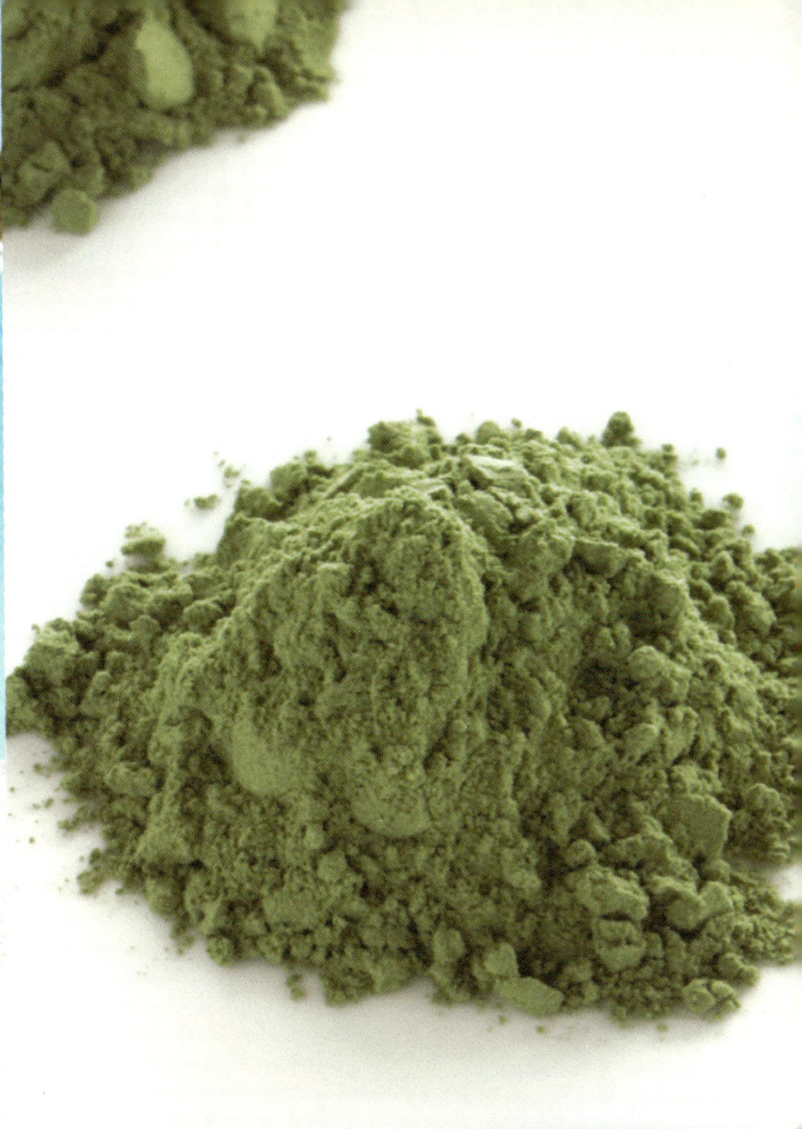

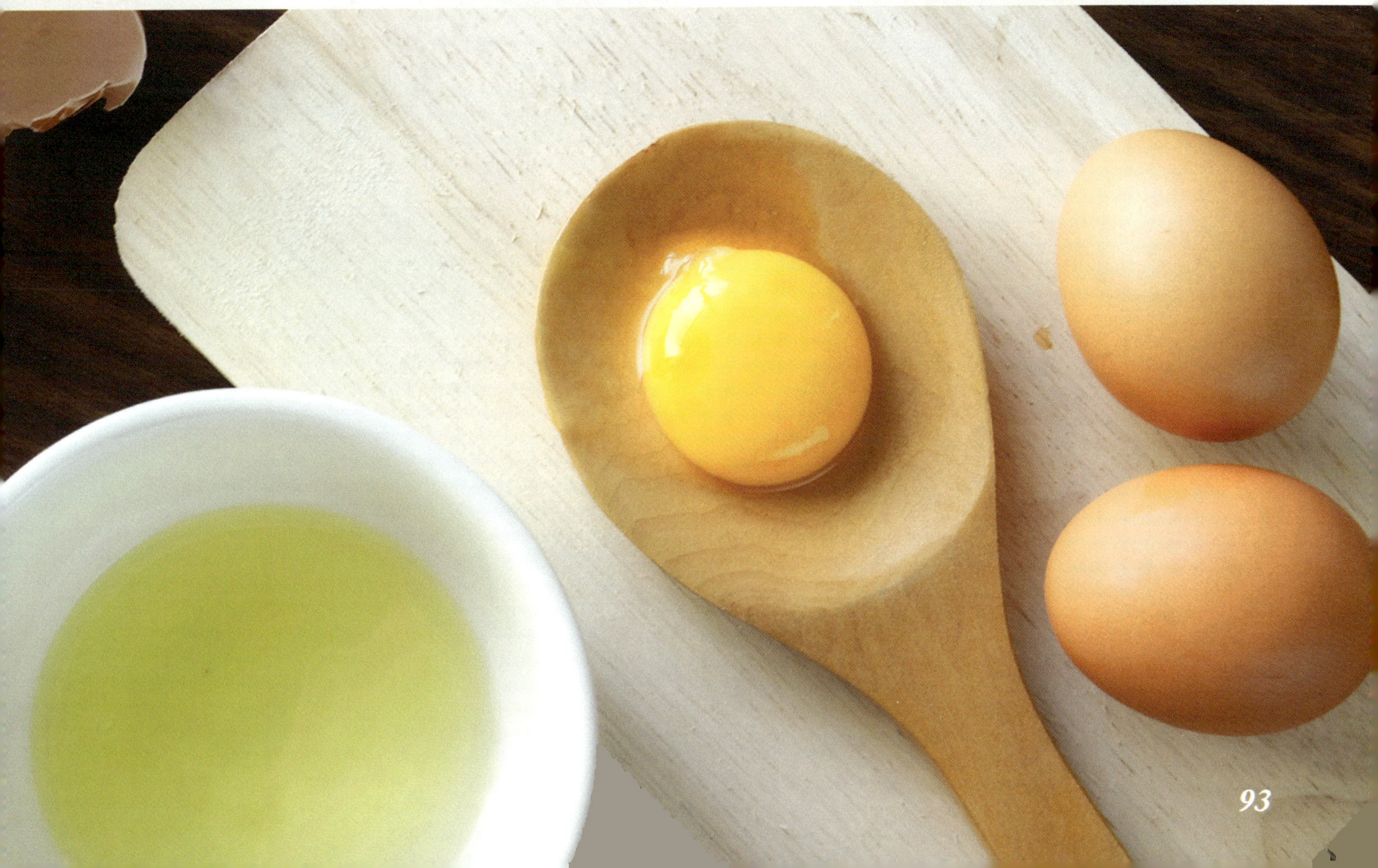

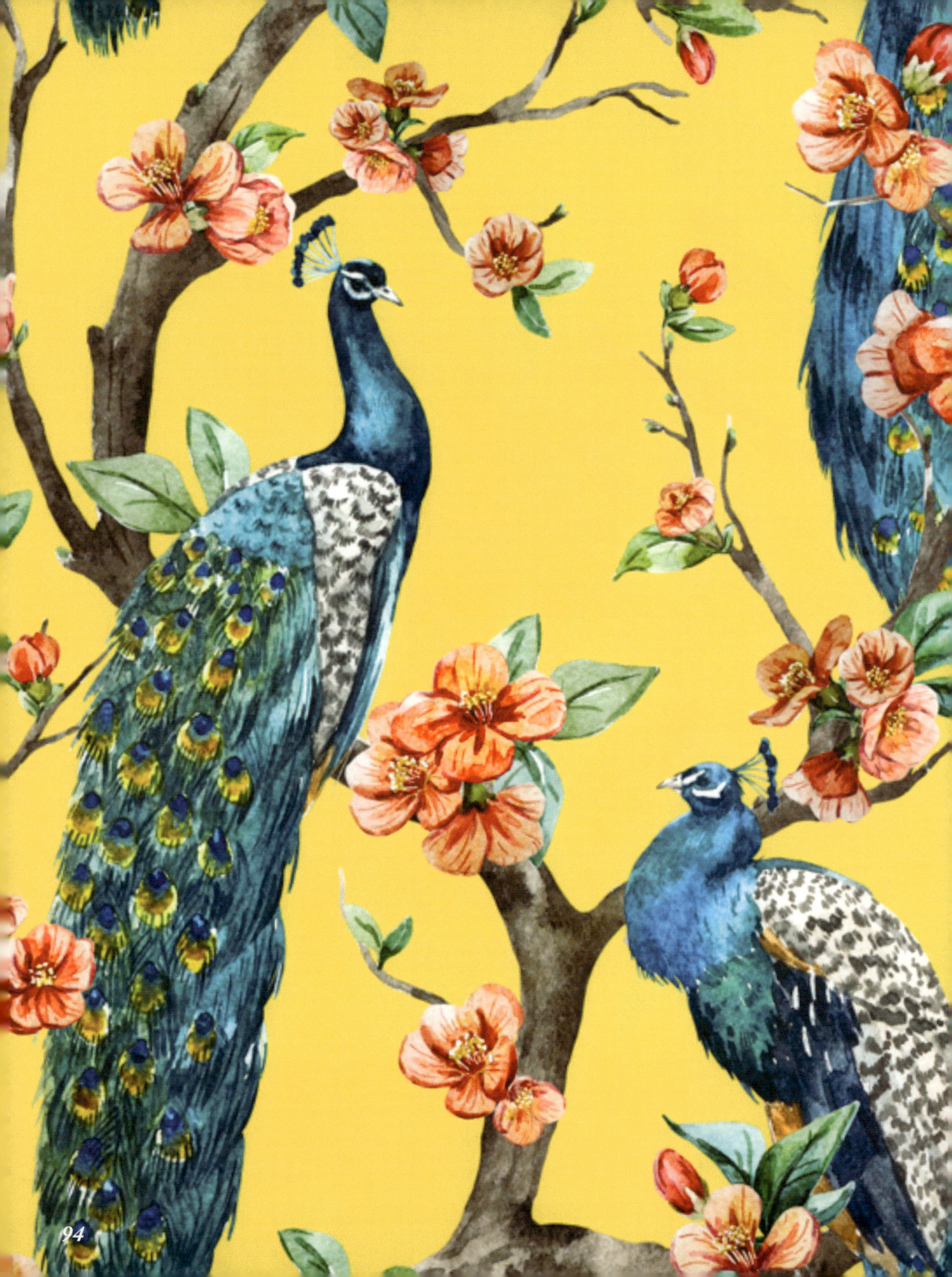

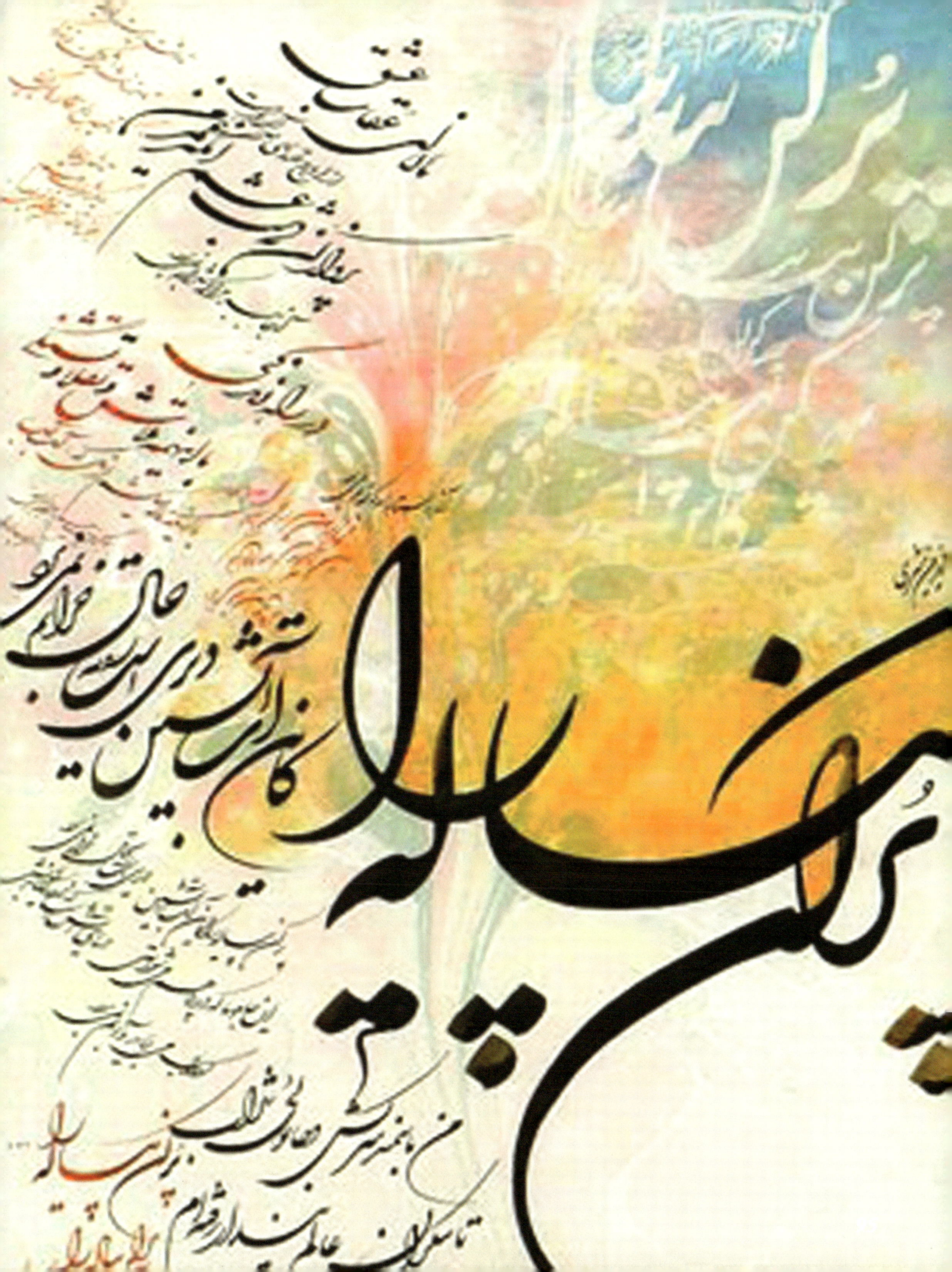

YOUTHFUL EYES

Erase under-eye puffiness

1 Organic carrot
1 Natural cotton ball
1 Small cheese cloth

Grate, blend or juice carrot. Put the mash or juice in the freezer for 5 minutes. Moisten cotton ball in the juice, squeeze then place it on the eyes. You can also place the grated carrots in a gauze and place it on your eyes. Lie down and relax for 20 minutes. Do it every day and the puffiness will disappear!

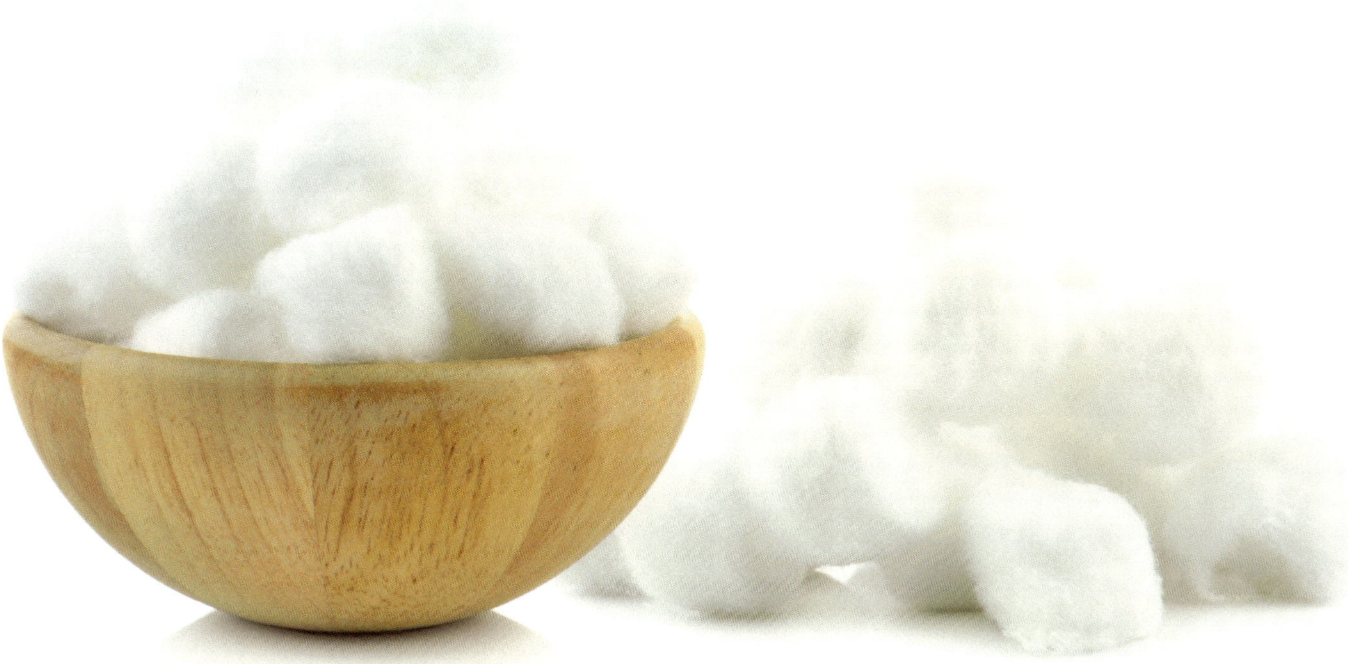

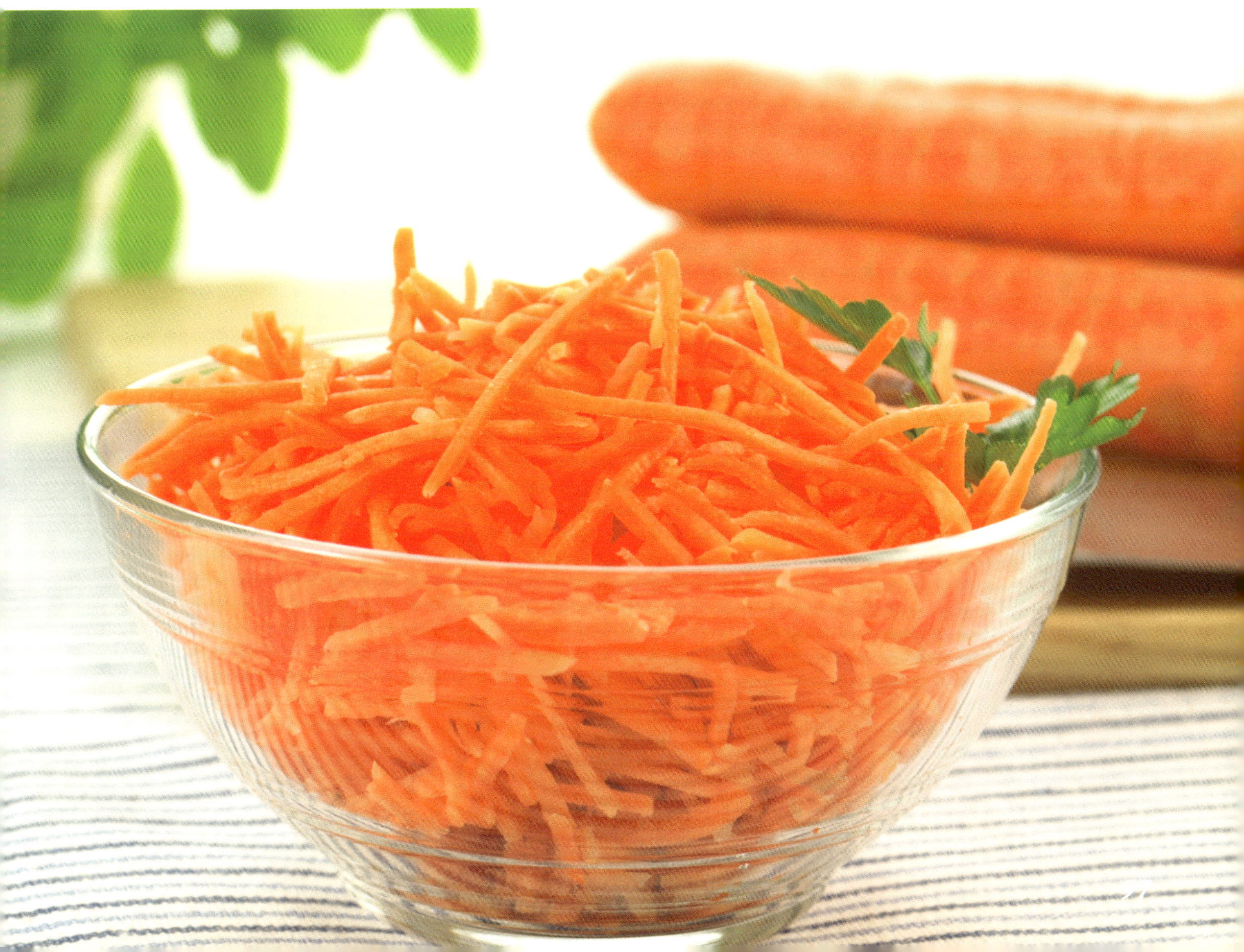

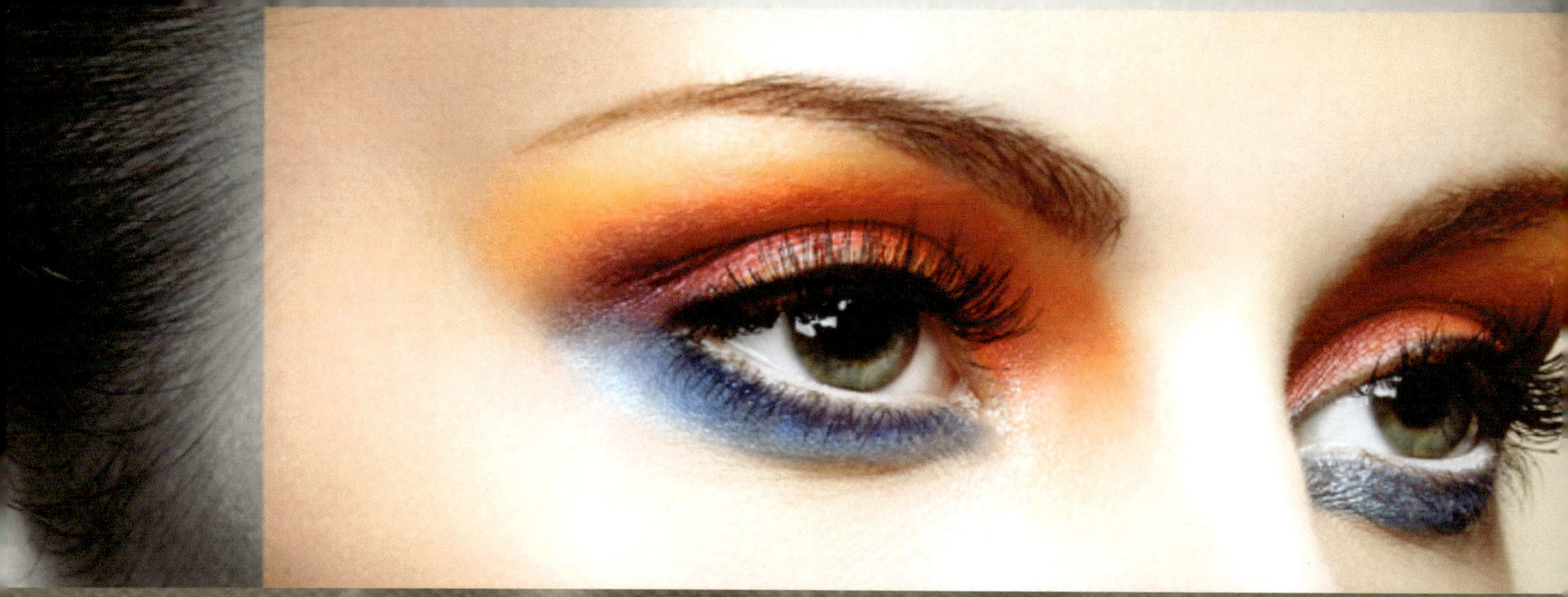

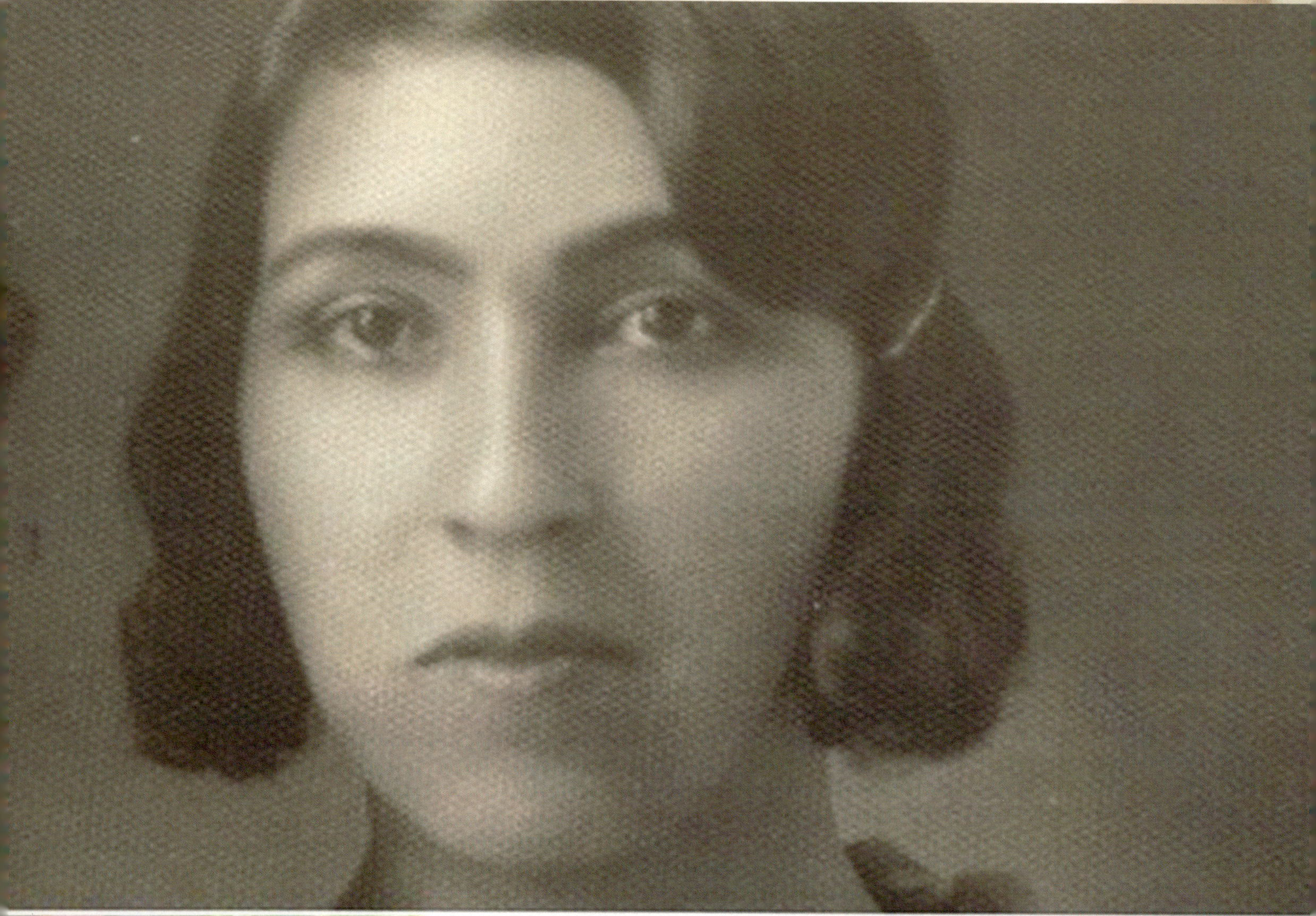

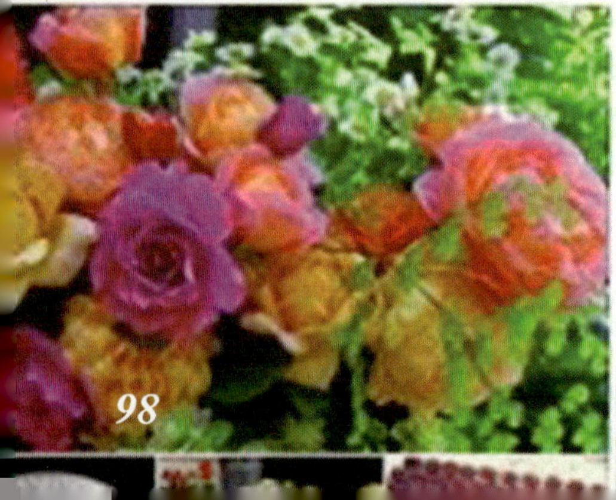

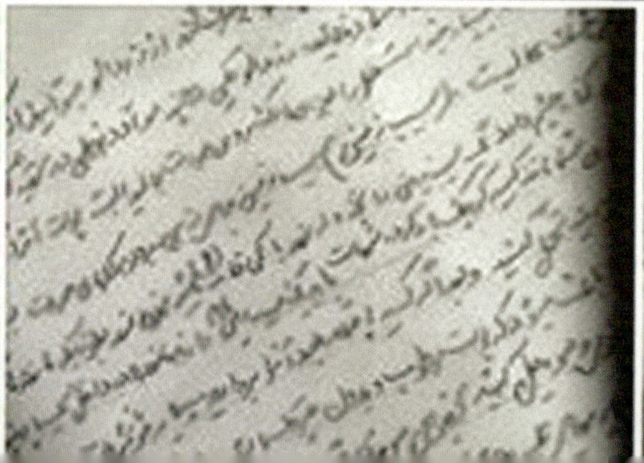

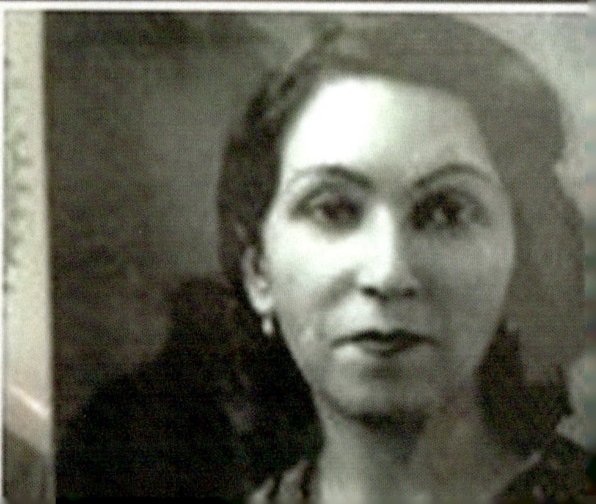

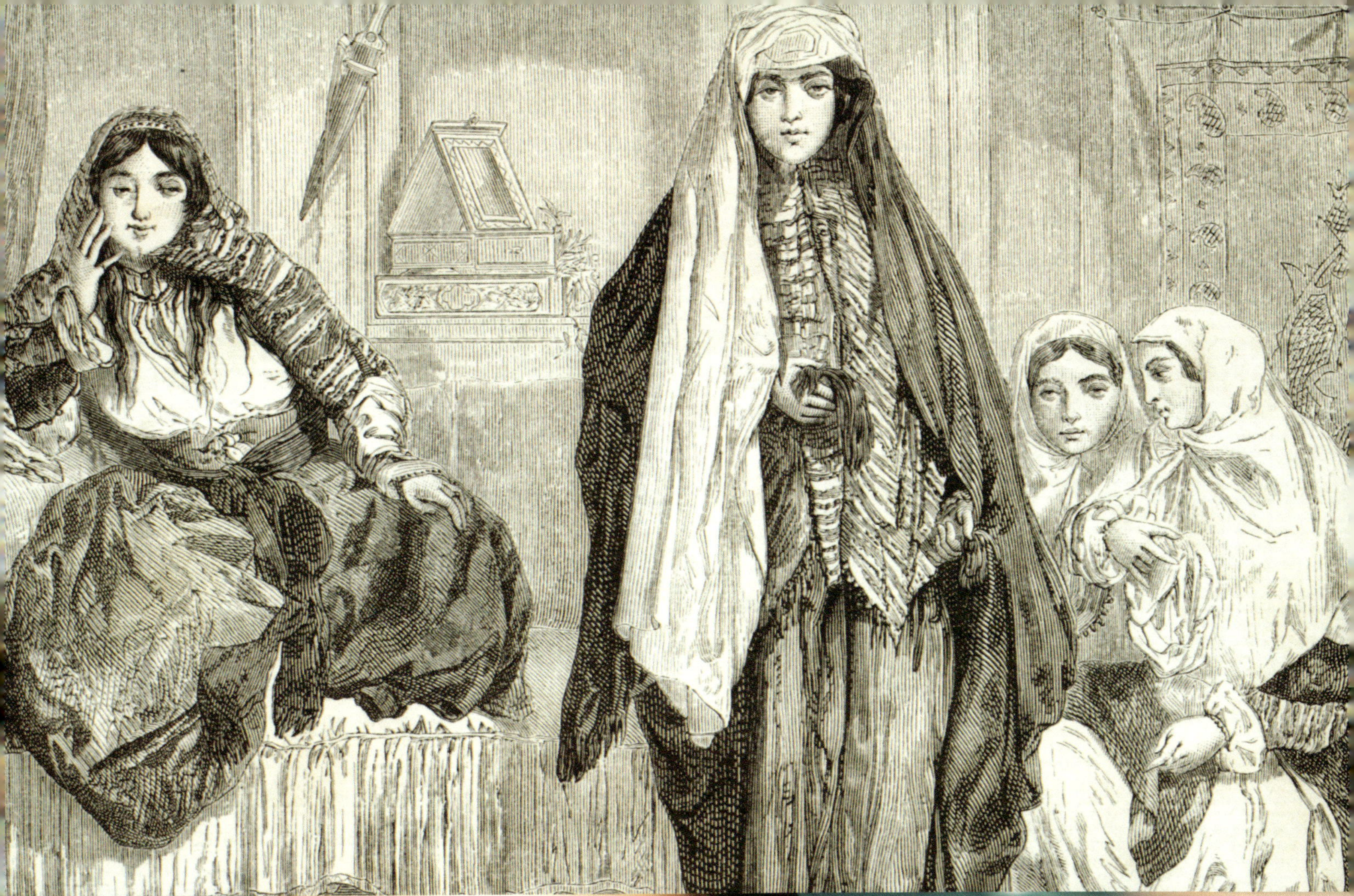

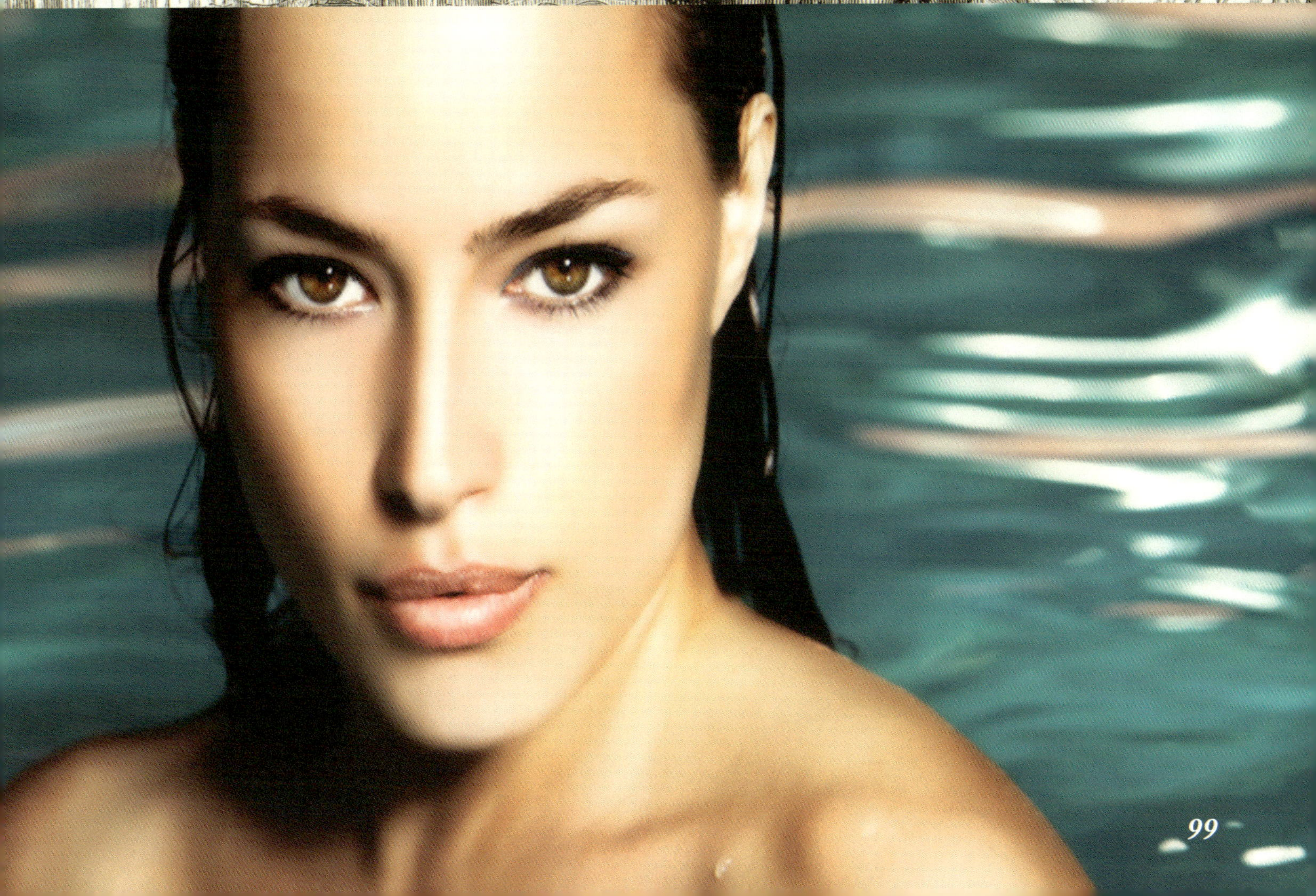

ERASE DARK UNDER-EYE CIRCLES

Catalase is an enzyme found in human organs such as the liver and kidneys, and is associated with the organs' roles of cleansing the body of toxins absorbed from ingested food. Catalase is also found in plants. Potatoes, particularly, contain high amounts of catalase and are used in high-end cosmetic creams to diminish dark under-eye circles.

1 Medium organic red potato
1 Natural cotton ball
1 Small cheese cloth

Juice, blend or grate potato. Place in freezer for 5 minutes. Moisten cotton ball in the juice or add the mashed or grated cold potato to a small cheesecloth and place under the eyes. Or, if your eyes tend to get puffy place over the entire eye covering upper and lower lids. Lay down and relax for 20 minutes. Do it every day for 10 to 20 minutes. Rinse with ice-cold water followed with nourishing under-eye cream. This will not only reduce the puffiness and dark circles it also tightens the skin of the eyes.

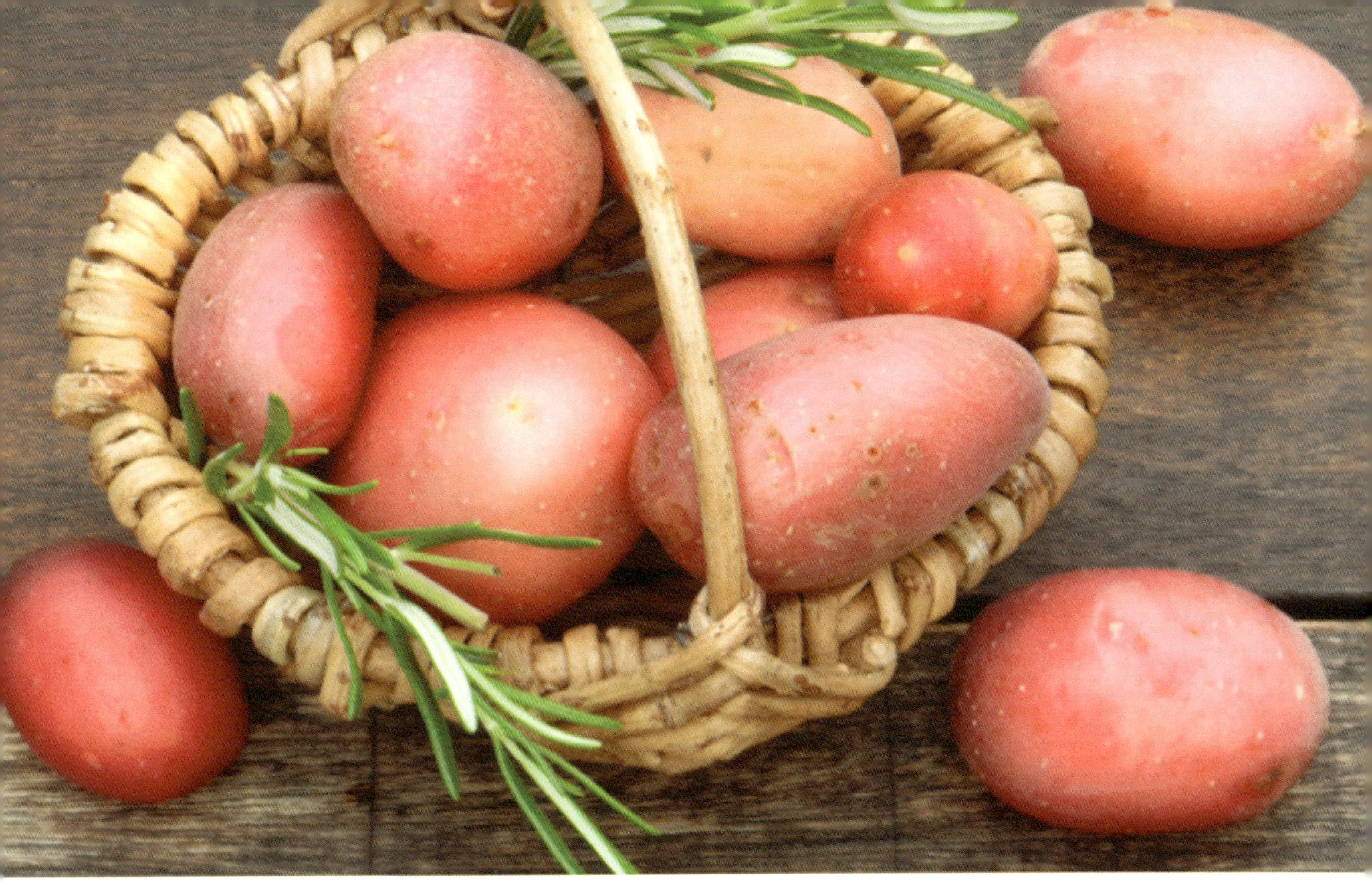

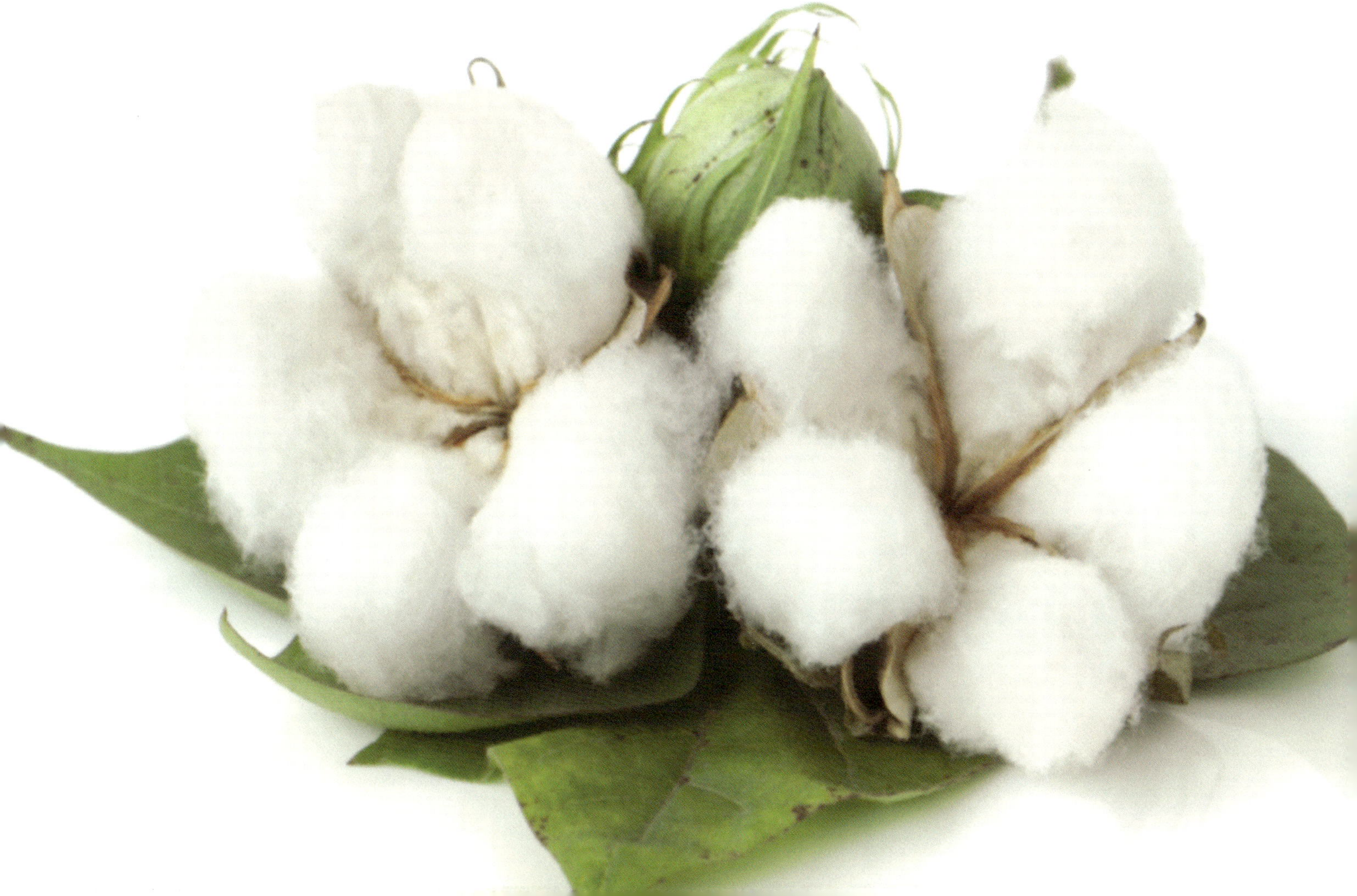

IMPROVE EYESIGHT

This amazing juice doesn't only improve eyesight, it also helps people who suffer from kidney disease, gastrointestinal tract problems, female reproductive organ inflammation, hemorrhoids, tuberculosis and cardiovascular issues.

6.5 Tablespoons aloe juice
4 Medium organic lemons
17.6 oz or 500 grams crushed walnuts
10.7 oz or 300 grams raw honey

It is best to make your own fresh aloe juice. (If you can't make your own buy fresh aloe juice in the refrigerated section of a health food store.) Remove the lower, middle and upper leaves, leaving the stem and remaining 3 - 4 leaves. Wash the leaves thoroughly with water which has been boiled and then cooled. Remove the spikes, chop the leaves, and strain the juice with double gauze.

Do not chop all the leaves at once but rather chop a few at a time, and squeeze out juice in batches. Then rewash the remaining leaves and continue with the procedure.

This method allows you to trigger biogen stimulators which awaken the aloe cells.

Keep chopped aloe leaves refrigerated for 10 - 12 days. Place the aloe juice, lemon juice, walnut and honey in your blender till it turns to liquid. Consume the solution half an hour before a meal, three times a day. Don't stop consuming it until you notice improvements in your vision.

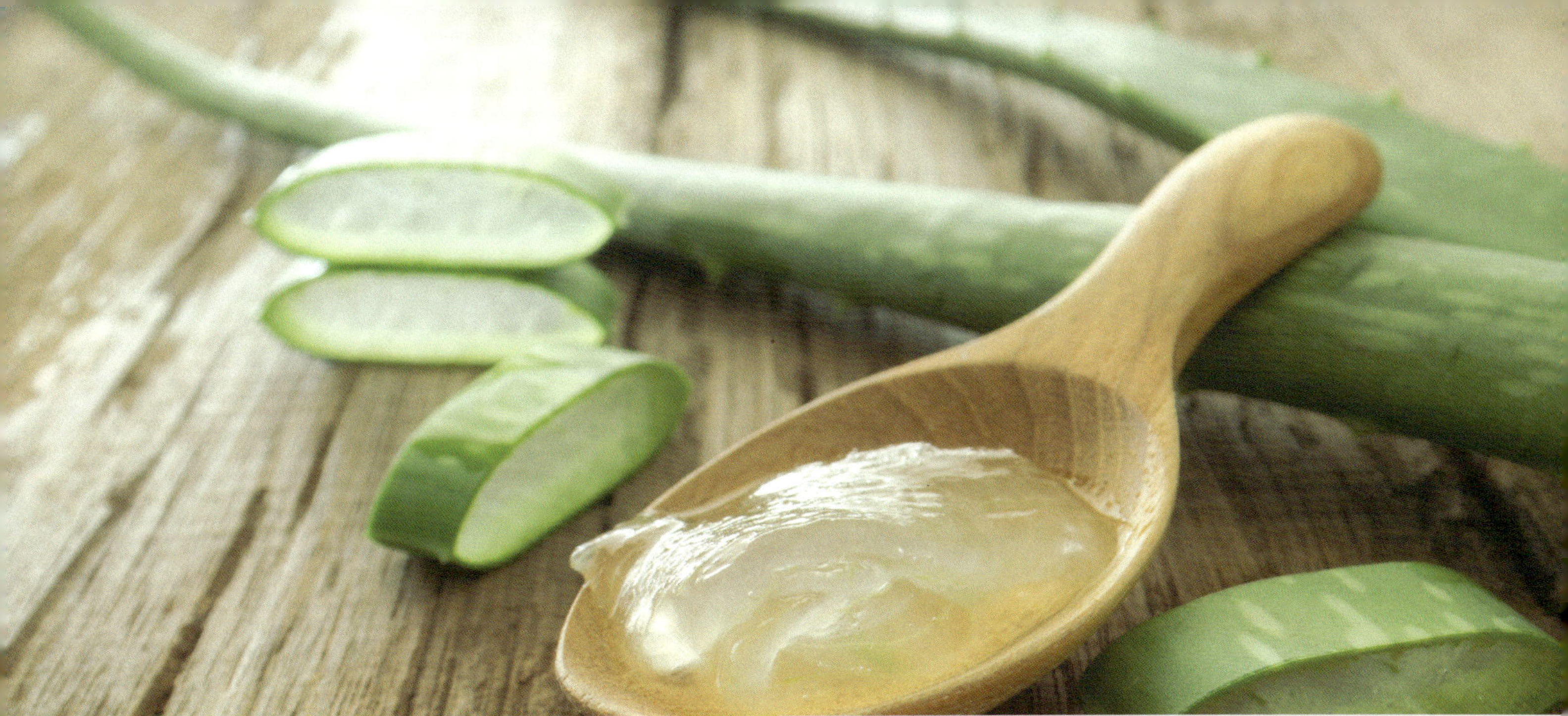

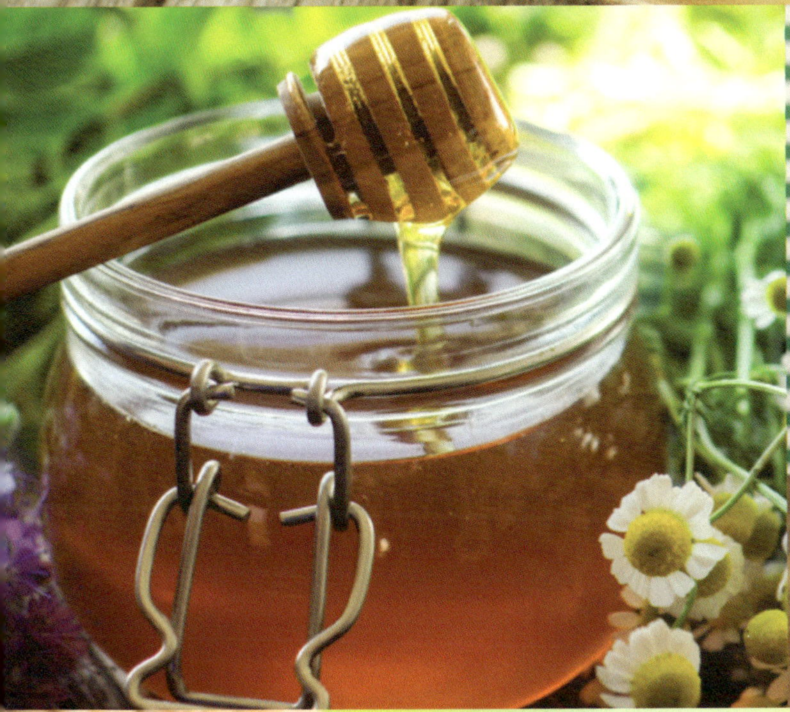

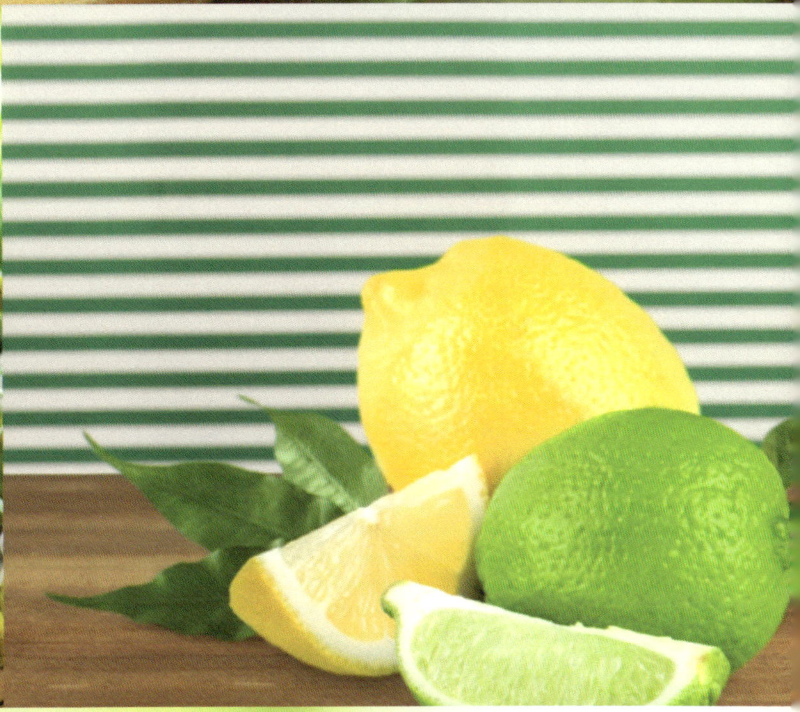

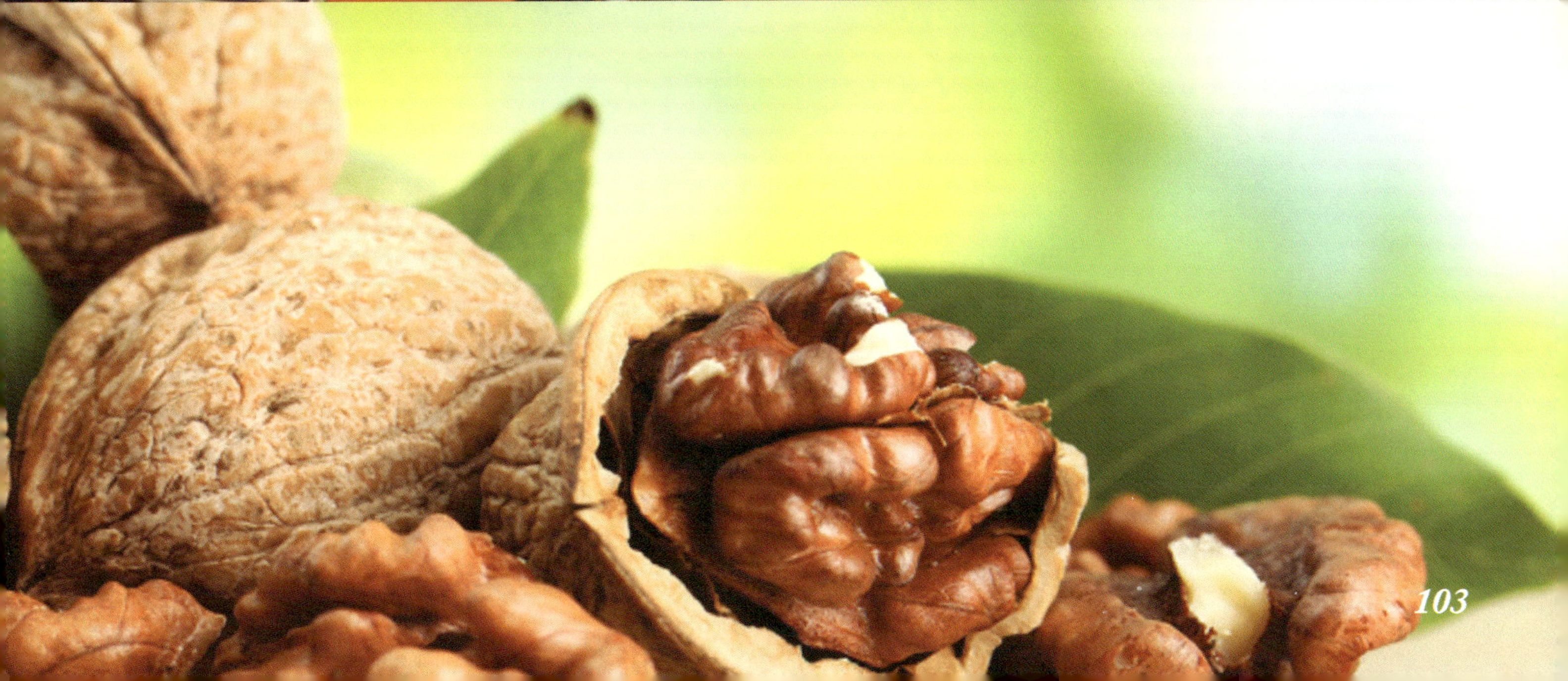

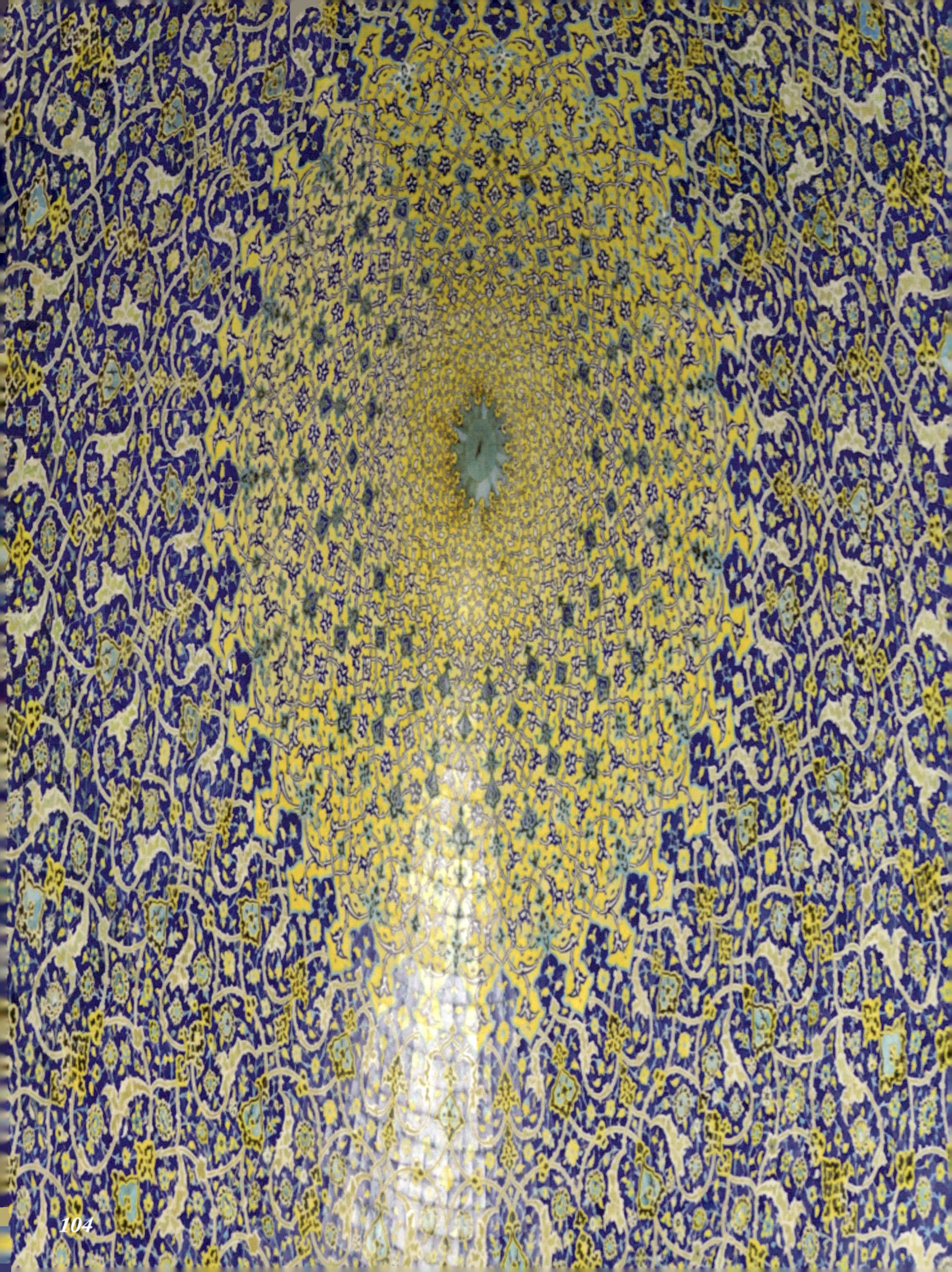

FACE

BEE VENOM MASK

Note: This product might not be suitable for those with a bee allergy.

One of the all-natural products being touted as a safe and organic facelift alternative is bee venom. This product is currently being used at certain spas and in some places is even available over-the-counter. The product is made from real bee venom, although if you want to ensure that a specific product is organic check out the ingredient list.

The bee venom is applied to the face just like a regular facial mask. After rubbing it onto the skin the venom stimulates the production of elastin and collagen. These substances help to give the face a smoother texture by reducing the appearance of wrinkles and fine lines. For many individuals, bee venom could be a good alternative to injectable dermal fillers or Botox.

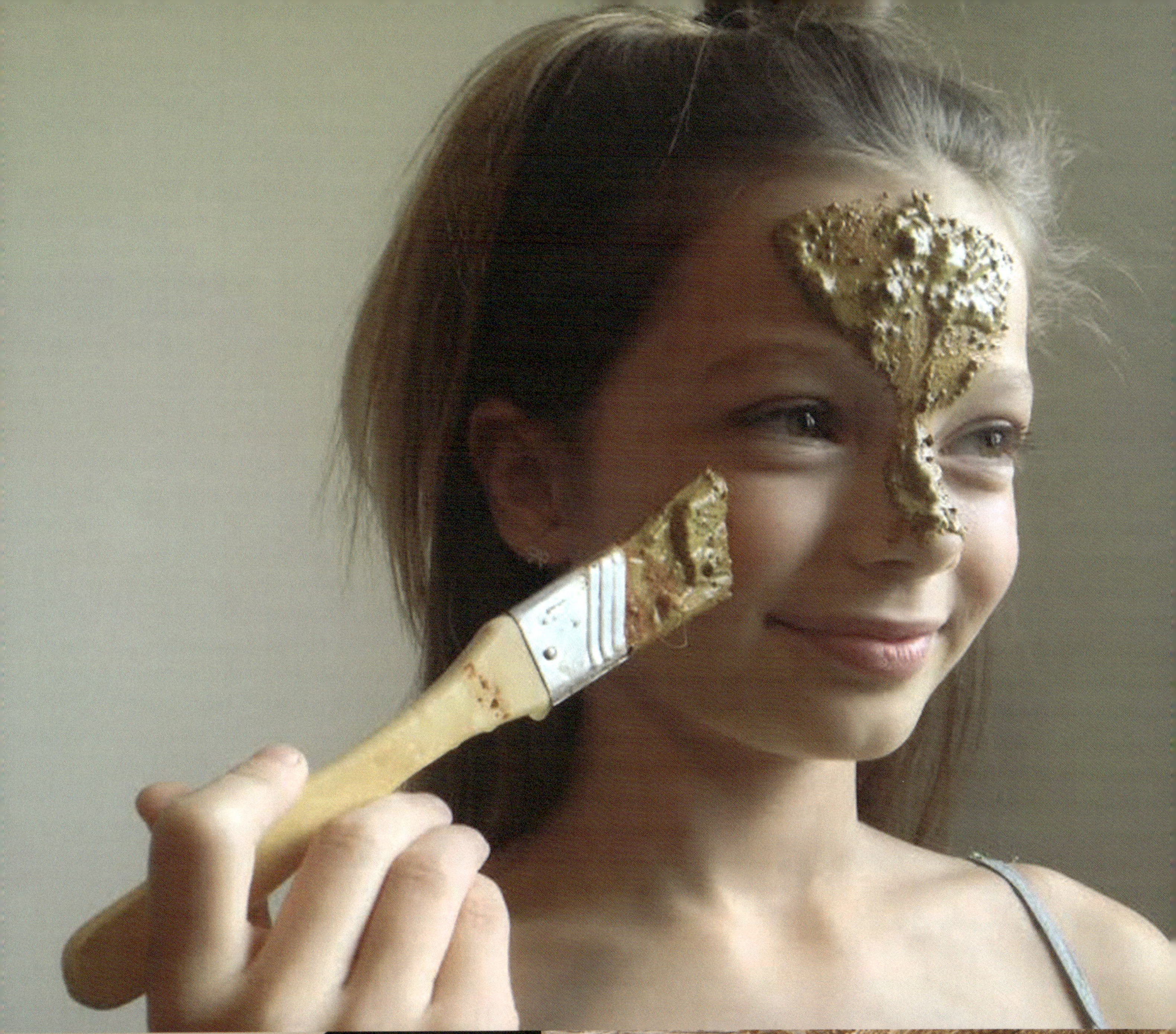

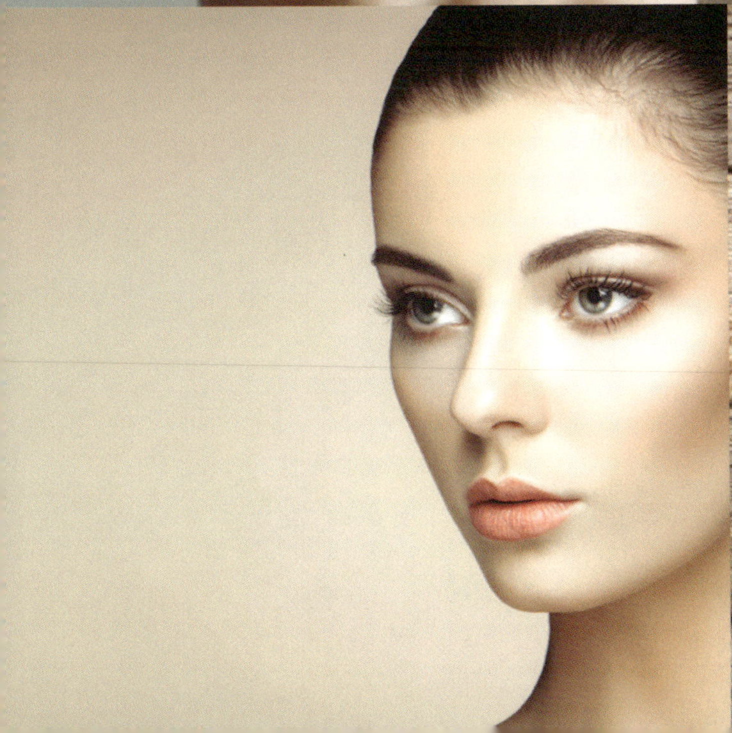

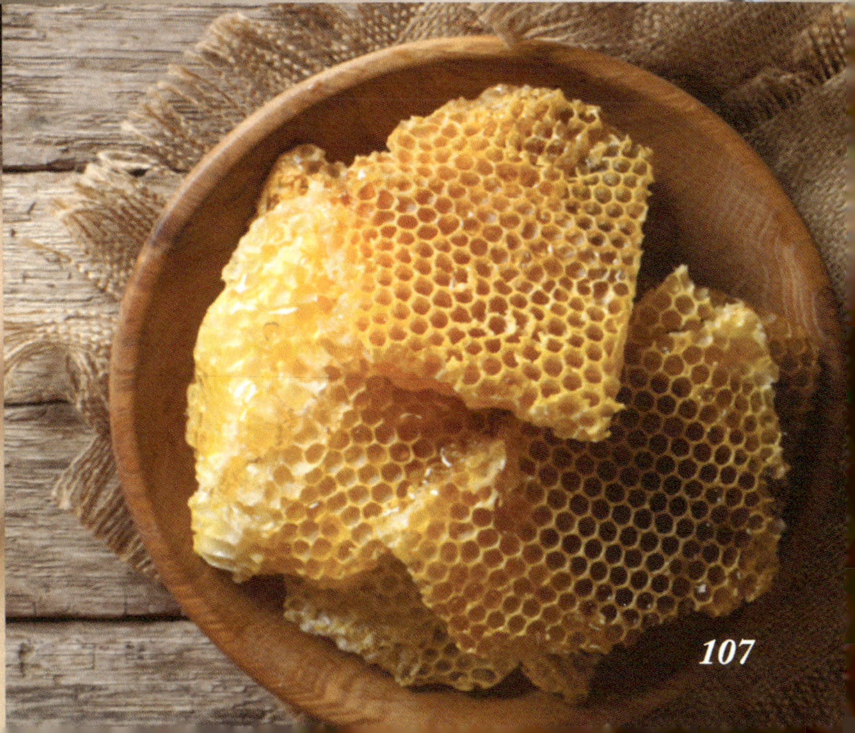

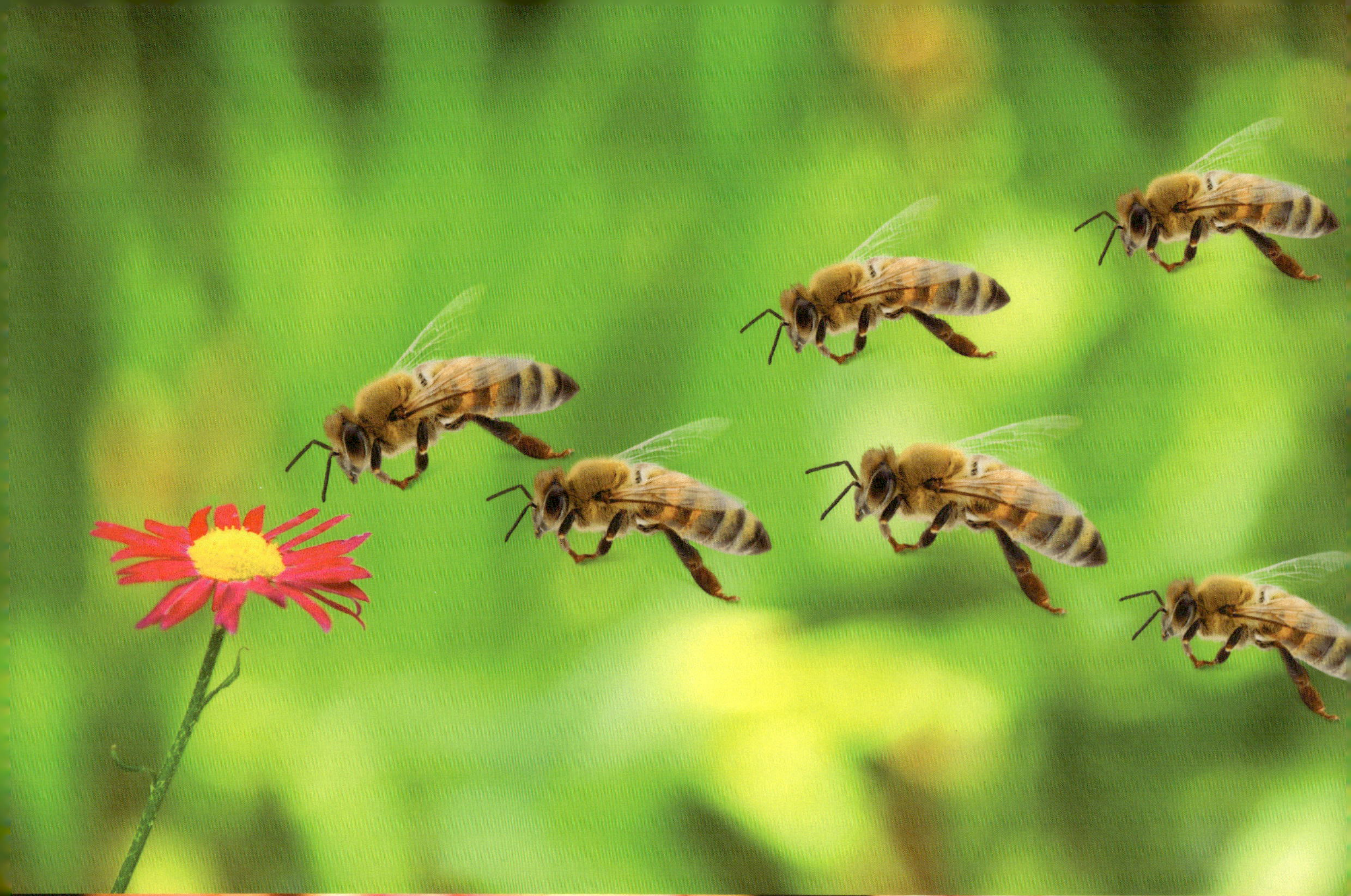

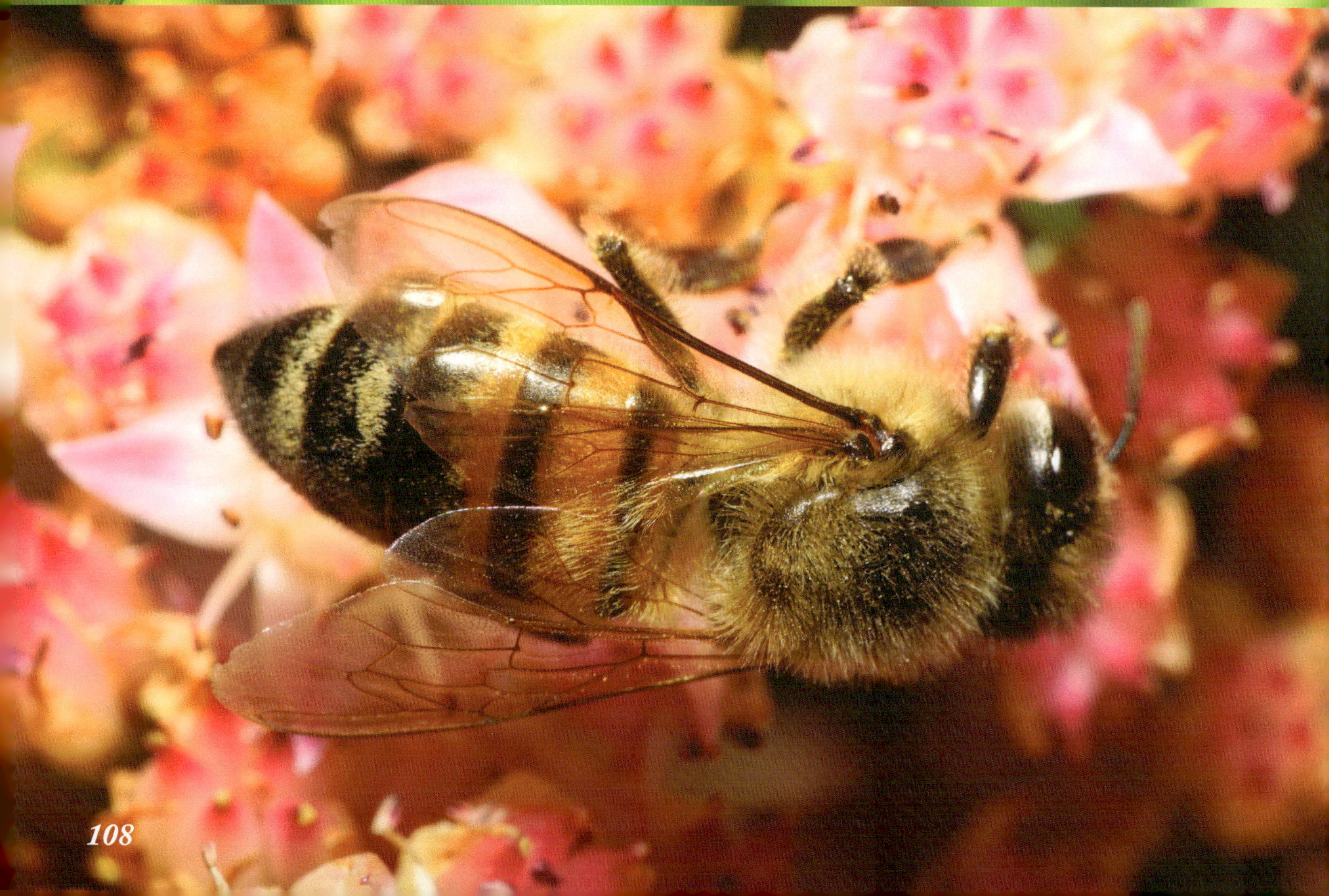

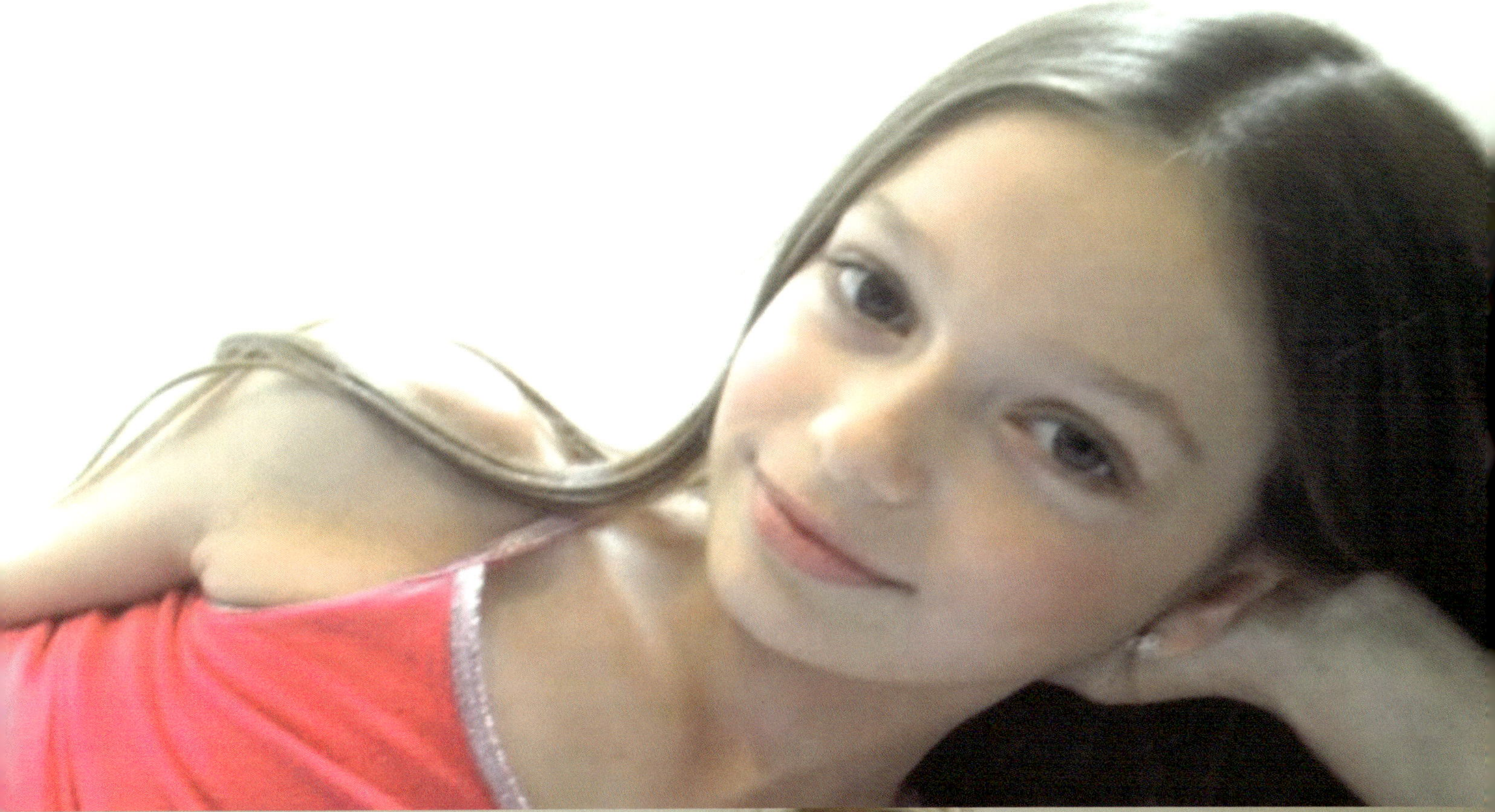

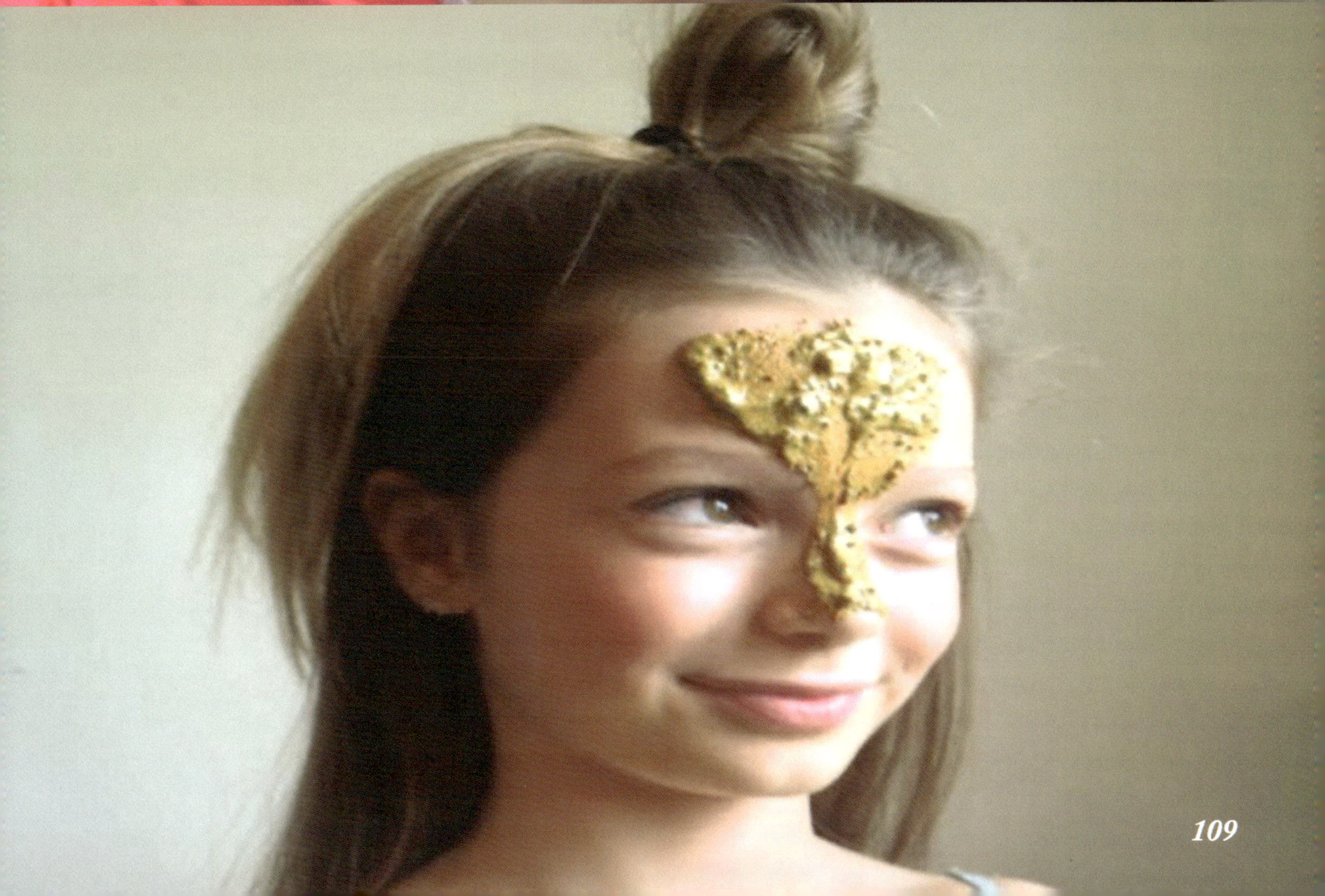

TURMERIC GOMMAGE

To remove skin pigmentation

1 Teaspoon turmeric powder
1/4 Teaspoon coconut oil
5 drops distilled rose water

Mix into a paste, then apply to your face using a circular motion with your fingers. Let it sit for 25 min, then clean with a washcloth dipped in lukewarm water. Follow with cold water, pat dry and apply your moisturizer. (Make sure to wear a dark tee shirt as turmeric stains.)

TURMERIC EXFOLIANT

A great exfoliant and mask to get rid of dark pigmentation, revitalize and brighten the skin.

1 Teaspoon turmeric powder
1/3 Teaspoon coconut oil (organic)
2 Drops of apple cider vinegar
1 Tablespoon distilled water to make a nice paste
(Make sure you are wearing an old tee shirt as turmeric stains.)

Apply it all over face neck and décolleté using a rotating motion to massage into the skin, leave on 20 minutes then wipe off with warm wash cloth and rinse with cold water and dry. Apply a dry gauze to make sure all the color has come off! To erase dark spots repeat 4 times a week.

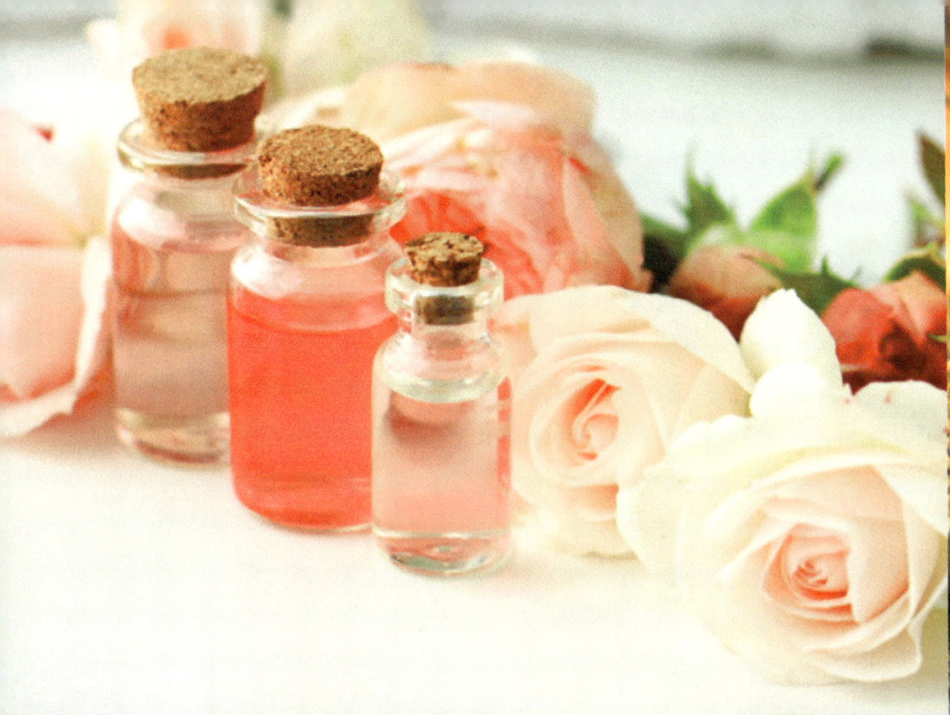
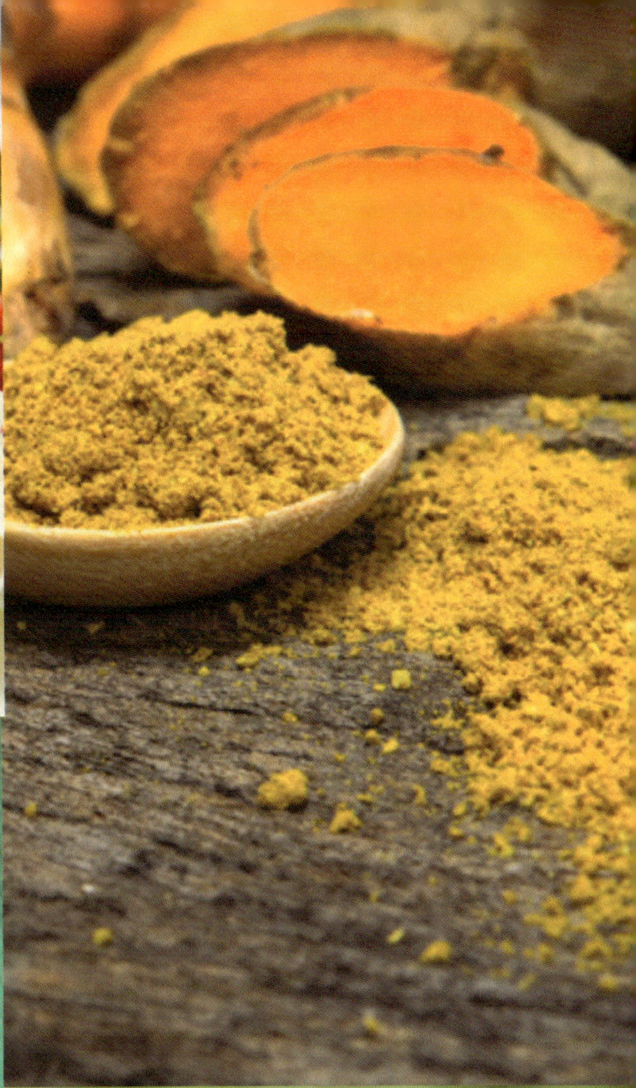
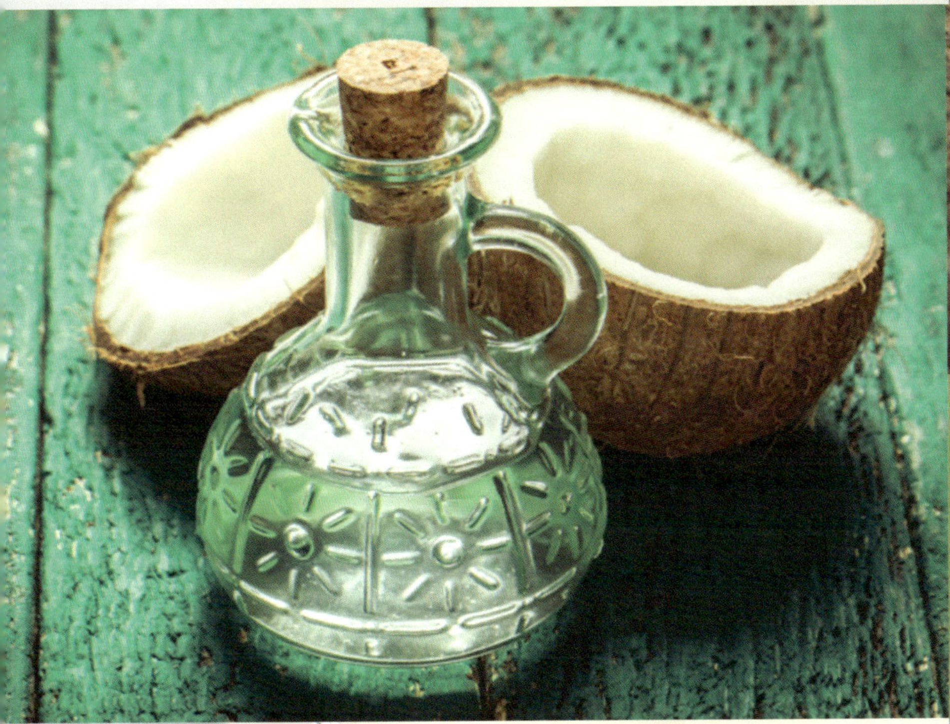
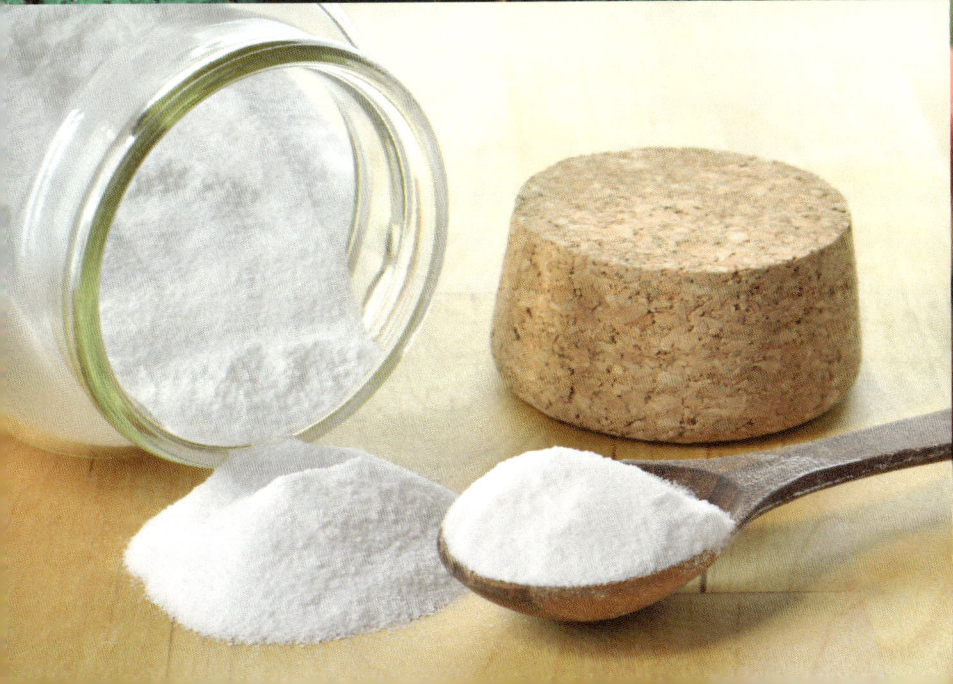
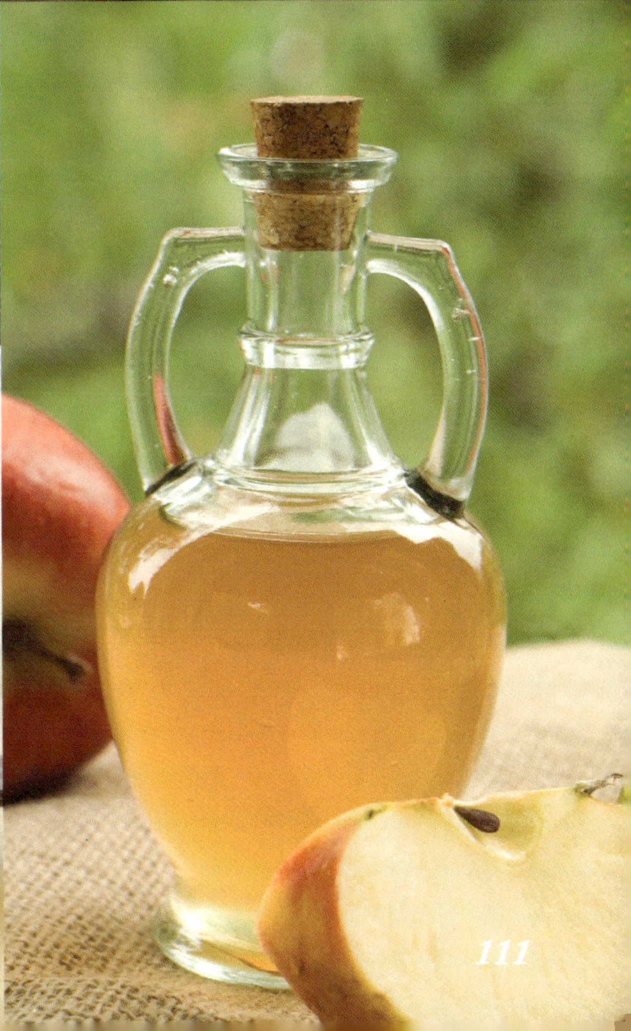

DEEP EXFOLIATING AND WHITENING MASK

Good for acne, but also for all skin types

4 Tablespoon full fat organic yogurt
1 Teaspoon natural baking soda

Mix together. You will see that the yogurt fizzes. Apply a thick even layer and leave on for 20 minutes. Use a circular motion to scrub the skin and stimulate the circulation to draw out the toxins. Rinse with lukewarm water, then splash the face with cold water to close the pores.

Full fat yogurt consists of lactic acid and probiotics that balance good and bad bacteria. It also offers a quick way to reduce inflammation and get rid of redness (very effective for sunburns). Mixed with baking soda it is a superb mask for shrinking pores and calming acne.

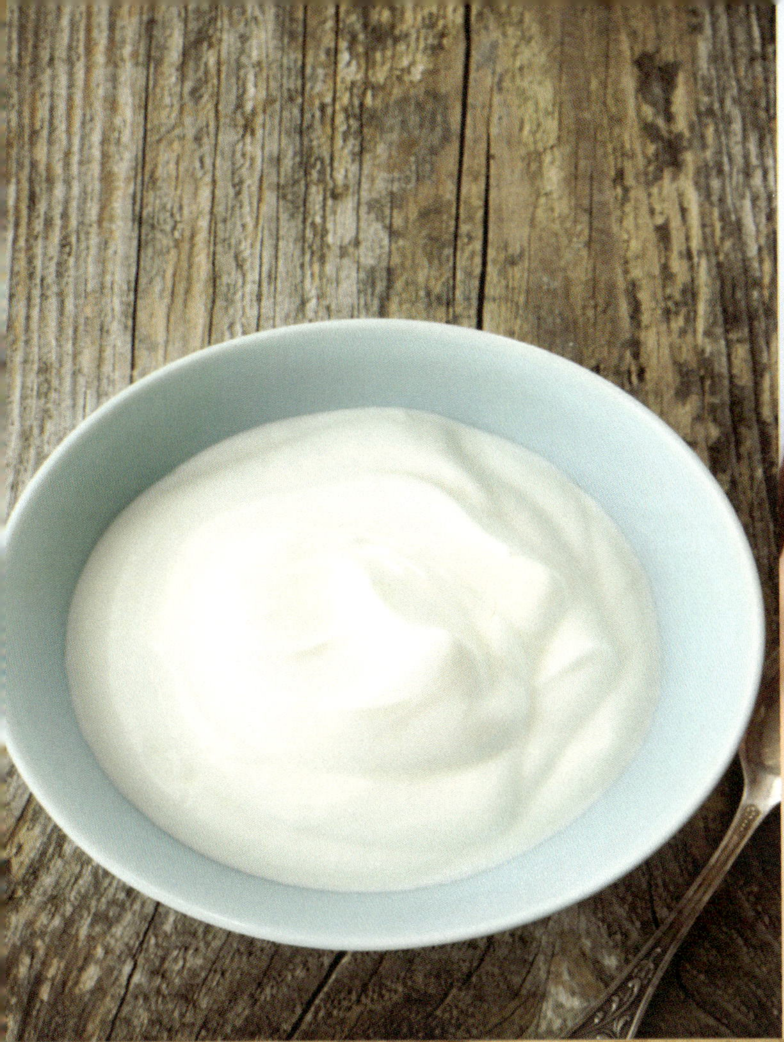
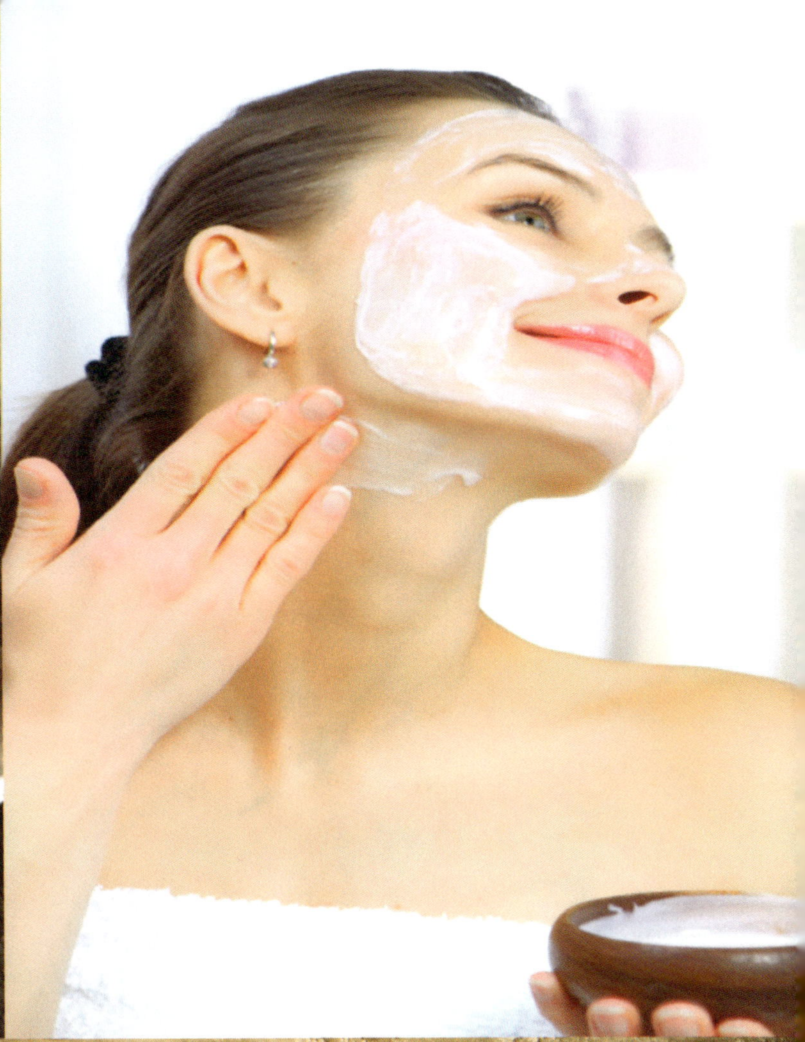
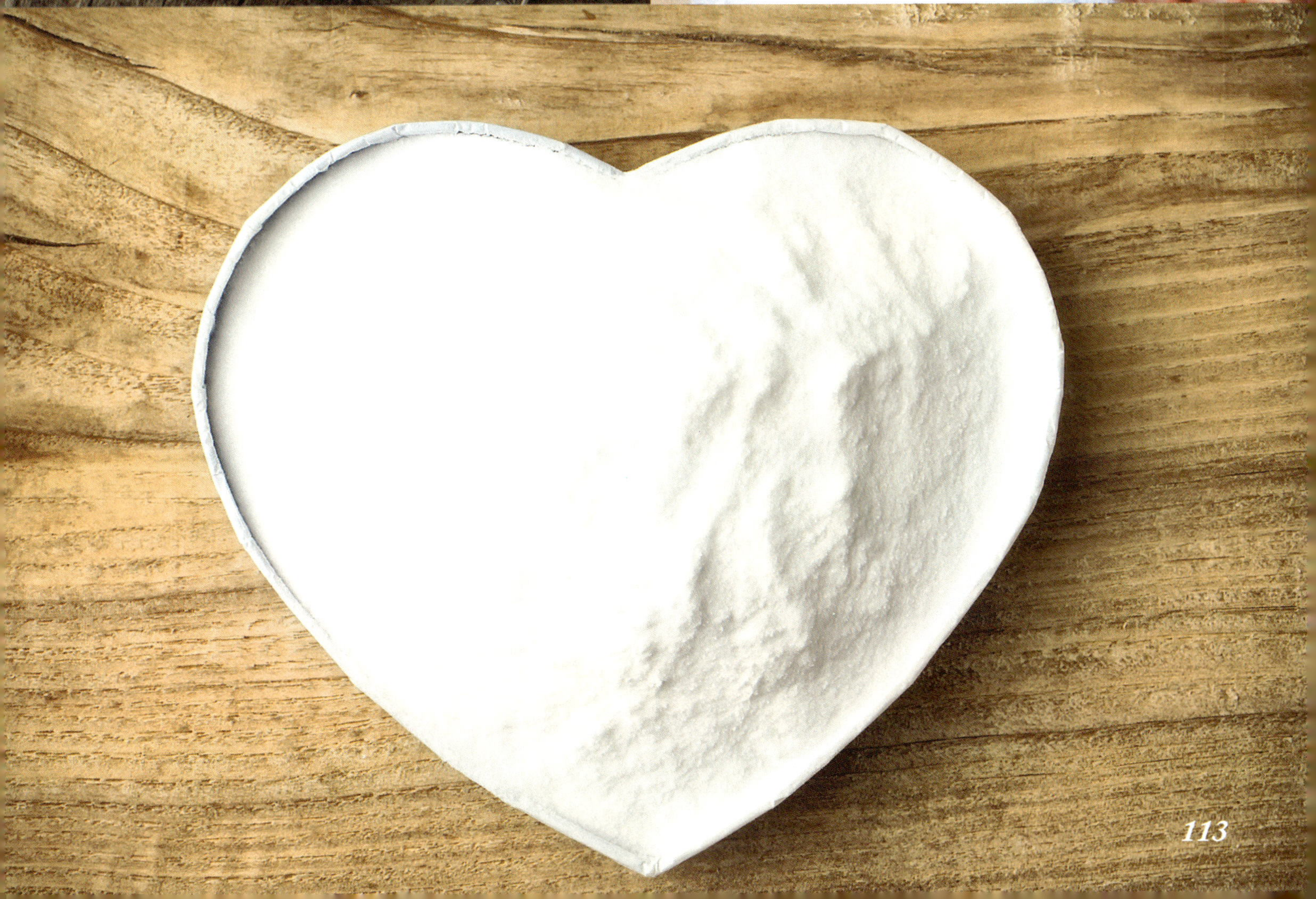

APPLE MASK

For youthful skin

1 Tablespoon fresh apple juice
1 Teaspoon coconut oil
1 Teaspoon cornstarch or oat starch
1/4 Teaspoon baking soda

Mix the ingredients to a smooth paste, brush on the face to cover the skin with a thick even layer. Lay down and relax for 25 minutes. Rinse well with cold water pat dry then apply your moisturizer of choice.

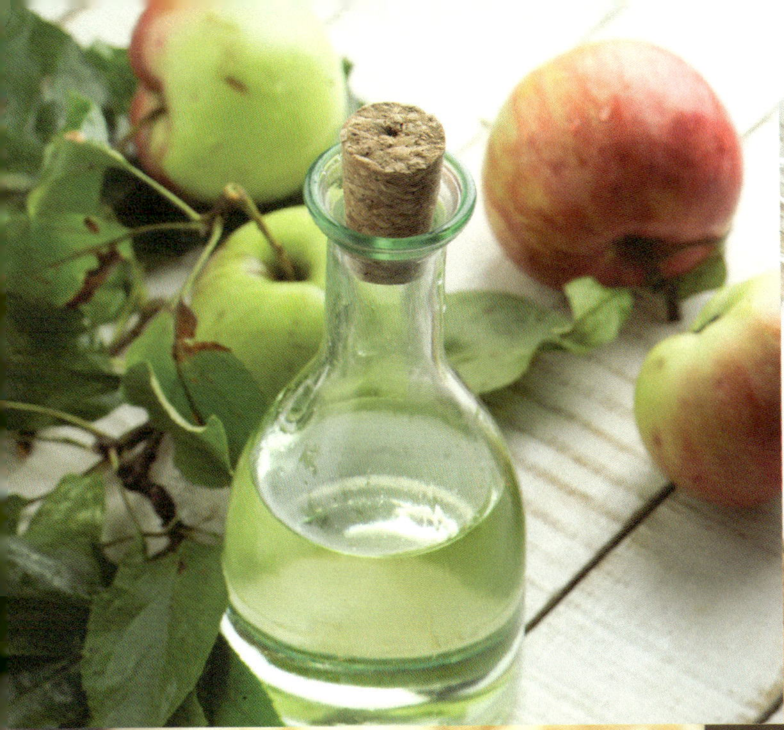
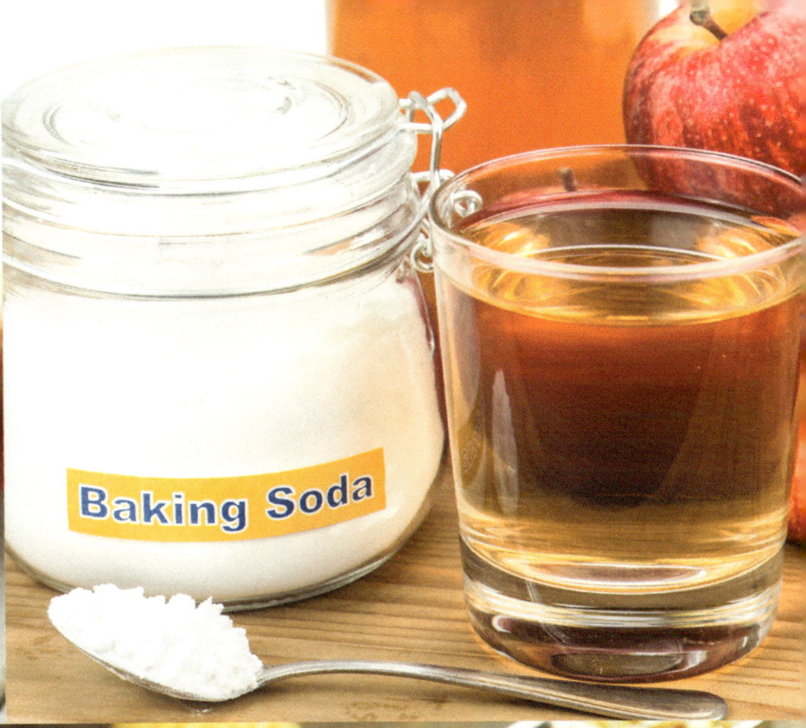
Baking Soda
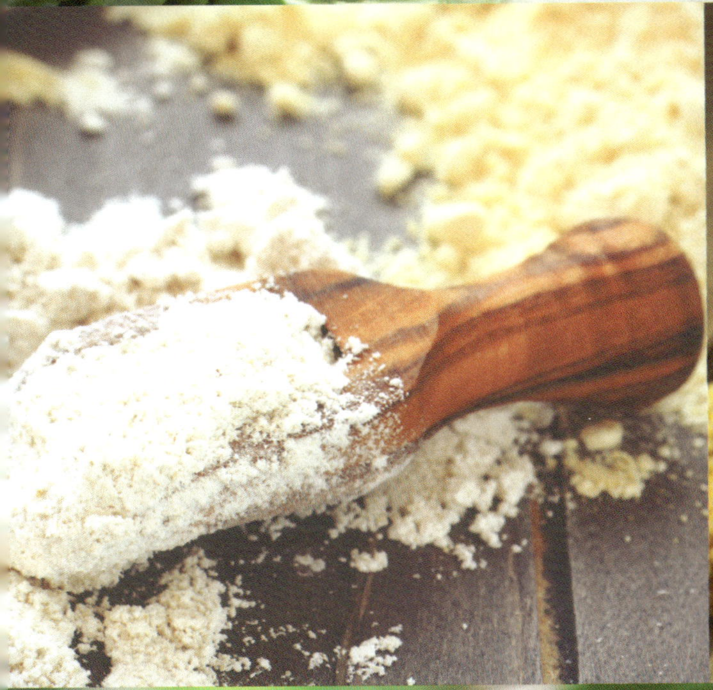
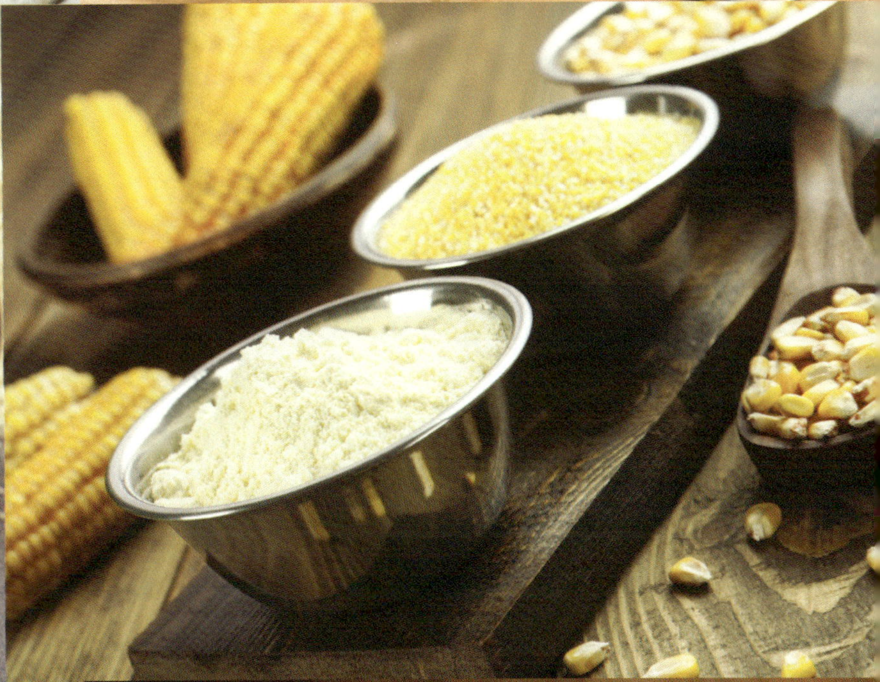
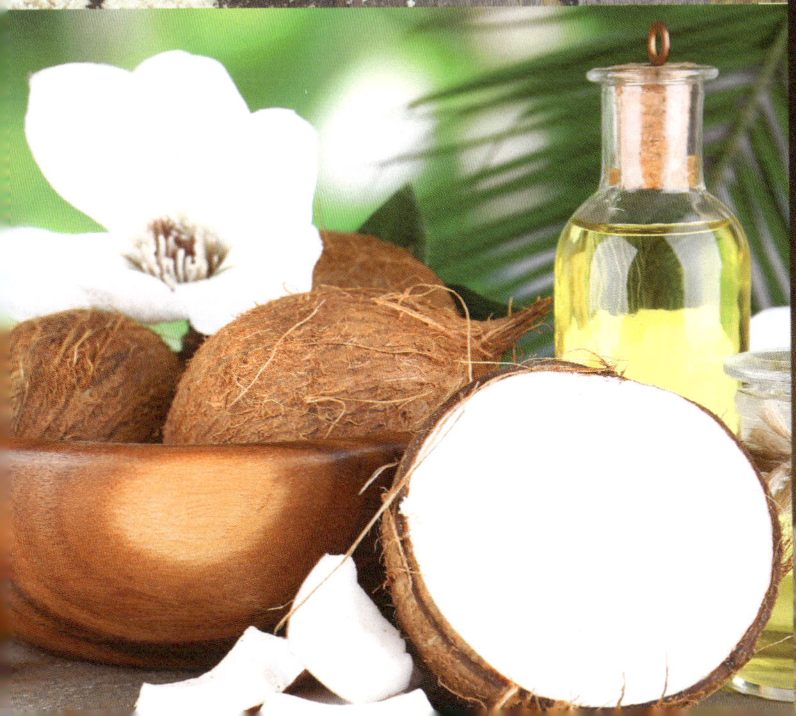
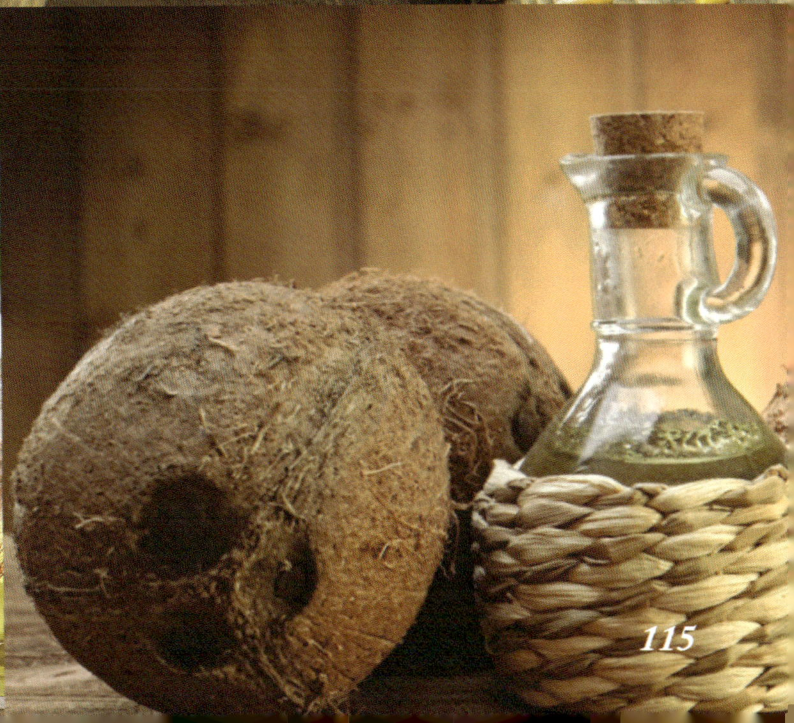

SKIN PIGMENTATION

The cause of skin pigment discoloration or melanin disorder can be external or internal or both. According to ancient Persian folk medicine it is due to the overheating and congestion of the kidney, liver and/or intestinal tract.

It is also especially common for people with dark skin tones. External causes include exposure to chemicals, hormonal imbalance, Betaxolol and overexposure to sunlight. Ultraviolet rays cause freckles and spots that can cause temporary or permanent discoloration -- common on skin areas such as hands and face that are exposed to the sun.

HYPERPIGMENTATION REMEDY

2 Teaspoons organic lemon juice
1 Teaspoon turmeric powder

Stir lemon juice slowly into the turmeric powder to a smooth paste. Apply on any affected area and leave on for 25 minutes. Remove with a warm wash cloth then rinse thoroughly with cold water and apply your moisturizer.

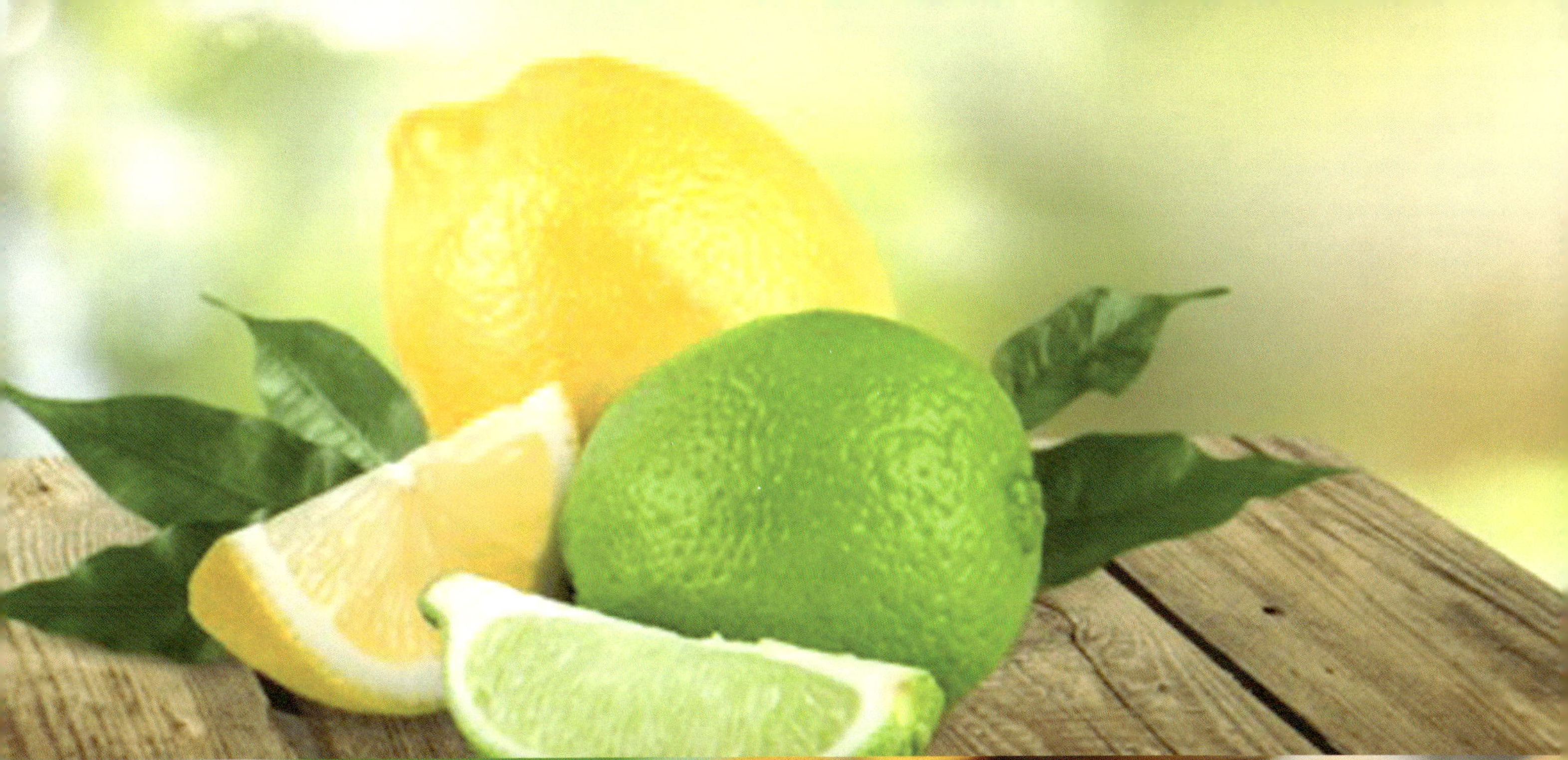

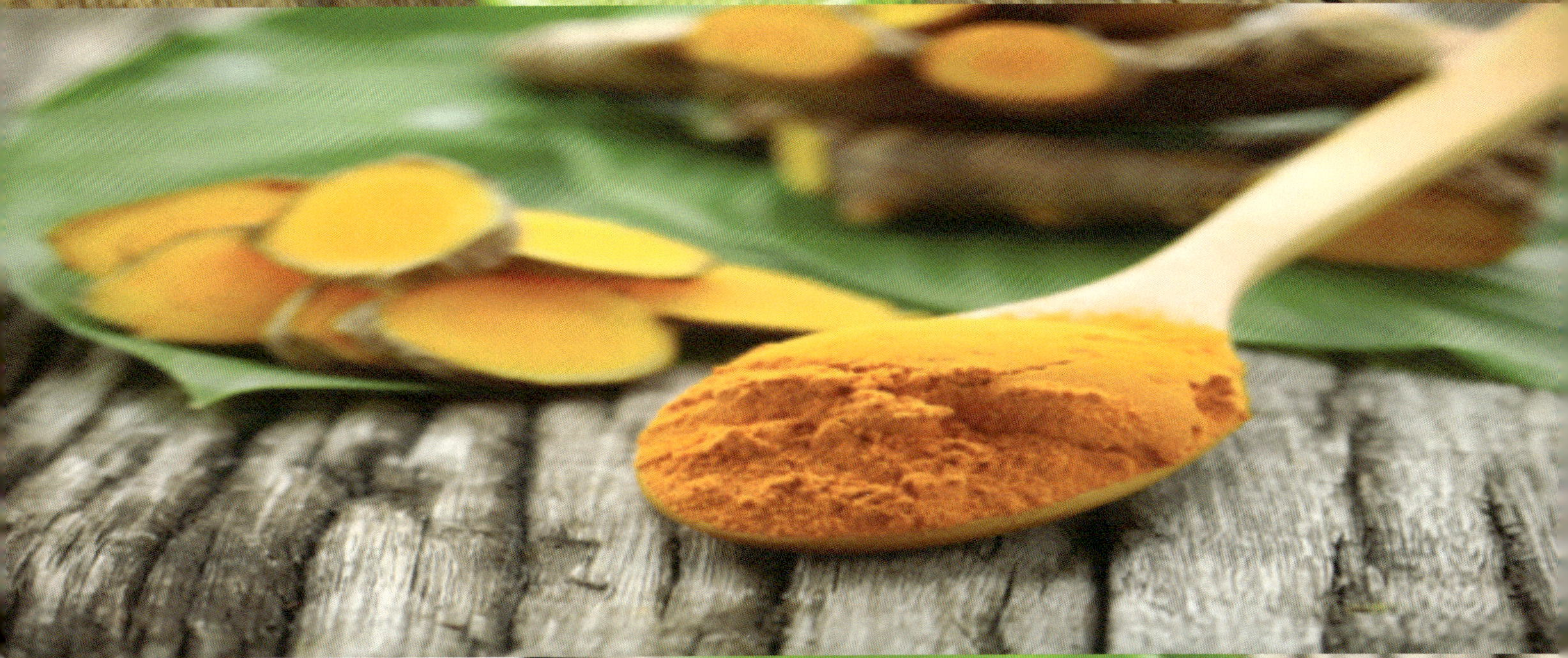

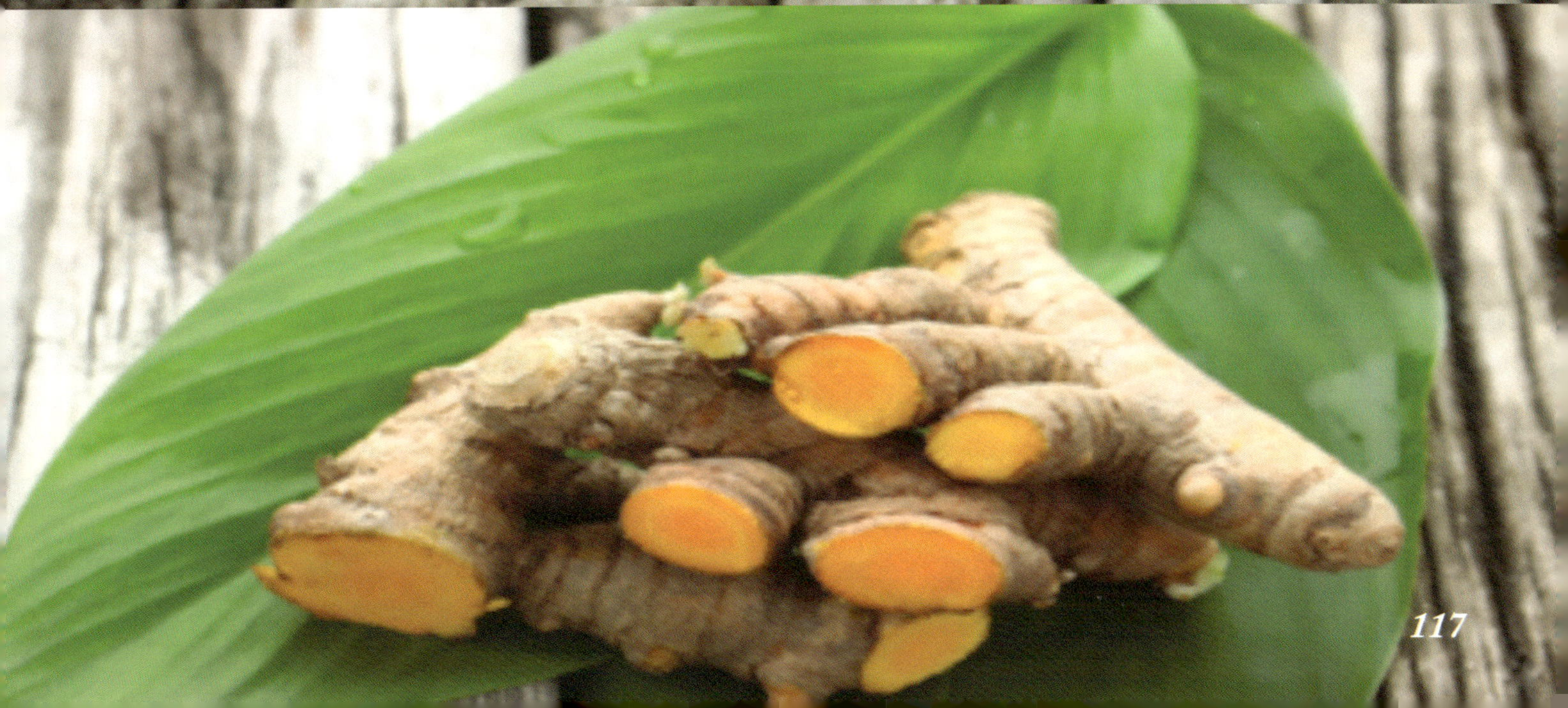

WATERMELON MASK

For dark pigmentation and dull skin

1 Teaspoon watermelon juice
1 Teaspoon fresh tomato juice
1 Teaspoon coconut oil
1 Teaspoon cornstarch
1/4 Teaspoon baking soda
1 Small fan brush (Makeup brush)

Mix the ingredients well to a smooth paste, then brush onto the face covering the dark spots. Lay down and relax for 25 minutes. Rinse with cold water, pat dry then apply your moisturizer of choice.

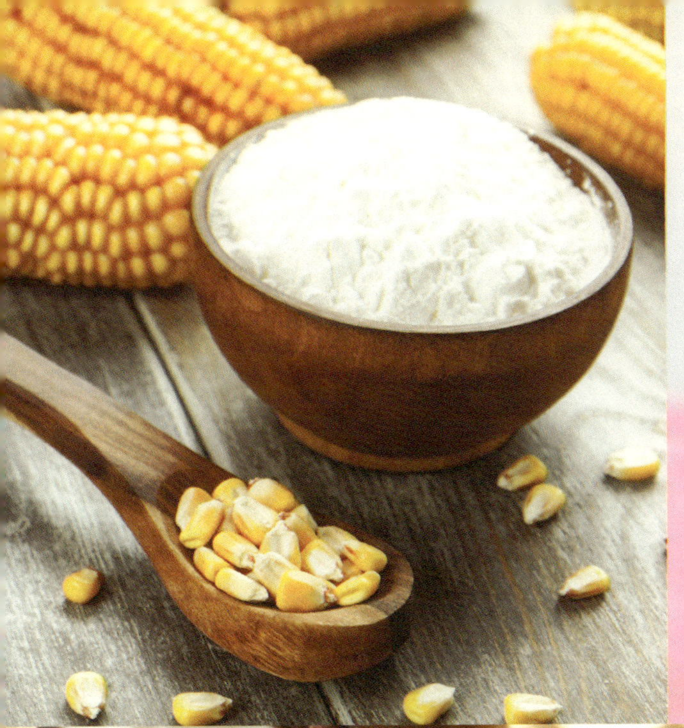

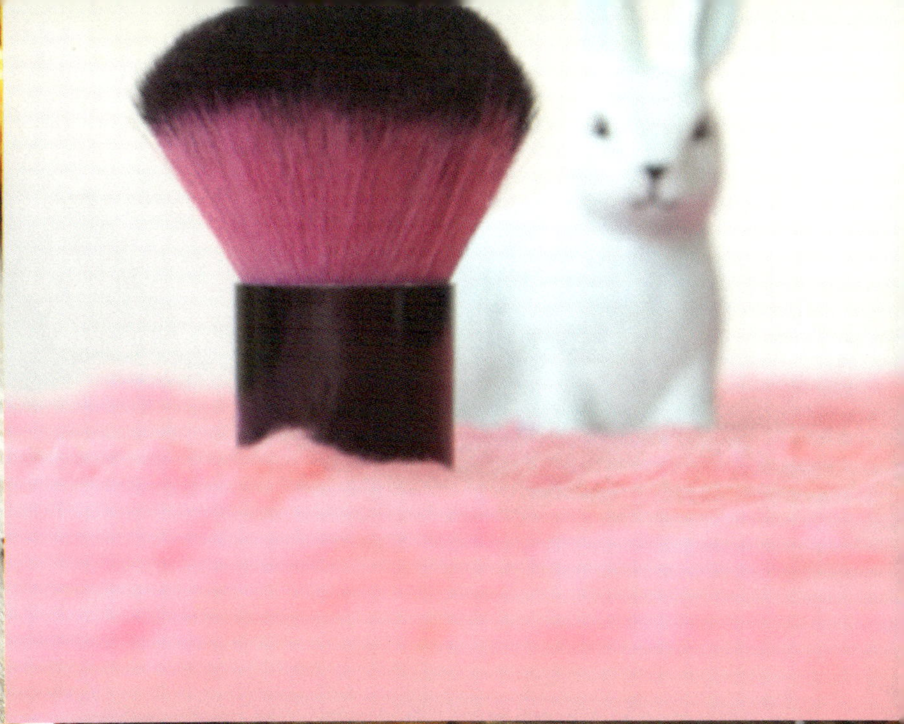

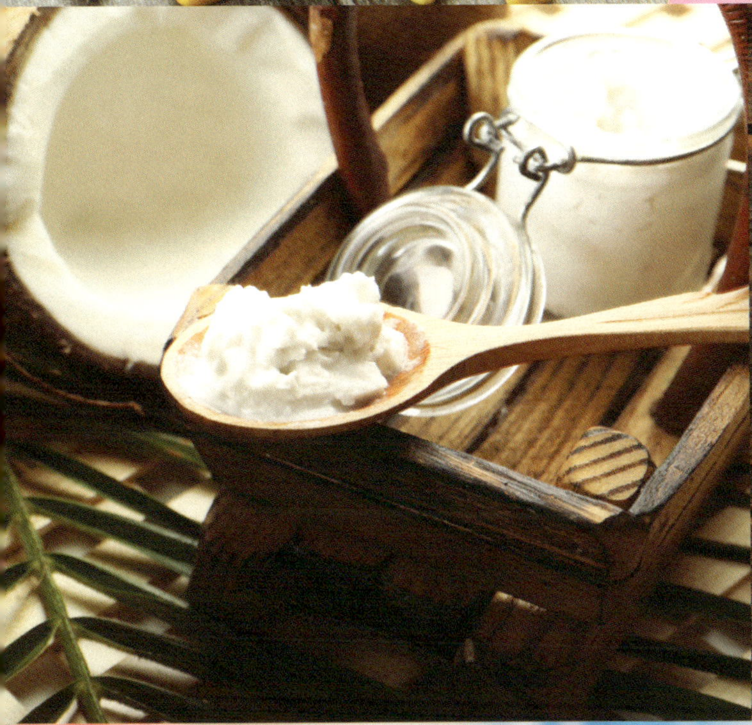

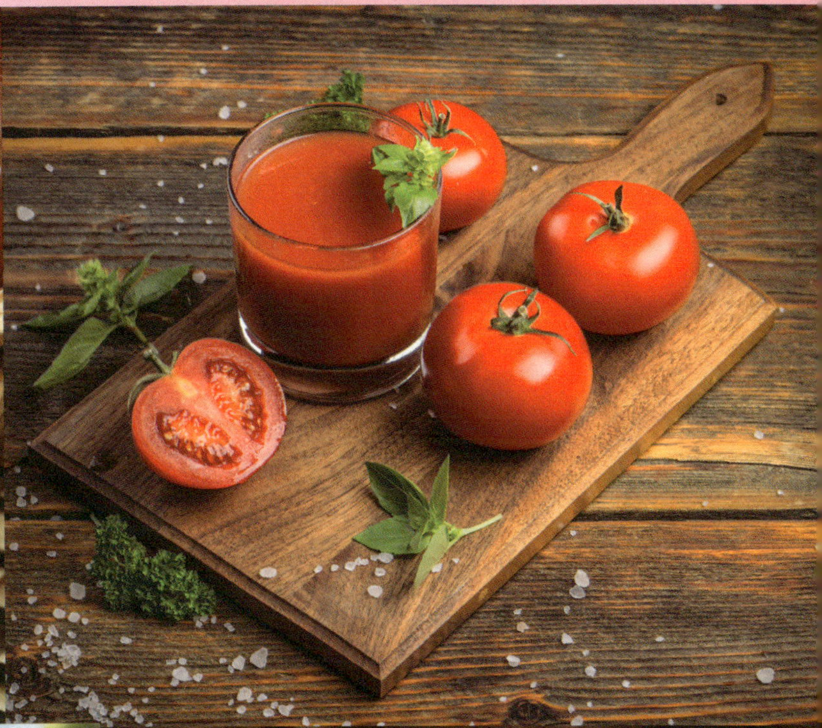

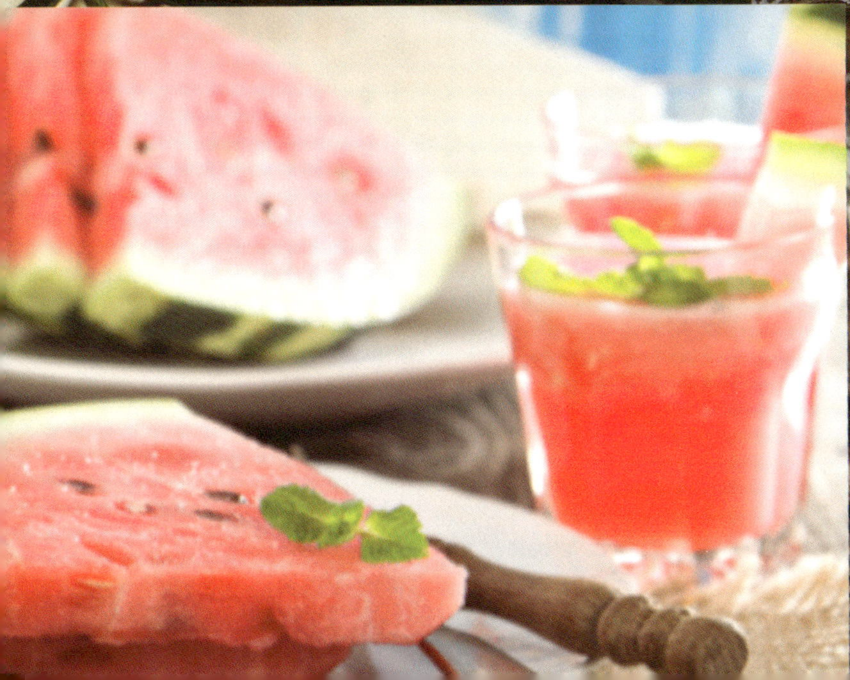

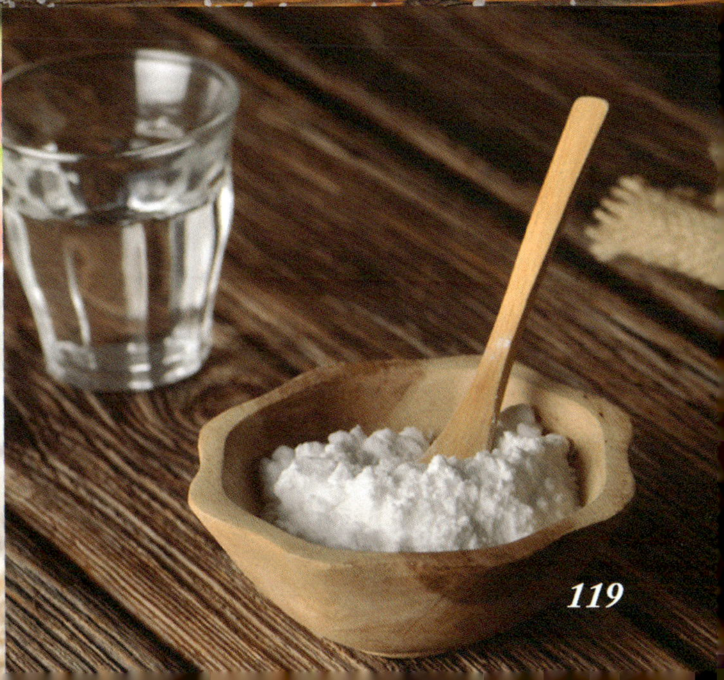

CARROT MASK

To shrink pores

3 Medium organic carrots
1 Teaspoon coconut oil
1 Teaspoon oat starch
1/4 Teaspoon non-GMO baking soda
5 Drops rosewater

Steam carrots, then mash. Add coconut oil, oat starch and baking soda and mix well, then add the rose water till it is a nice smooth paste. Apply evenly to face and lay down for 20 minutes. Rinse with cold water, pat dry then apply your moisturizer of choice.

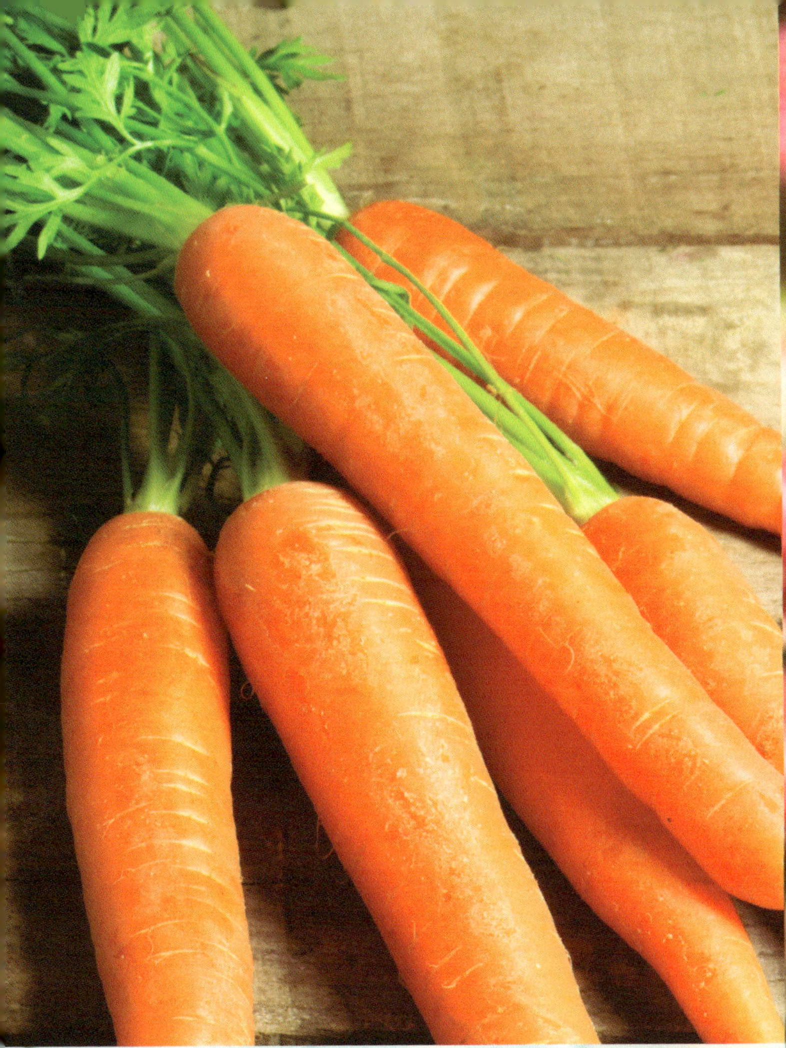

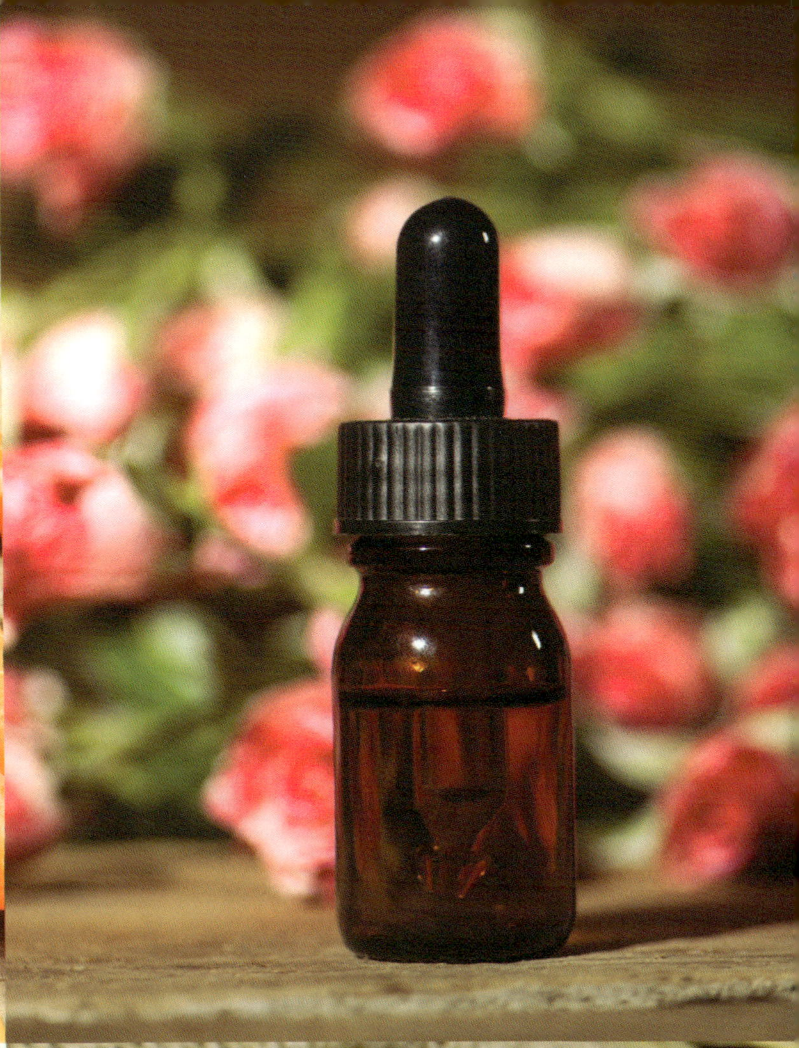

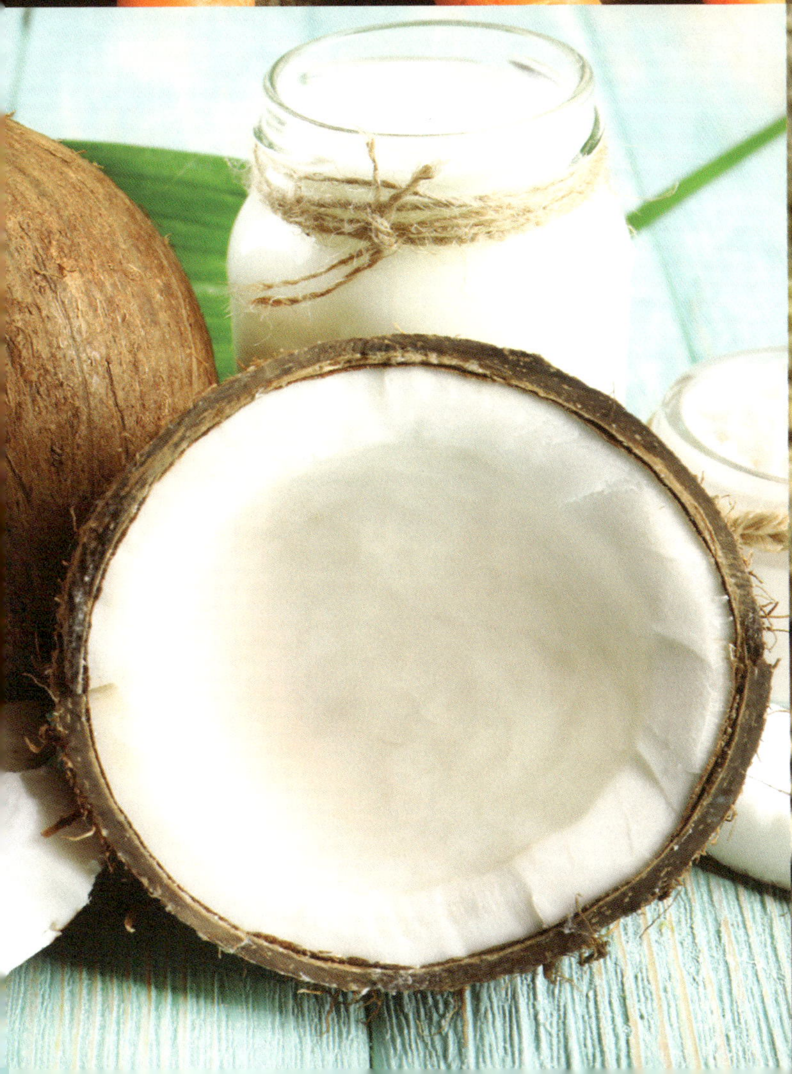

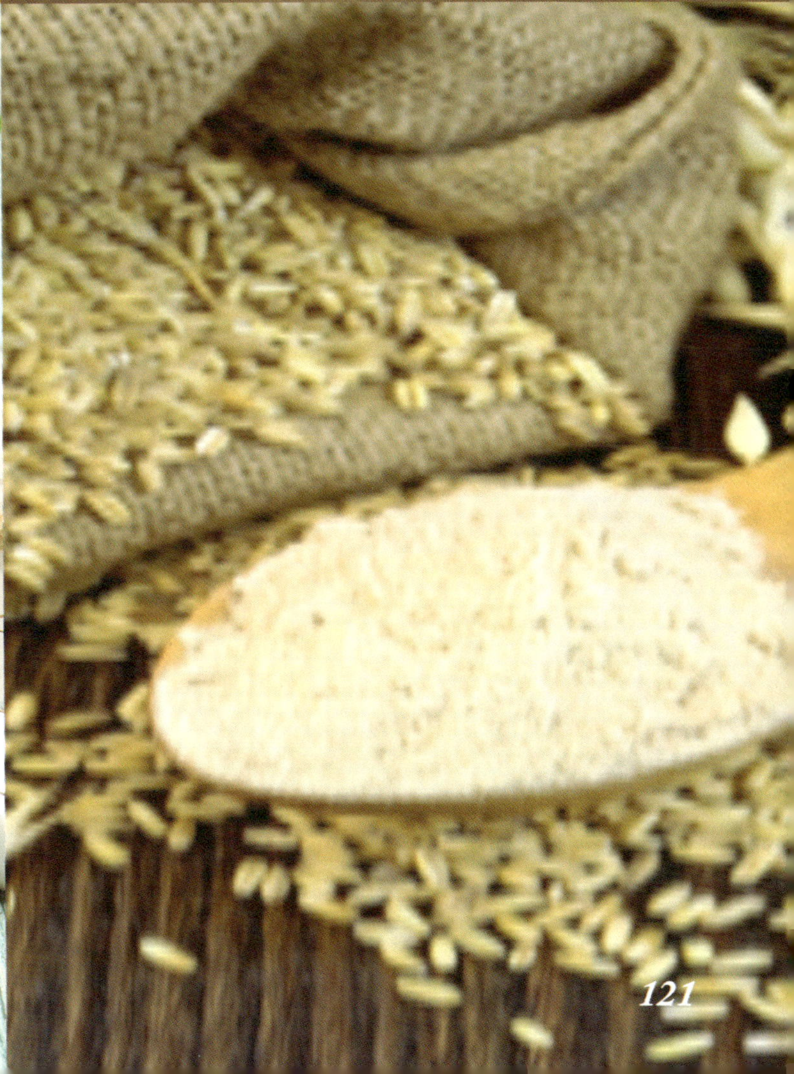

BANANA PIGMENT REMOVAL MASK

1 Skin of unripe banana
1 Teaspoon virgin coconut oil

Mix the banana peel and coconut oil in a blender then apply evenly to the face. Lay down for 20 minutes. Remove with wash cloth or tissue, then rinse with cold water, pat dry and apply your moisturizer of choice.

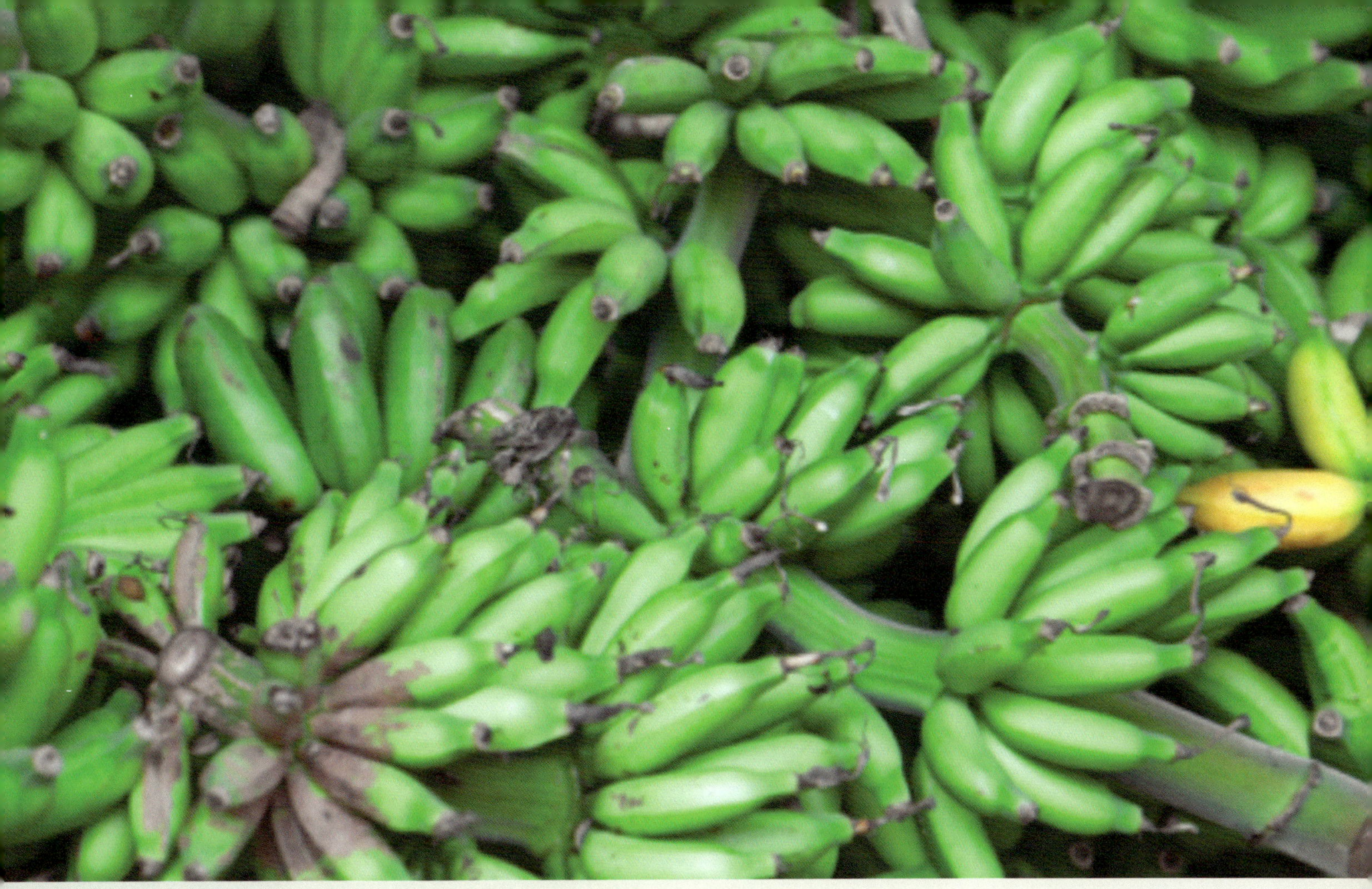

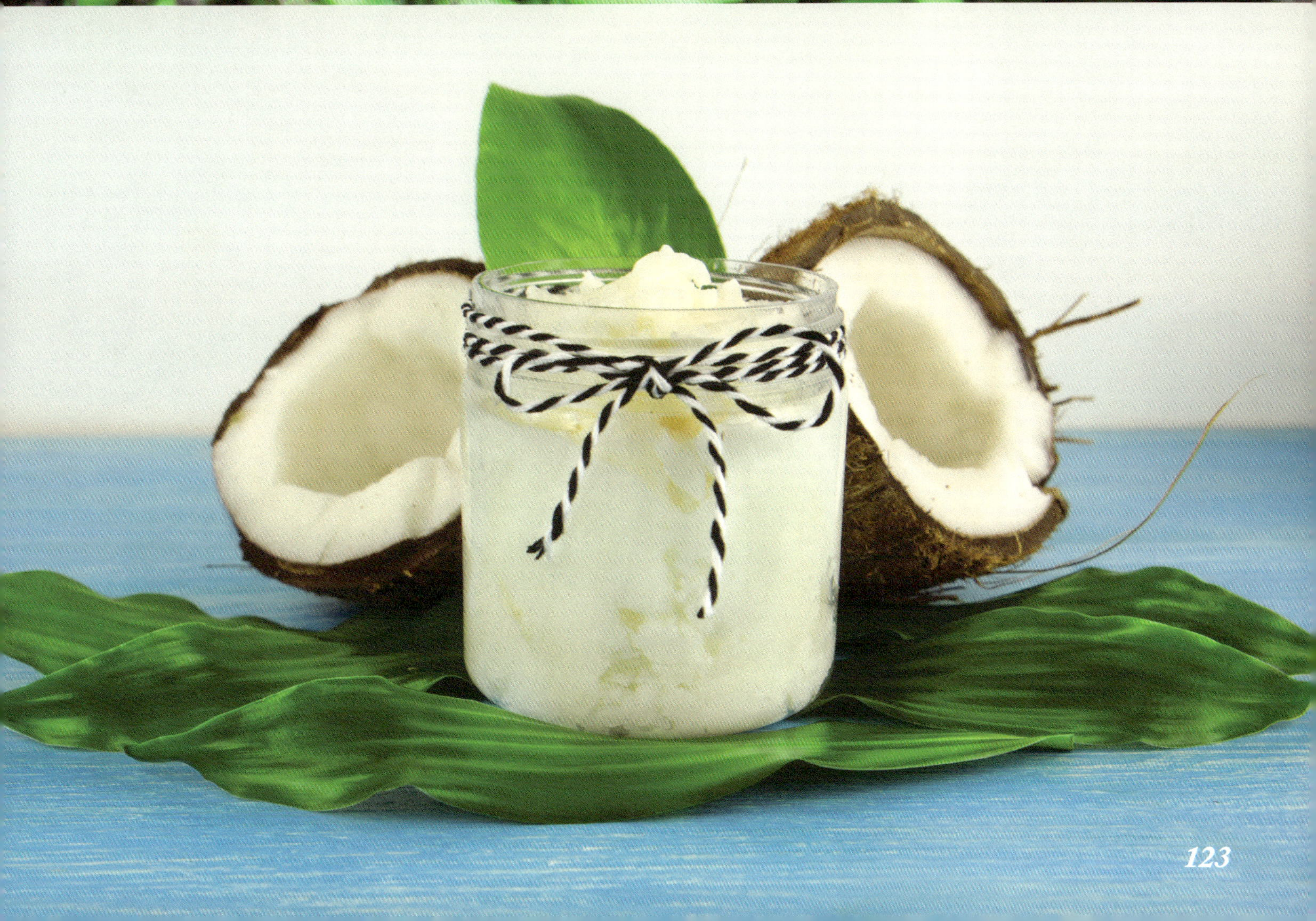

BANANA YOGURT BRIGHTENING MASK

Tightens skin, shrinks pores and reduces under eye circles

2 Tablespoons full-fat (preferably raw) yogurt
1 Unripe banana with its skin
2 Drops rosewater

Mix the banana with peel and full-fat yogurt in a blender. Apply evenly to the face and eyes. Lay down for 25 minutes. Once dry remove with warm moist washcloth or tissue then rinse with cold water, pat dry and apply your moisturizer of choice.

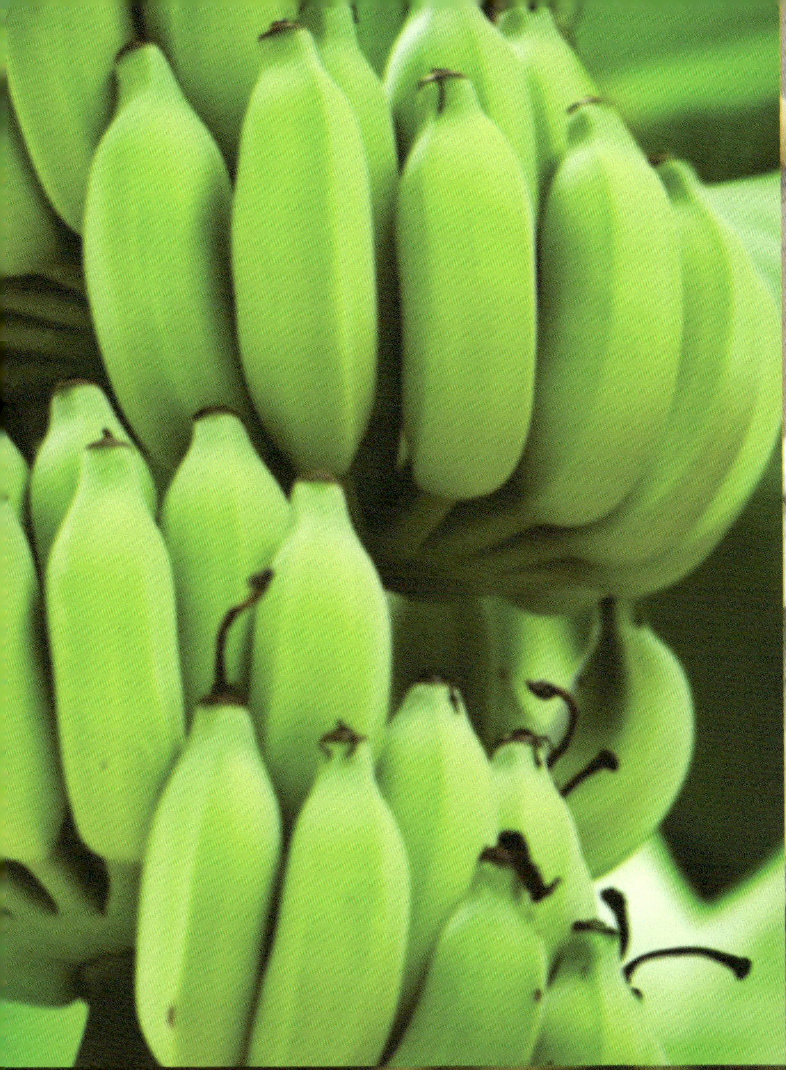
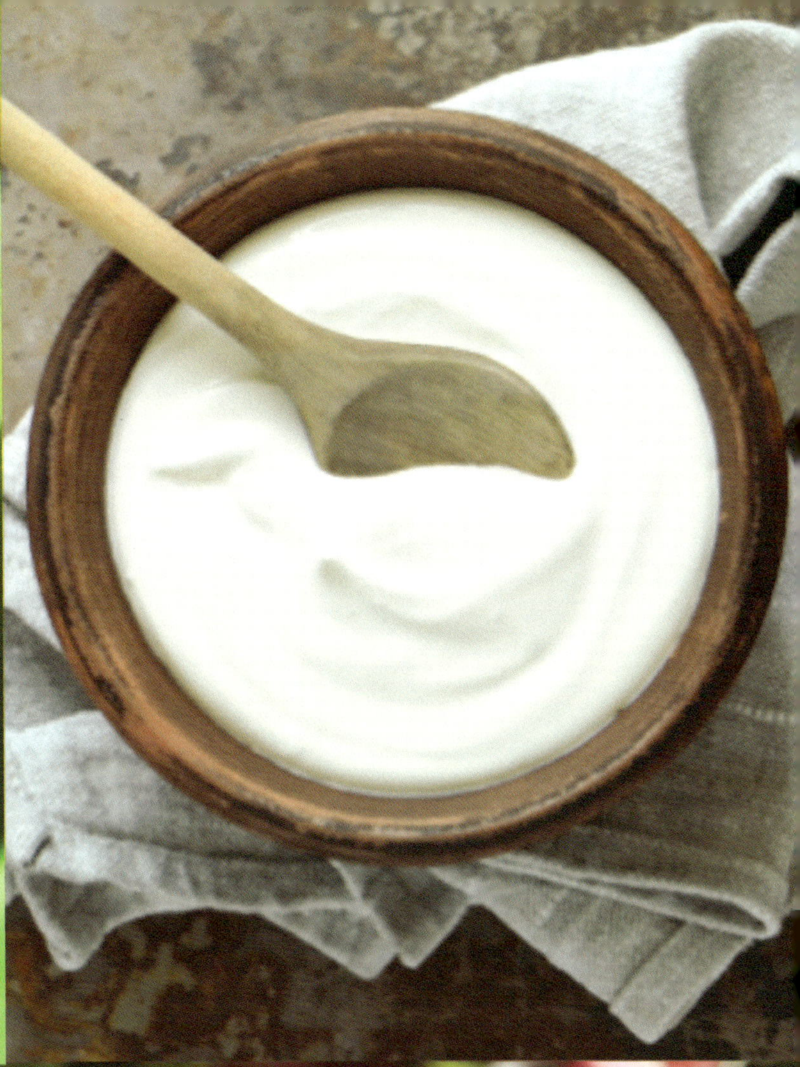
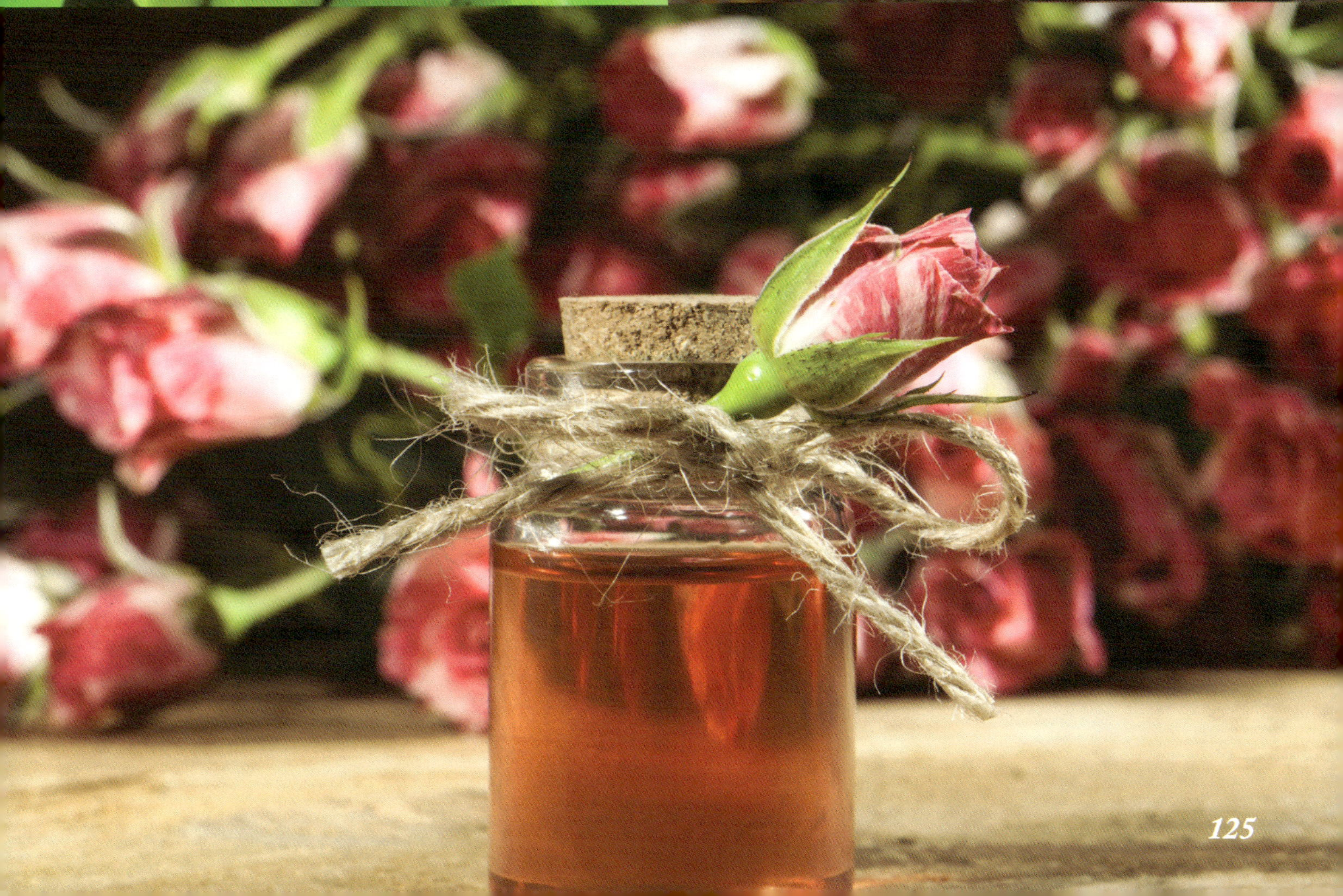

POMEGRANATE

Pomegranate is another heavenly fruit and is extremely high in such antioxidants as flavonoids and phenolics. It also has high levels of Vitamins A, E and C. Regular use of pomegranate helps to delay premature aging and can impart smooth, soft, glowing skin. Pomegranate also has anti-inflammatory properties. Pomegranate does a whole lot of good to all kind of skin problems – age spots, wrinkles, acne, hyperpigmentation, etc. Pomegranate firms up skin by aiding in collagen production. It is also believed pomegranates brighten and lighten skin tone.

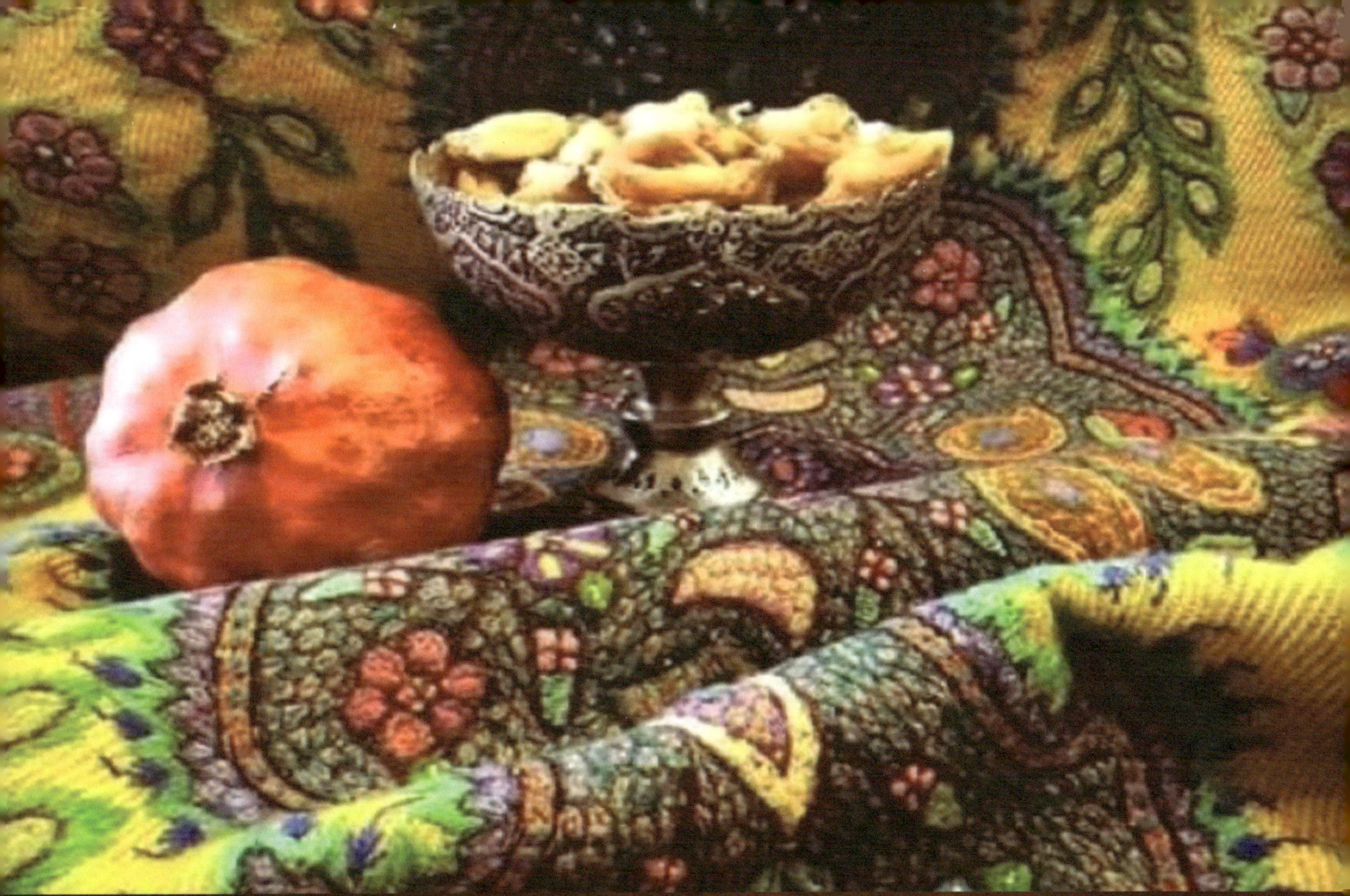

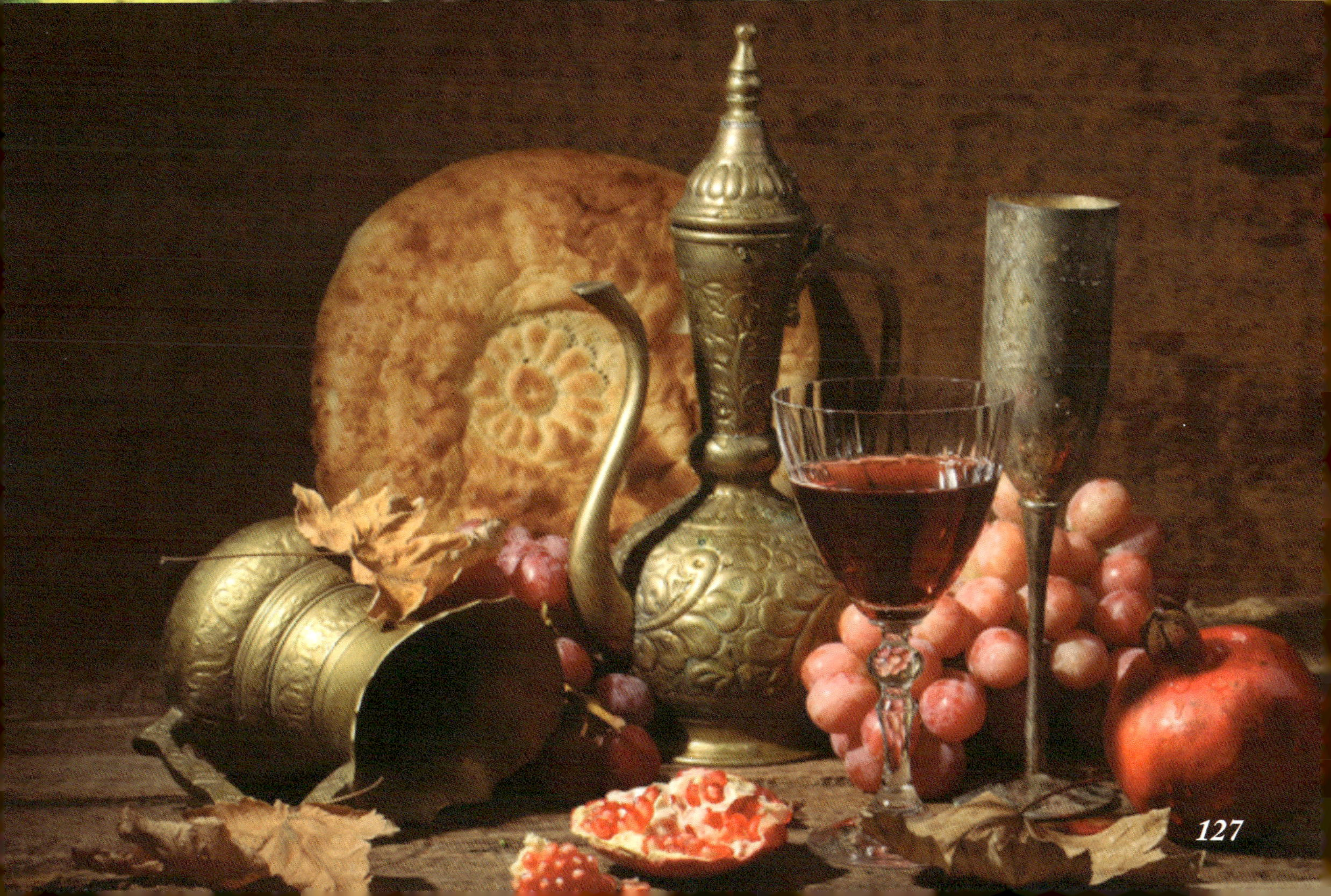

POMEGRANATE ELIXIR MASK

4 Tablespoons pomegranate seeds
1 Teaspoon coconut oil
1 Teaspoon raw honey
1 Tablespoon organic oats
2 Drops rosewater

Mix all ingredients in a blender and apply evenly to the face and eyes with a fan brush. Lay down for 25 minutes. Once dry remove with warm moist washcloth or tissue, then rinse with cold water, pat dry and apply your moisturizer of choice.

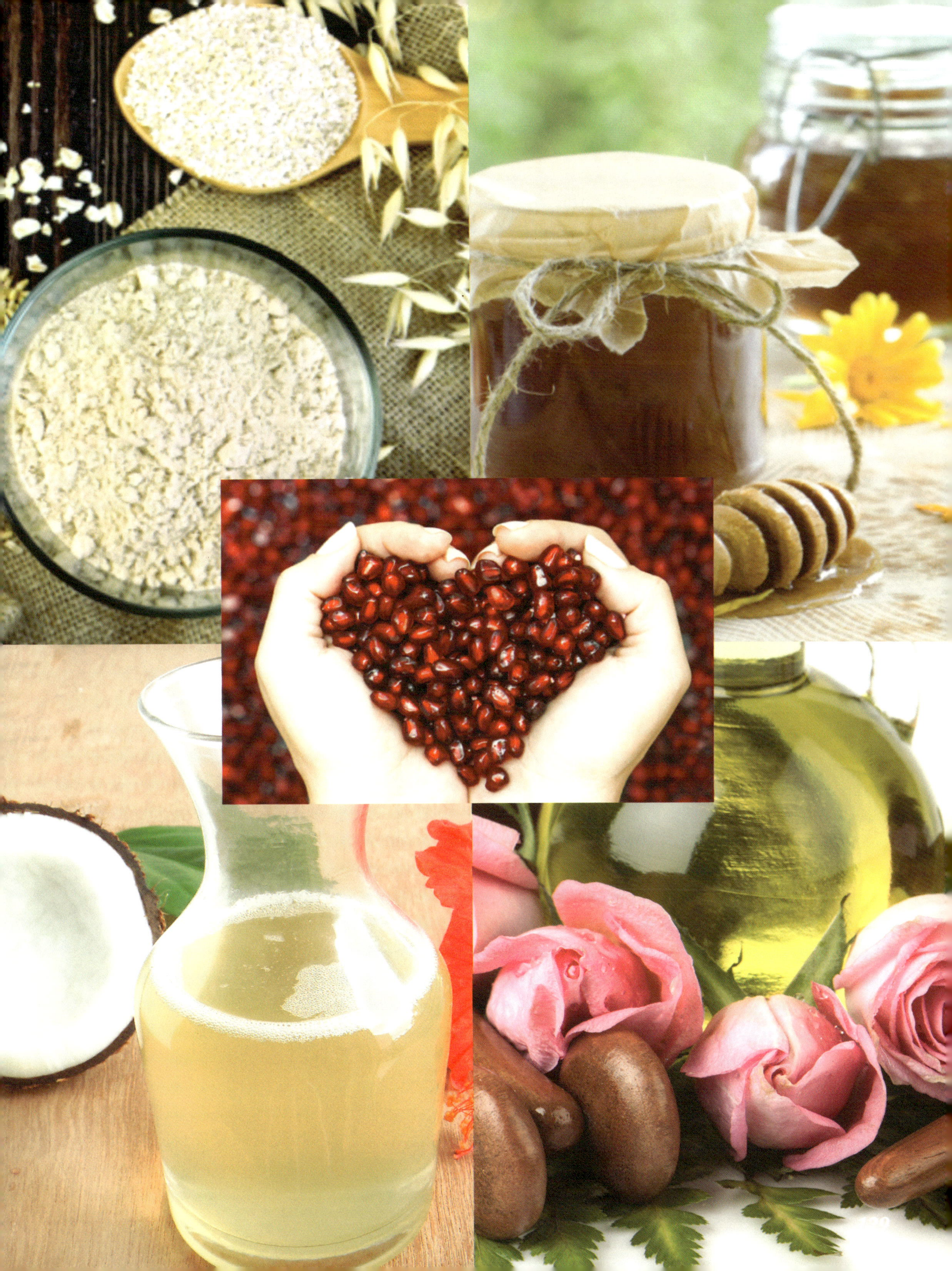

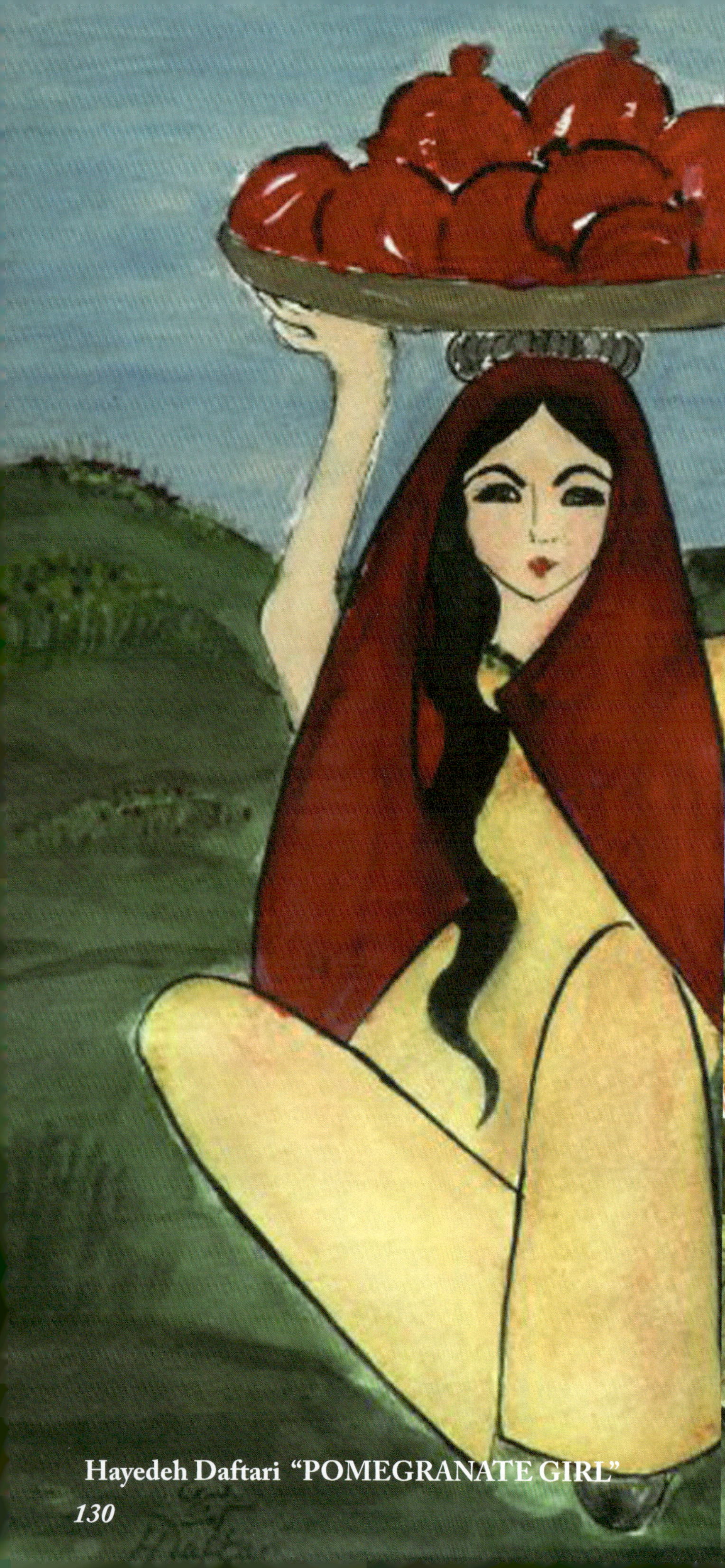

Hayedeh Daftari "POMEGRANATE GIRL"

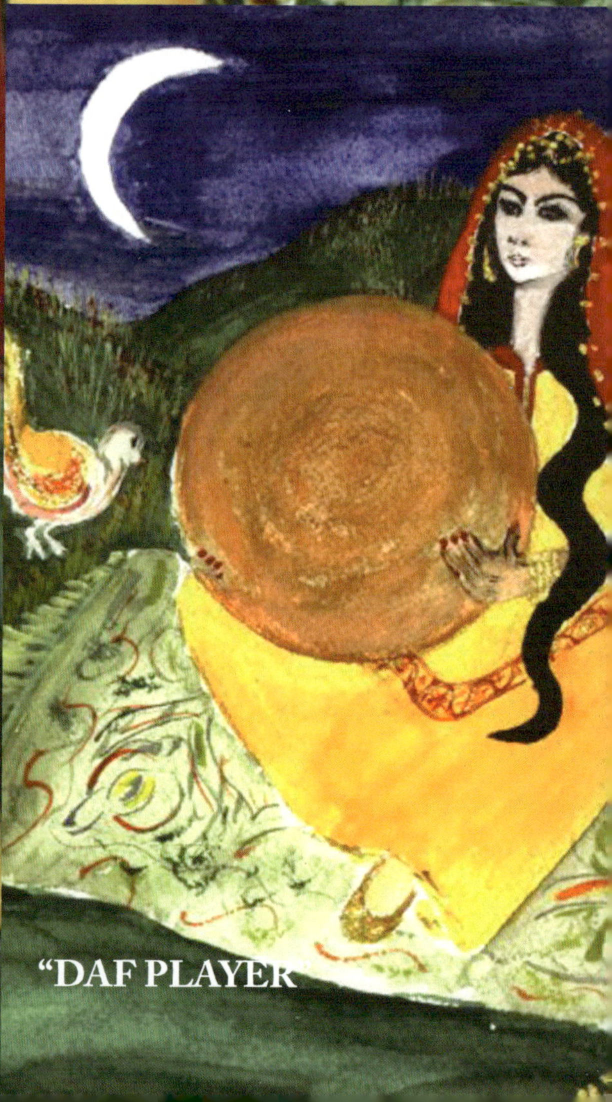

"DAF PLAYER"

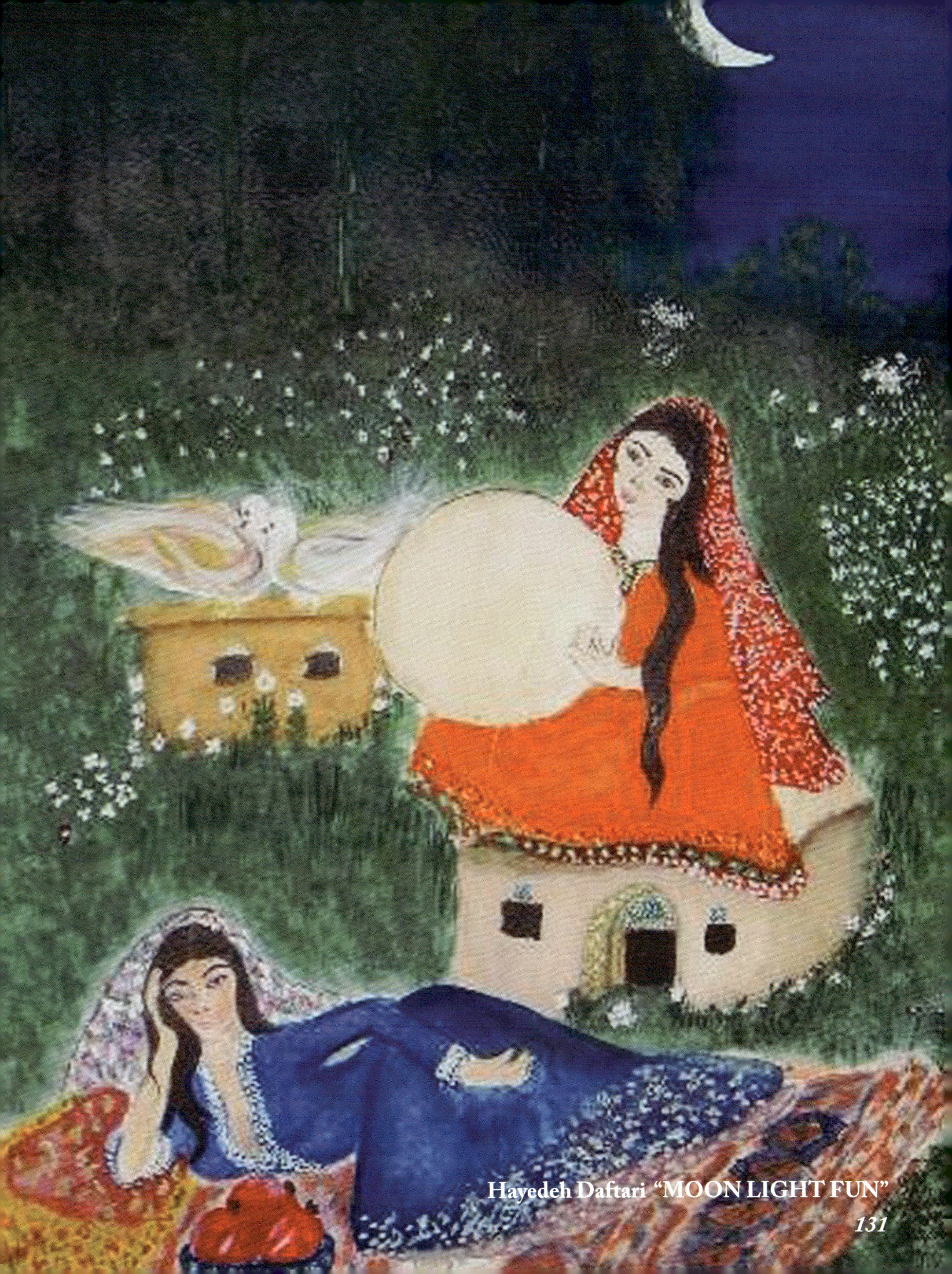

Hayedeh Daftari "MOON LIGHT FUN"

POMEGRANATE YOGURT MASK

To brighten and firm the skin

4 Tablespoons pomegranate seeds
2 Tablespoons raw yogurt
1 Teaspoon raw honey

Mix all ingredients in a blender and apply evenly to the face and eyes with a fan brush. Lay down for 25 minutes. Once dry remove with warm moist washcloth or tissue then rinse with cold water, pat dry and apply your moisturizer of choice.

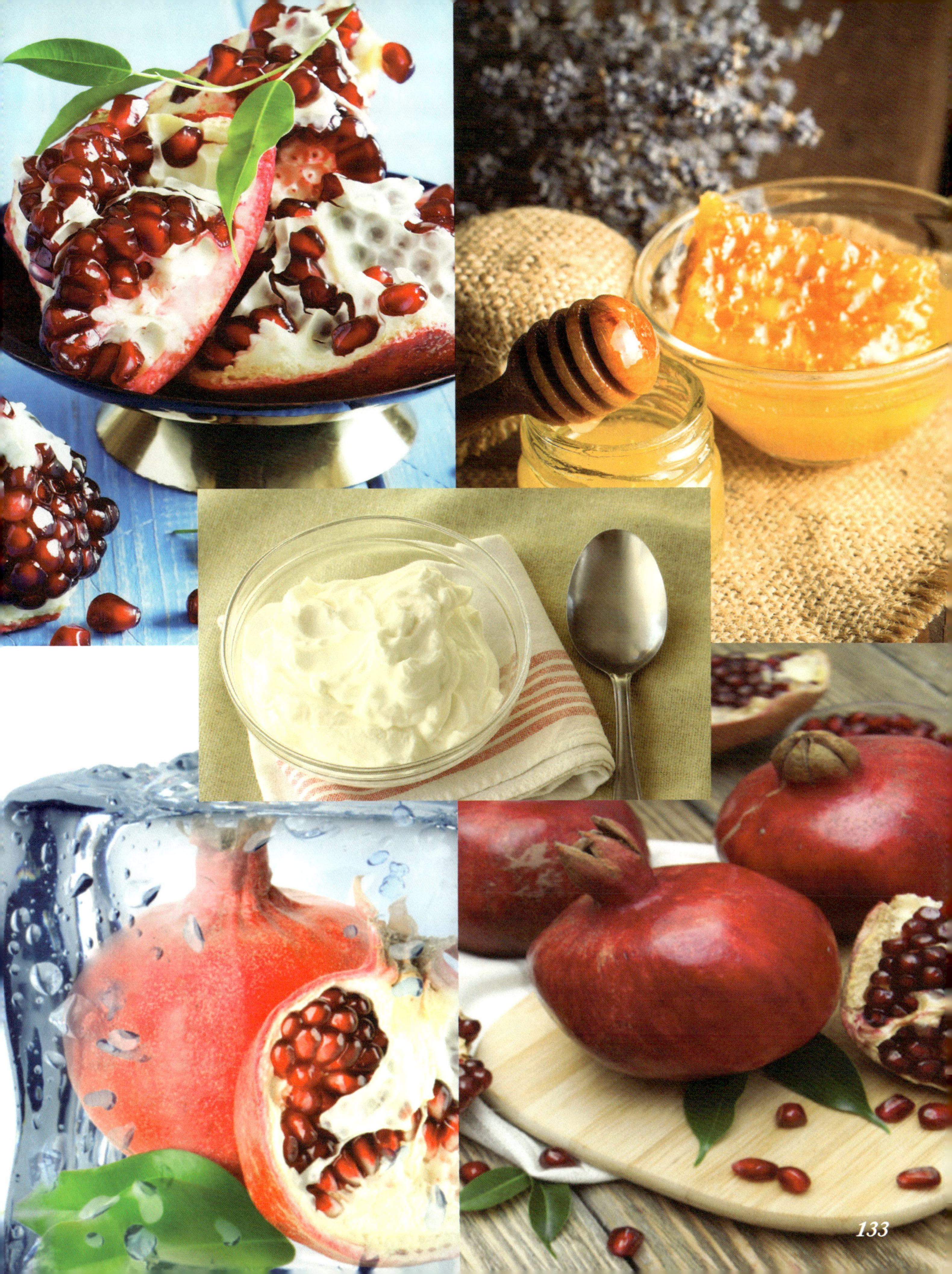

ACNE TREATMENTS

Acne is due to congestion, or as they say in Farsi "an overheated liver." Thus it's important to also drink the turmeric tea or turmeric juice a couple times a day, every day, so you are working from the inside out!

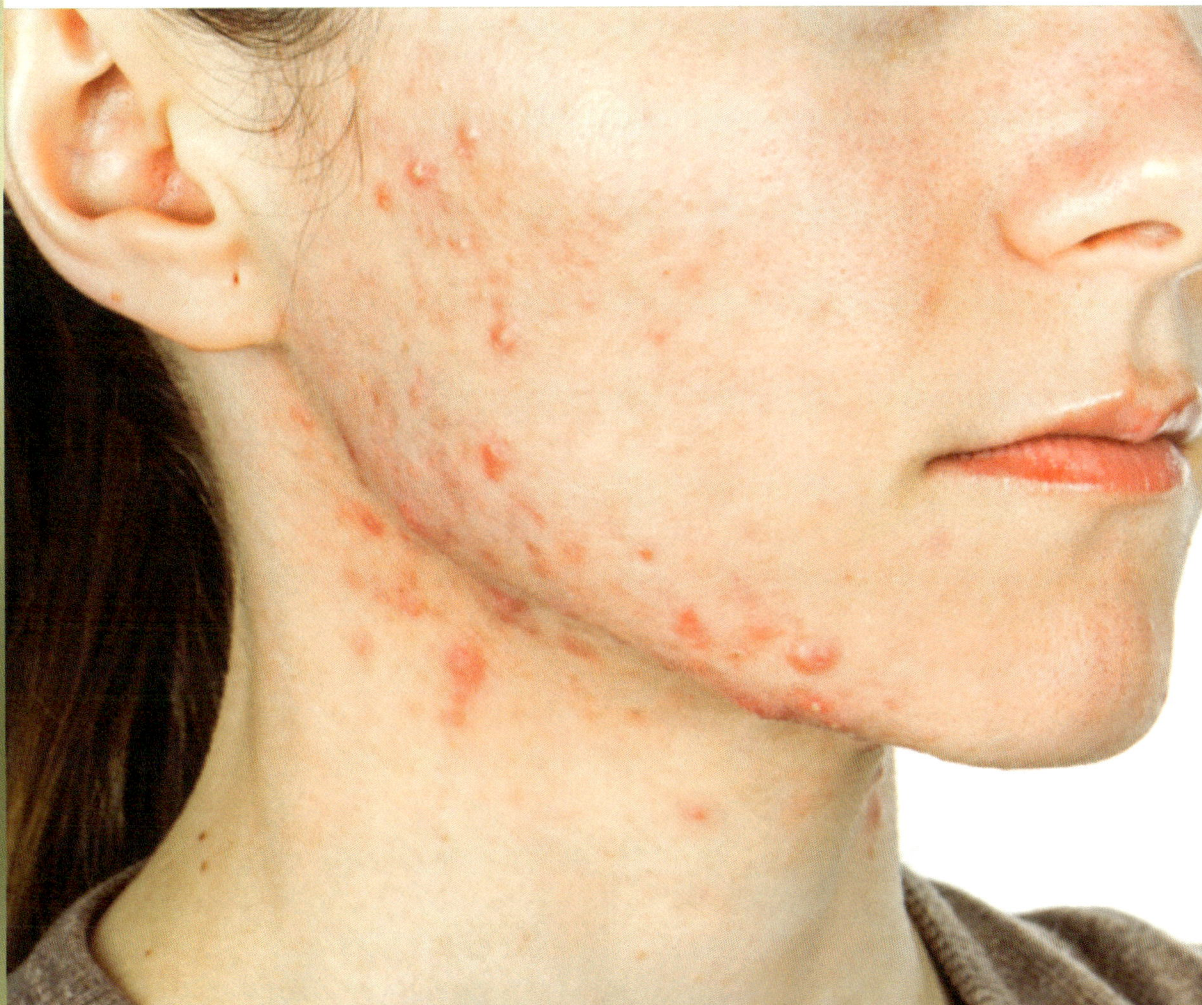

ACNE MASK

2 Tablespoons cold pressed virgin olive oil
1 Ripe banana with its skin
1 Teaspoon raw honey
5 Drops rose water

Mix well, place on face for 25 minutes, rinse off with lukewarm water. Repeat 3 times a week.

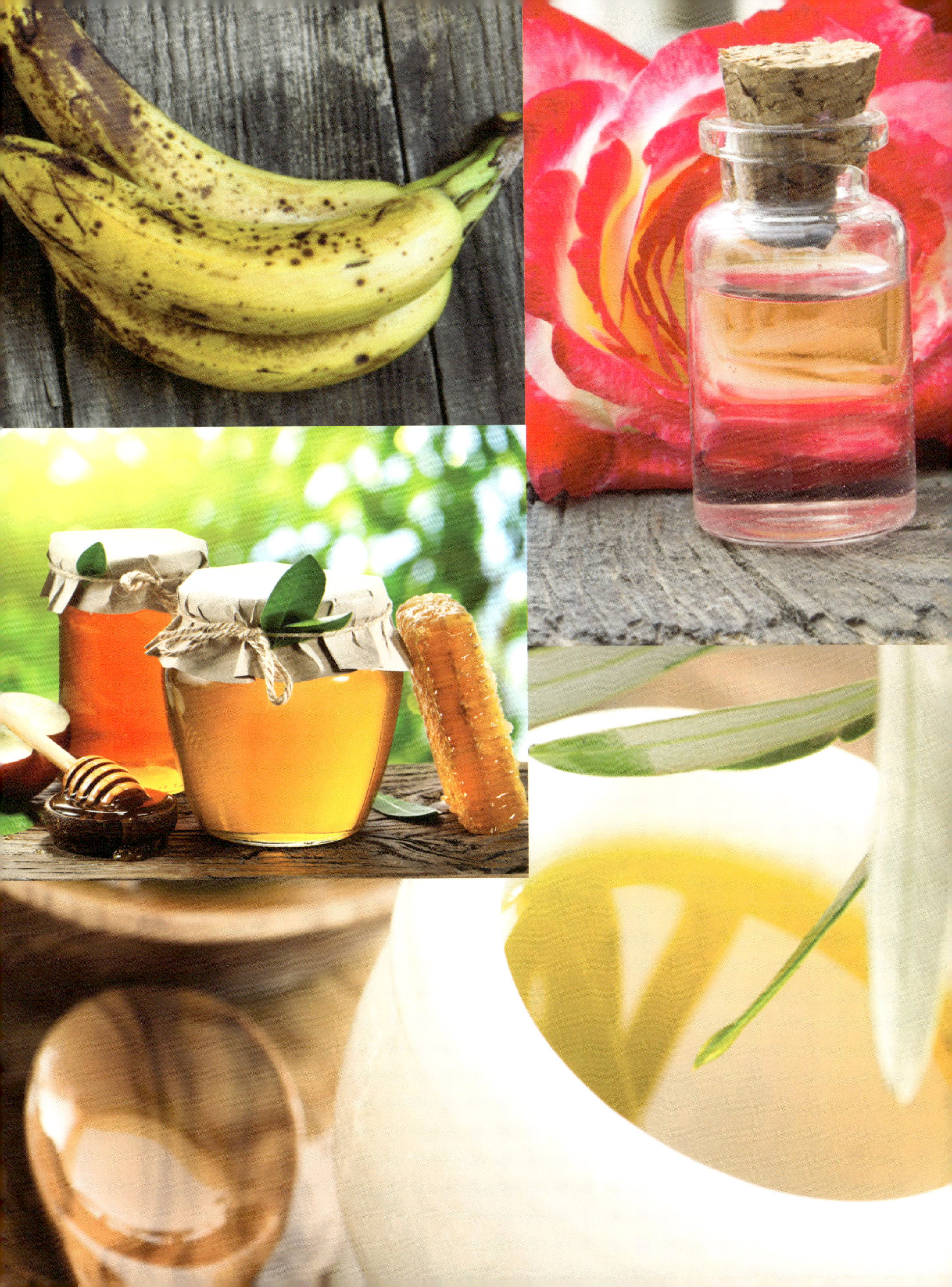

SKIN TAGS

As I like to say, as we get wiser we have challenges with skin tags. Skin tags are very common small, soft skin growths. They are harmless but can be annoying. They tend to occur on eyelids, neck, armpits, groin folds, and under breasts.

1 cotton swab (Q-Tip)
1 Teaspoon organic apple cider vinegar (Braggs)

Dip the swab in vinegar and pat on the skin tag making sure it is completely soaked let dry.

Apply 3 times a day .

In a few days you will see the skin tag has disappeared without having to burn or laser it .

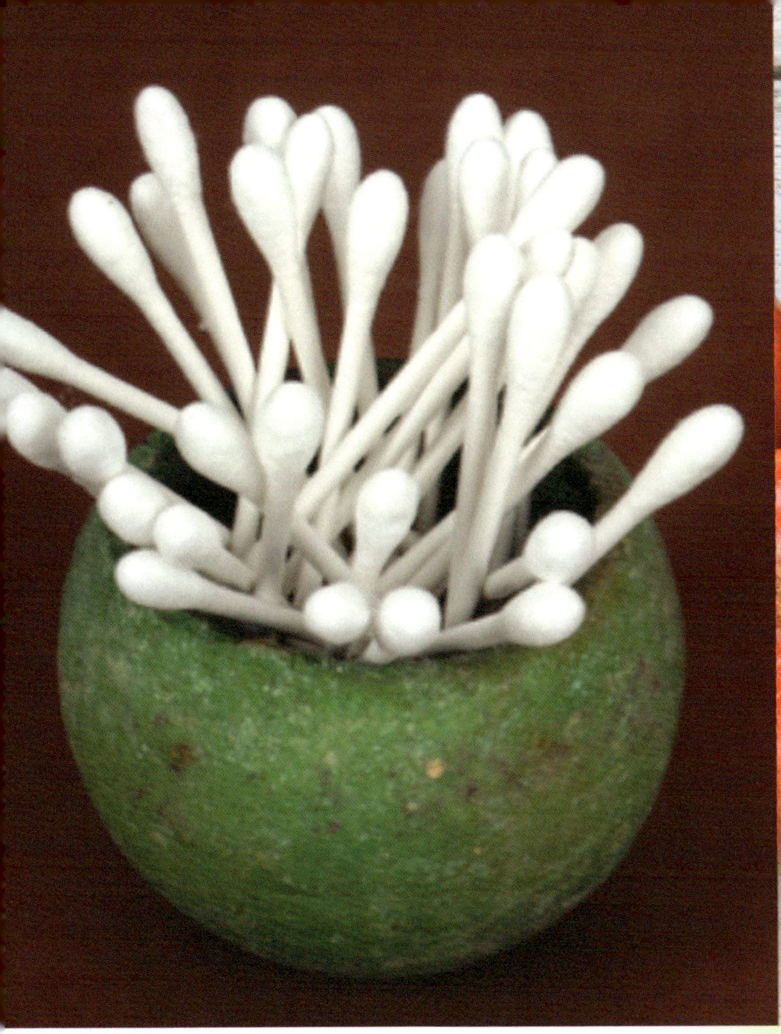
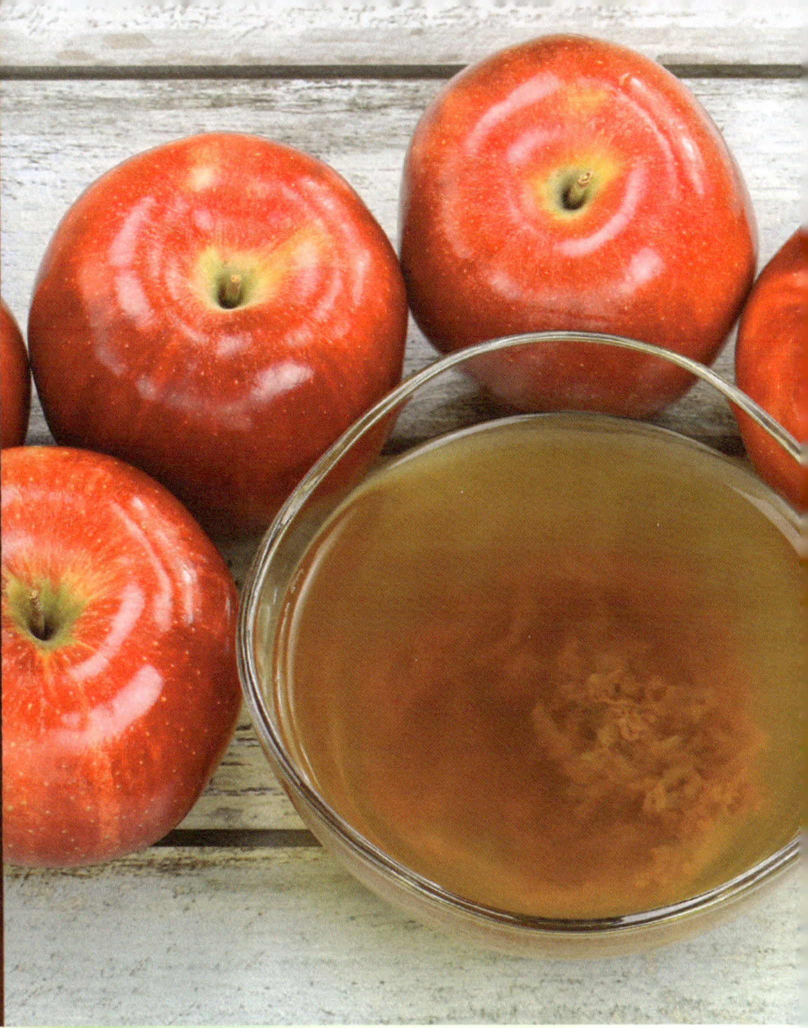
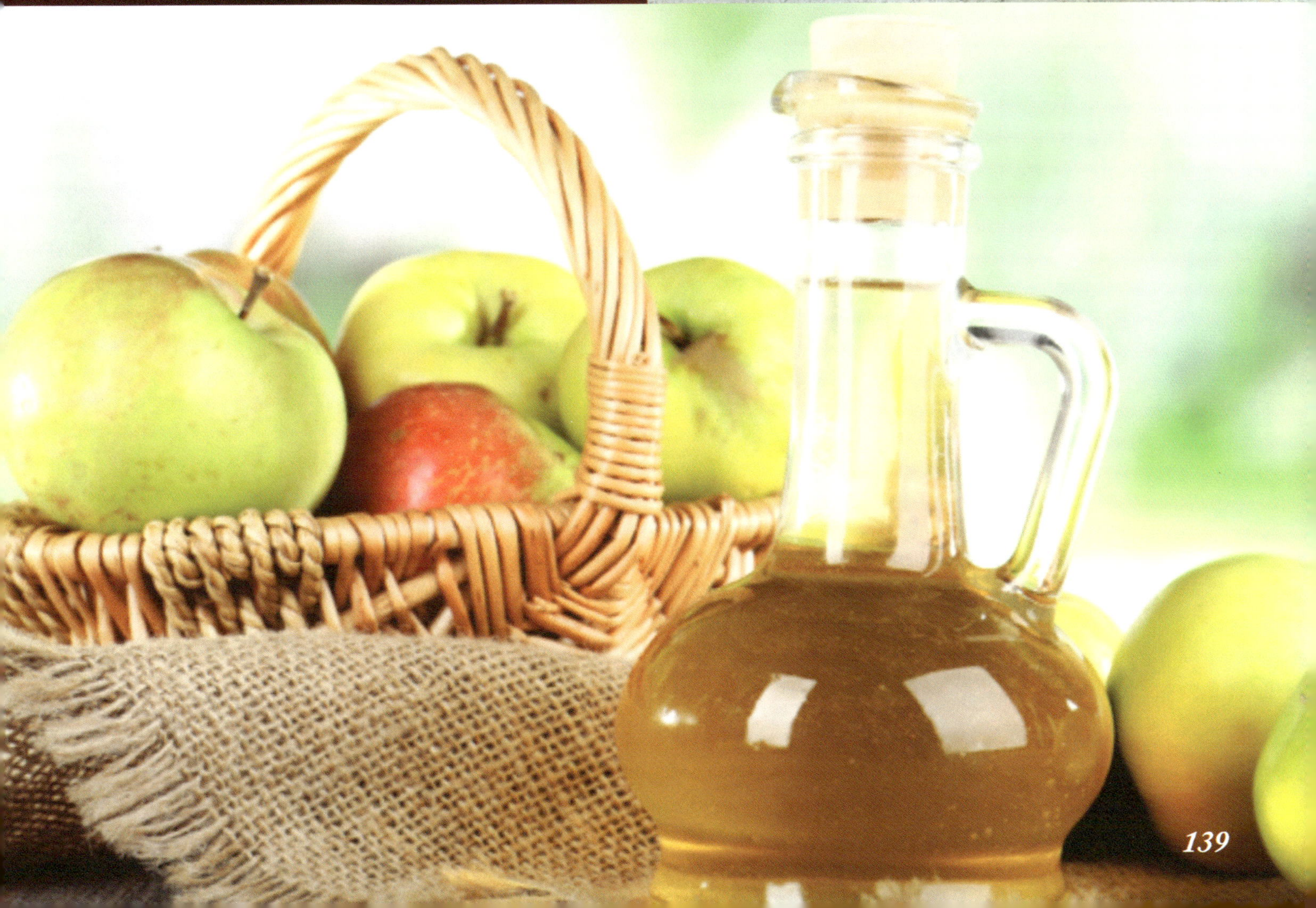

BLACK HEADS

For all recipes be gentle to your skin. Never pinch, scrape, poke, press or squeeze too hard!

Prepare a mixture of equal parts of baking soda and water and rub it onto your face or other body areas prone to blackheads. Leave it on for 15 minutes and then rinse it off with warm water.

TOMATO

Tomatoes have natural antiseptic properties that dry up whiteheads and blackheads. Peel and mash a small tomato. Apply the tomato pulp to your blackheads and whiteheads before going to bed. Leave the tomato pulp on your face while you sleep and then wash your face in warm water in the morning.

LEMON

Wash your face in warm water. Then squeeze the juice of one lemon into a bowl. Add in a pinch of salt and stir the mixture. Apply the mixture to your blackheads and whiteheads. Leave the mixture on for approximately 20 minutes and then wash your face with warm water again.

LIME

You can also use equal parts of lime juice and cinnamon powder and apply this mixture to blackheads. Leave it on overnight and rinse it off in the morning.

CORNSTARCH

Mix about a three-to-one cornstarch to vinegar ratio into a paste. Apply it to your problem areas and let sit for 15 to 30 minutes. Remove the paste with warm water and a washcloth.

YOGURT

Mix three tablespoons of plain yogurt with two tablespoons of oatmeal. Add one teaspoon of olive oil and one tablespoon of lemon juice to the mixture. Stir the mixture thoroughly and apply it to the affected area of the face. Let the mixture sit for five to seven minutes then rinse off with cold water.

ALMOND MEAL OR OATMEAL

Mix either oatmeal or almond meal with just enough rose water to make a spreadable paste. Apply it to your problem areas with your fingertips first and then apply it to the rest of your face. Let it set for about 15 minutes and then rinse your face with cold water.

RICE

Soak raw rice in milk for 5 hours and then grind in a blender until it is paste-like in consistency. Use the paste as a scrub on affected areas of the body, to remove the blackheads.

HONEY

Honey is also good for removing blackheads. Spread honey on the affected area and remove it after 15 minutes.

POTATOES

Grate raw potatoes and then rub the area with the mixture. Wash it off after 15 minutes.

FENUGREEK LEAVES

Crush some dried fenugreek leaves and mix with water to form a paste. Put this on the face for 15 minutes and then remove it. Do this every night to keep your face free of blackheads.

CORIANDER (CILANTRO) LEAVES

Mix some coriander leaves and a little turmeric powder with water and form a paste. Use this as a mask to eliminate blackheads.

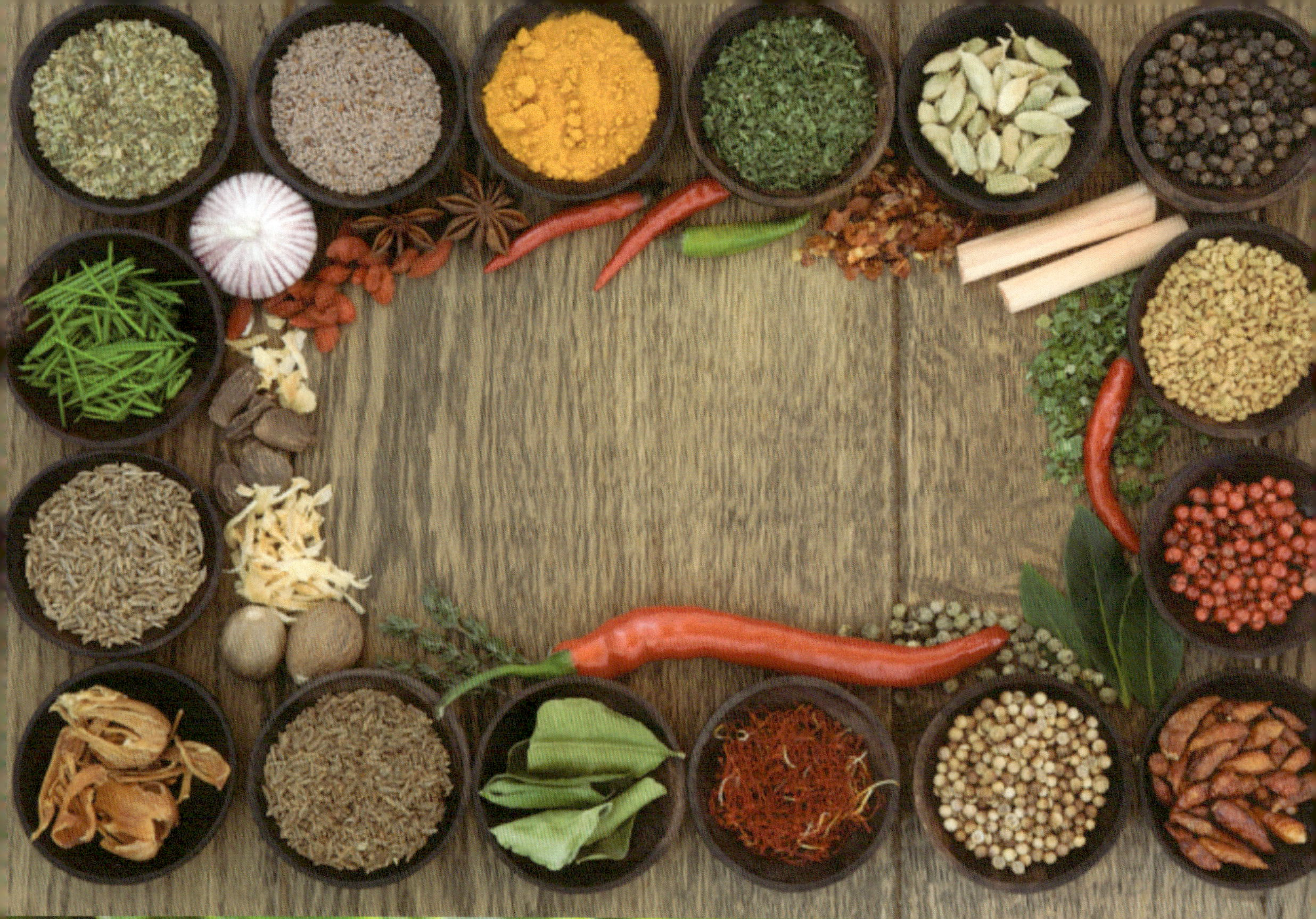

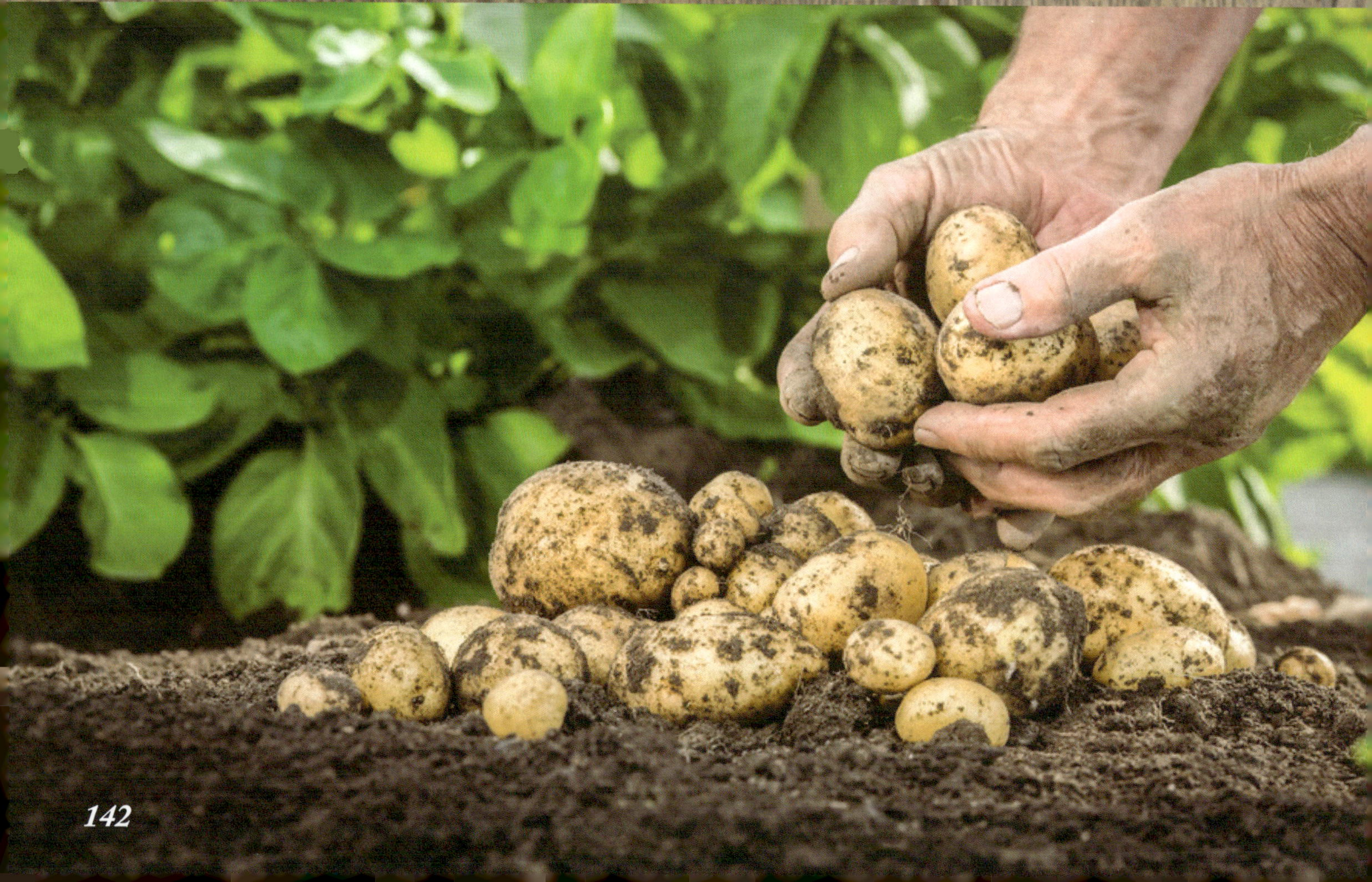

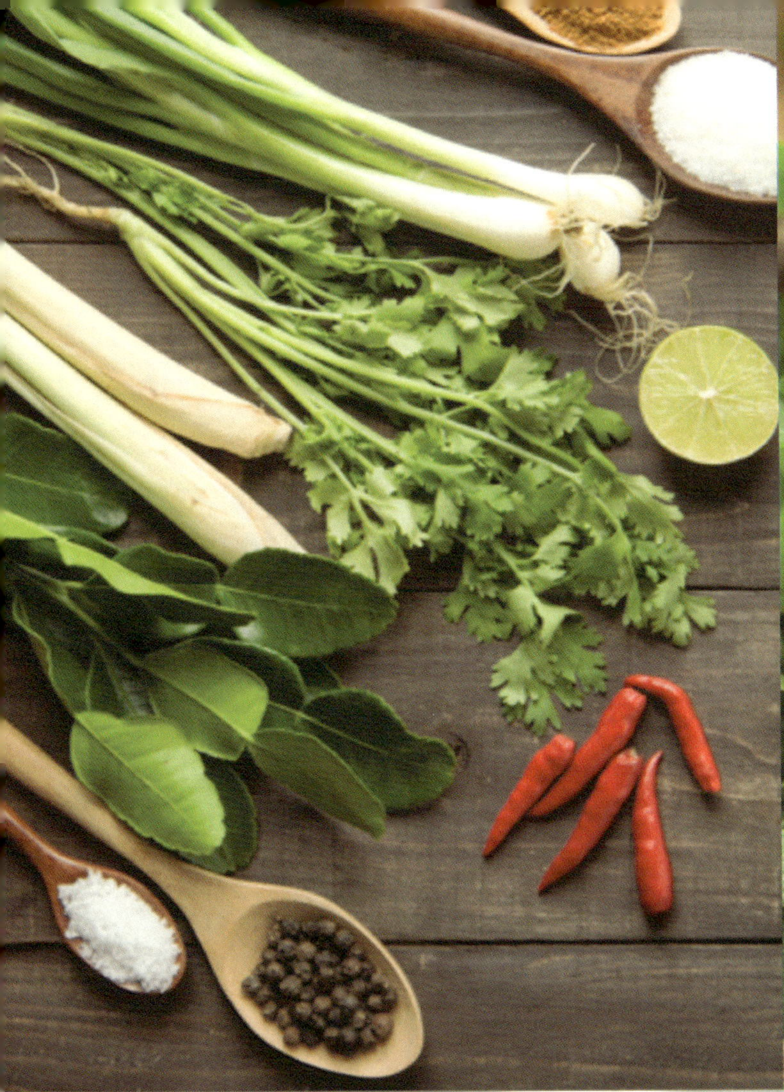

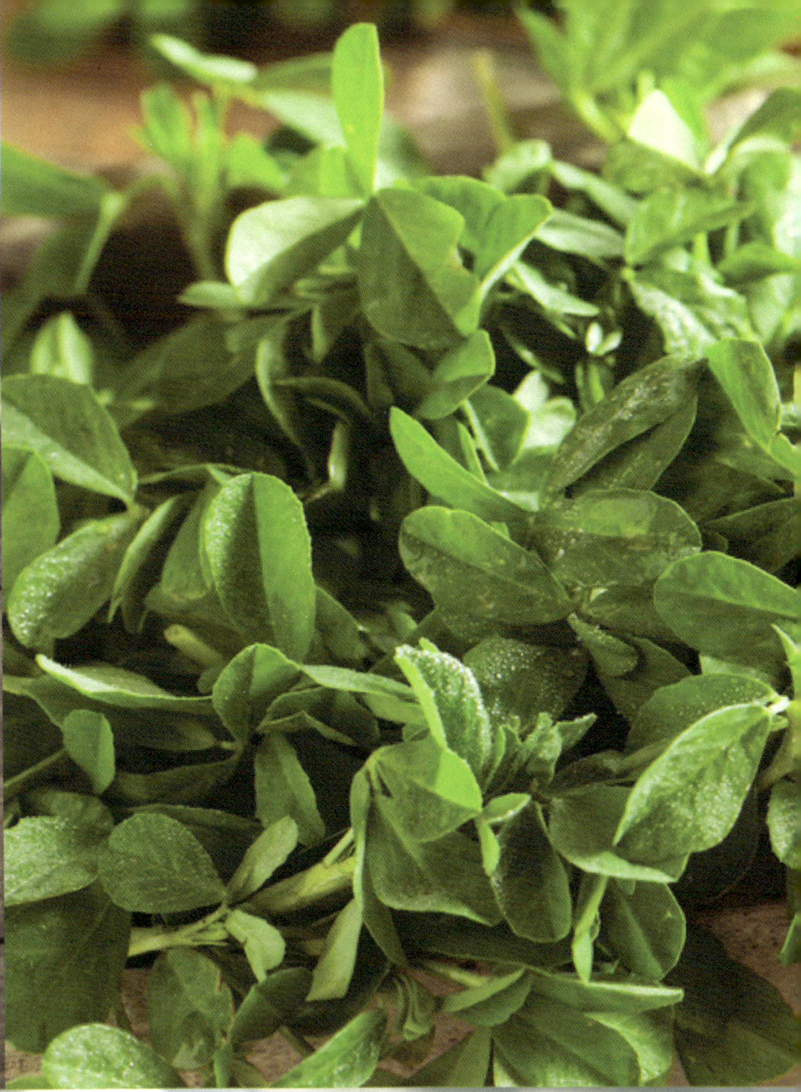

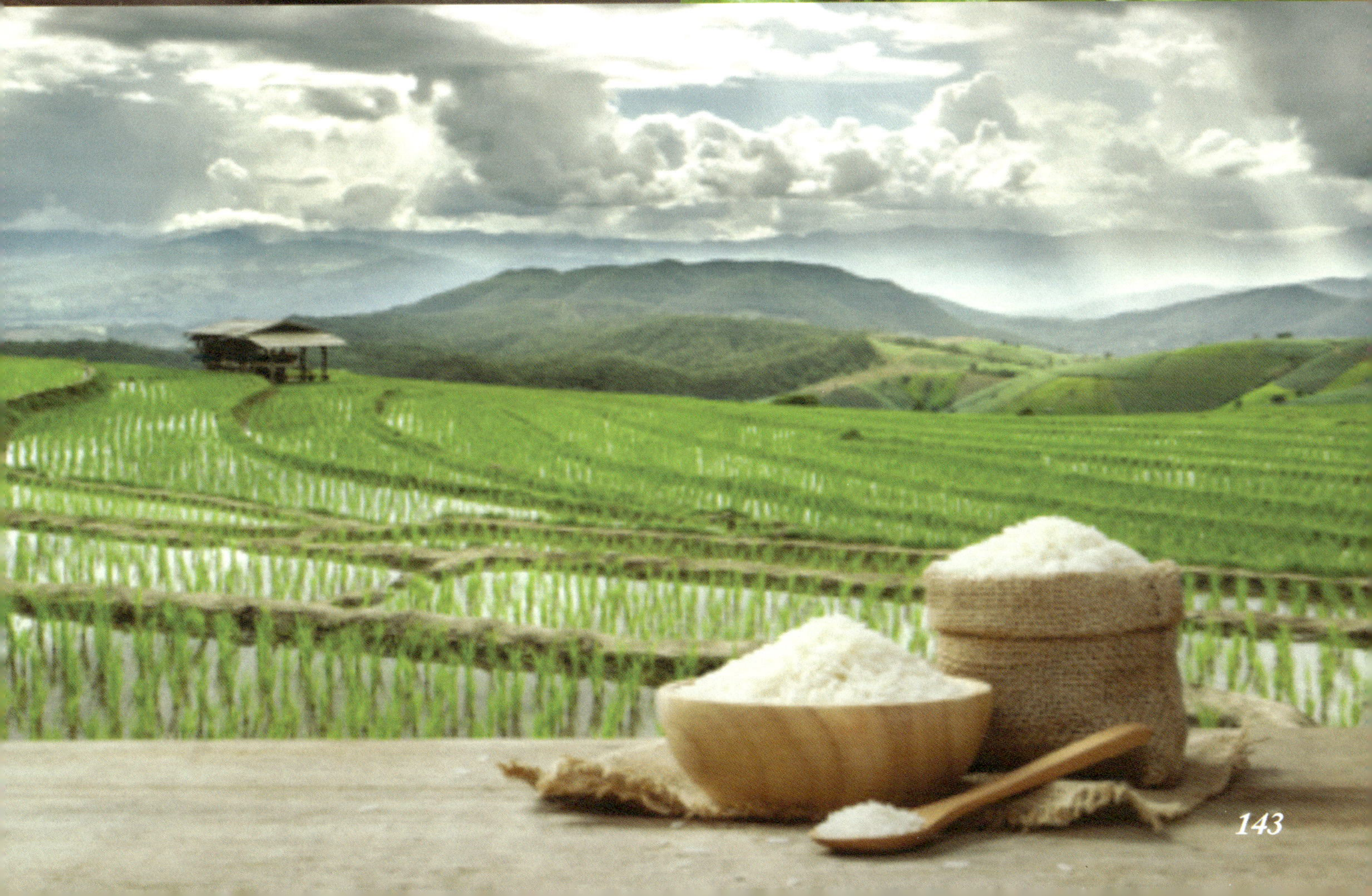

FACELIFT MASK

Amazing for sagging neck

1 Organic egg white
1 Teaspoon organic coconut sugar
1 natural face brush
1 teaspoon organic raw coconut butter

Mix egg white, coconut sugar and coconut oil and beat firmly until well mixed. Brush it evenly on your face, eyes neck, décolleté and around eyes (making sure not to get it in your eyes). Leave for 25 minutes then wash with cool water. This is a great refresher before you apply your makeup for a black tie event. Your skin will be calm, firm and luminous, and your makeup will glide on beautifully.

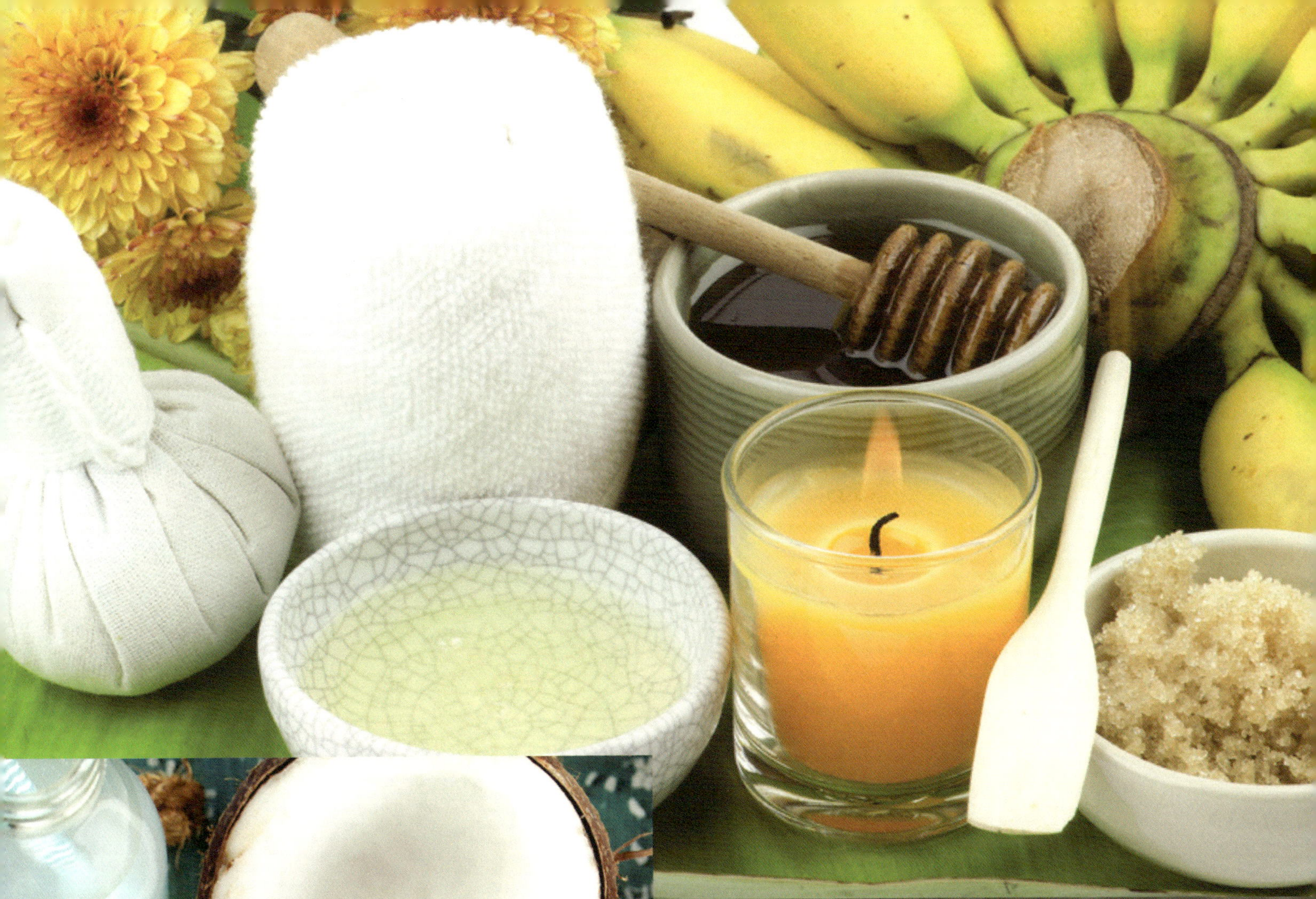

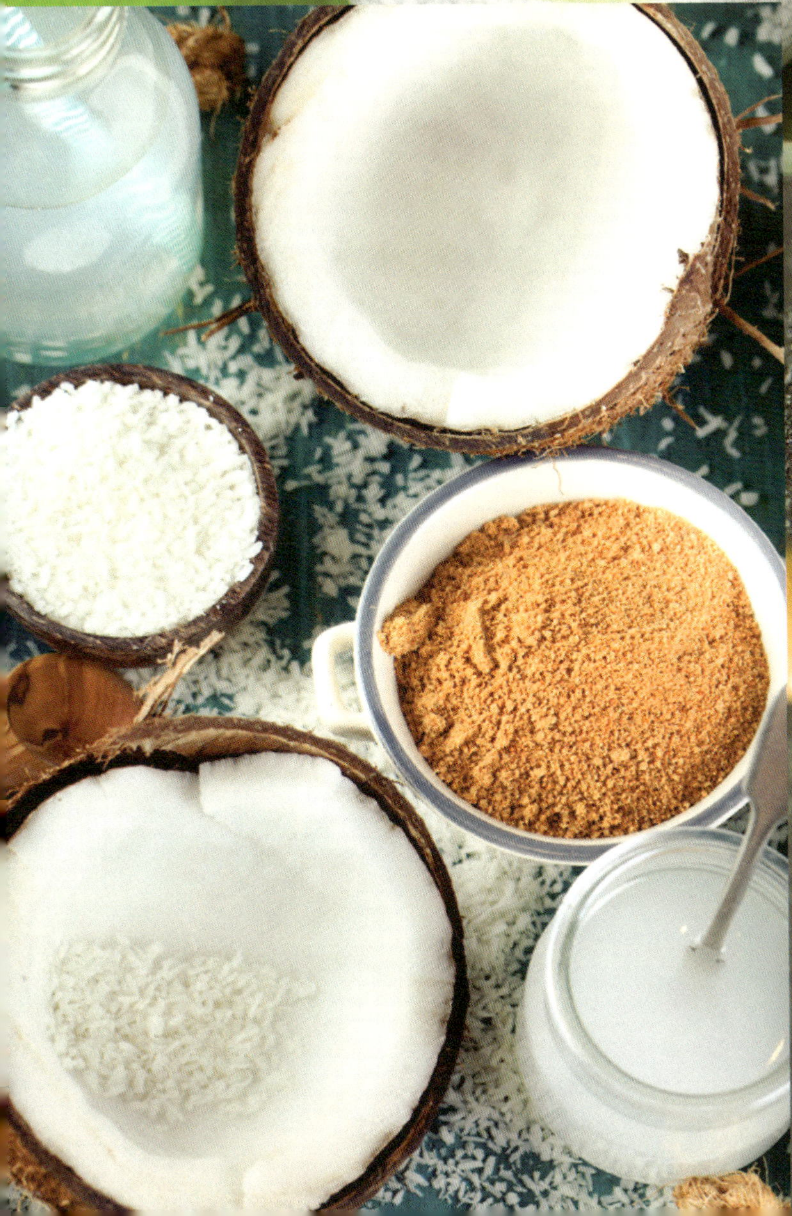

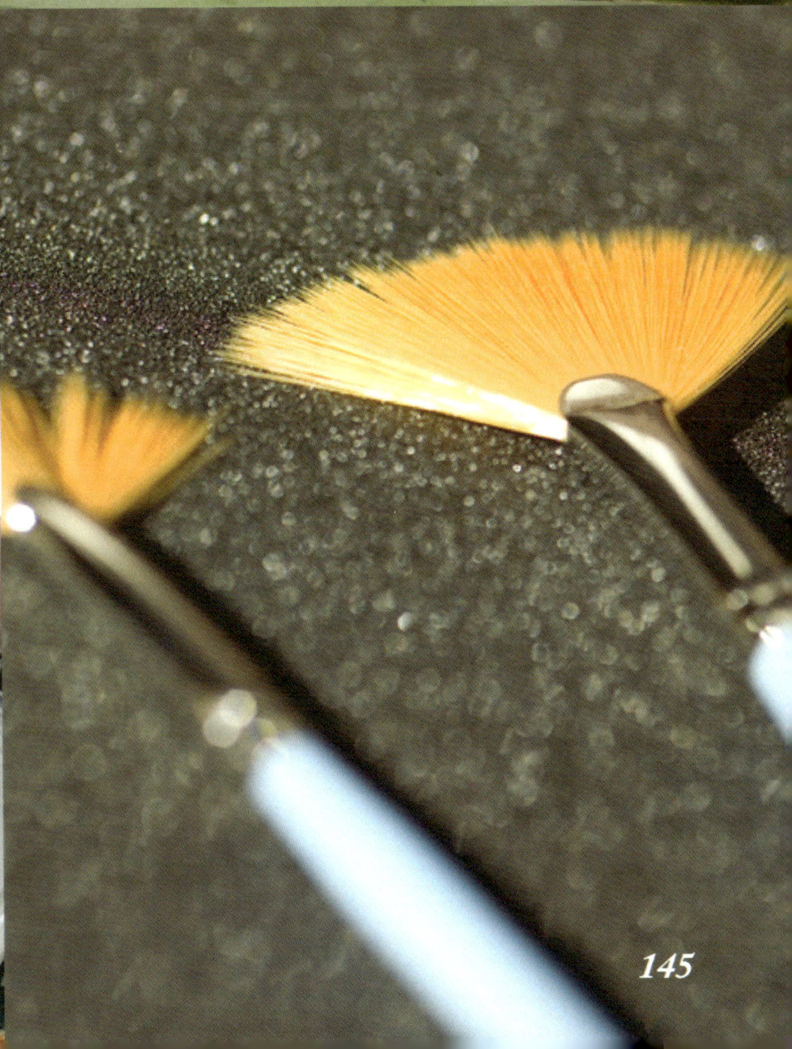

LUMINOUS SKIN

For bright tight luminous skin

1 Organic tomato
1 Tablespoon organic virgin coconut oil
3 Drops juniper oil (essential oil)

Mix in your blender and place in your freezer for 5 minutes. Brush it evenly on your face, neck, décolleté and around eyes (making sure not to get it in your eyes). Leave for 25 minutes then rinse with cool water.

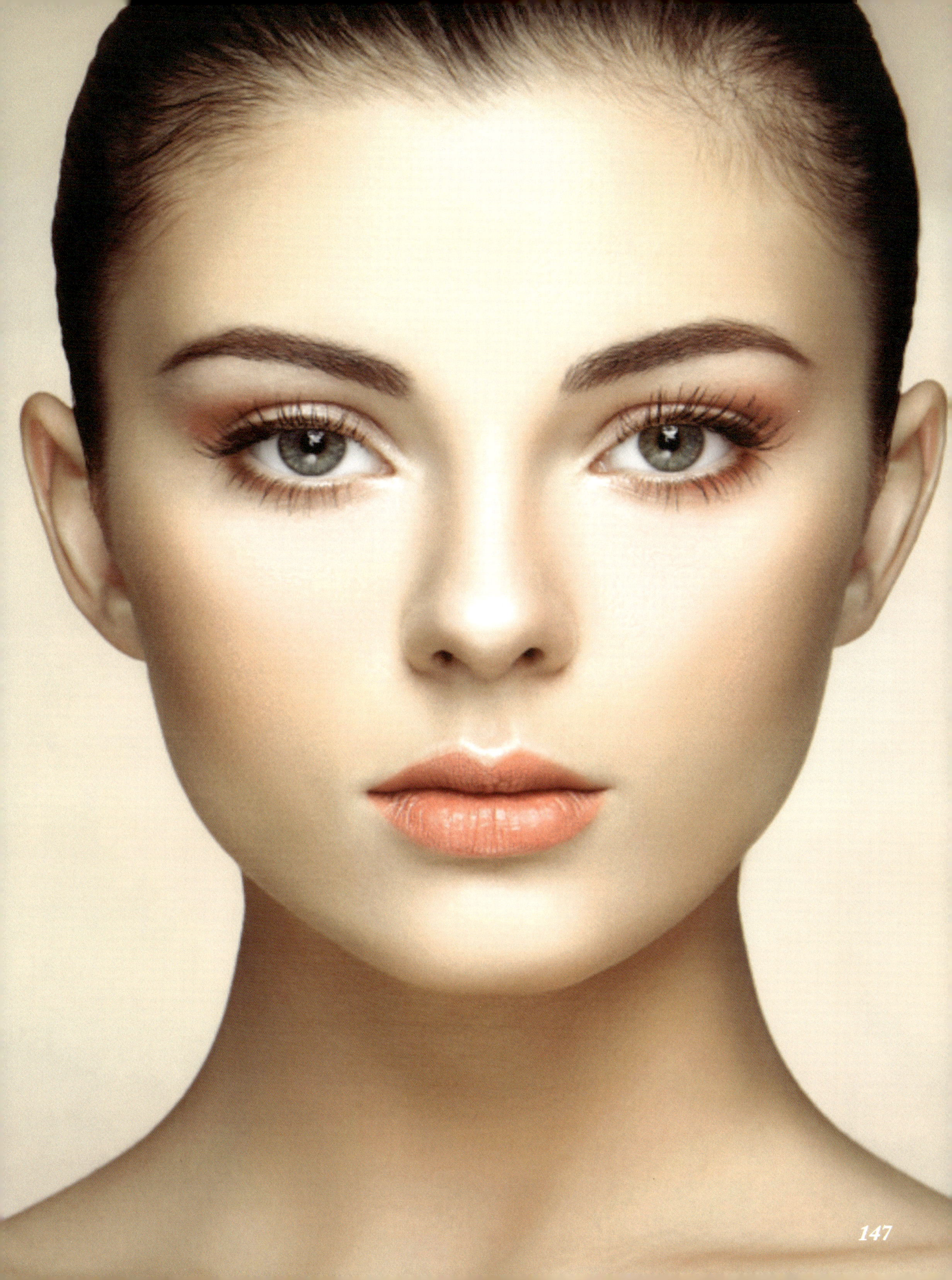

STINGING NETTLE MASK

Organic facelift and natural filler

1/4 Cup stinging nettles
1 Cup warm water
2 Tablespoons full-fat yogurt
1 Tablespoon raw honey

Let stinging nettles sit in cup of warm water for 20 minutes then mix in the yogurt and honey and apply to the face evenly. Lay down relax for 25 minutes. Wipe off with moist warm cloth, rinse with cold water, pat dry and apply your moisturizer.

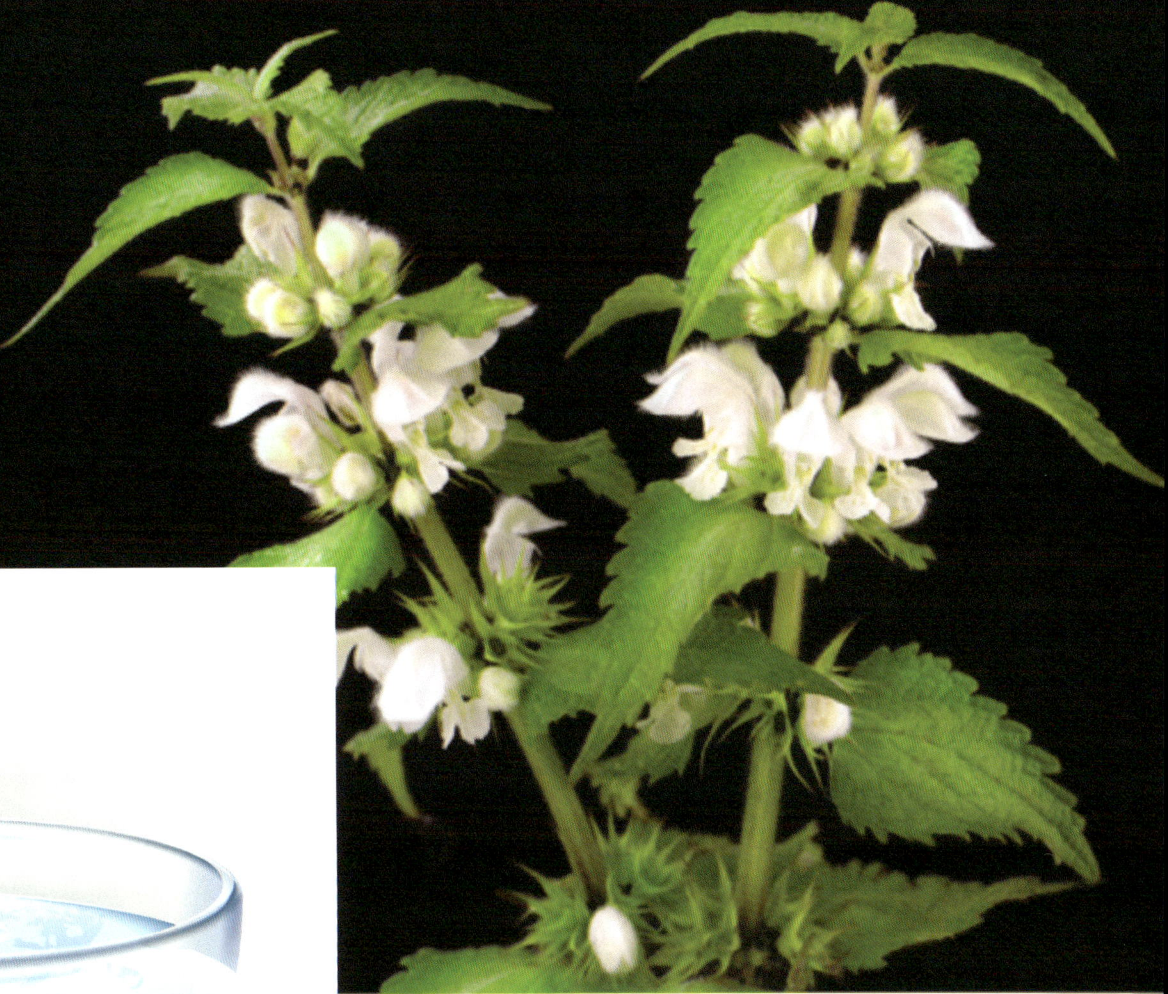

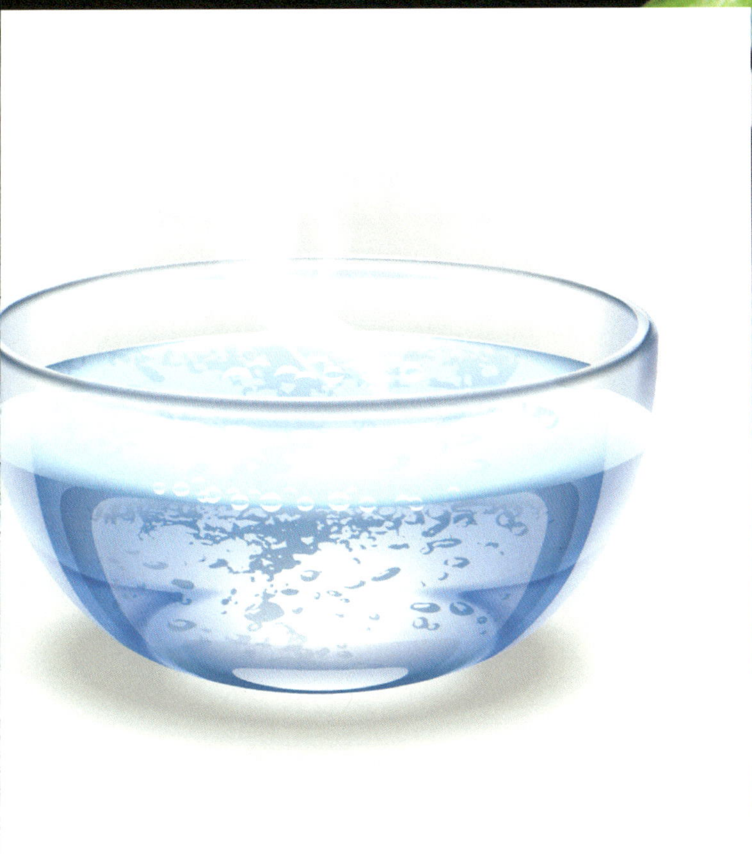

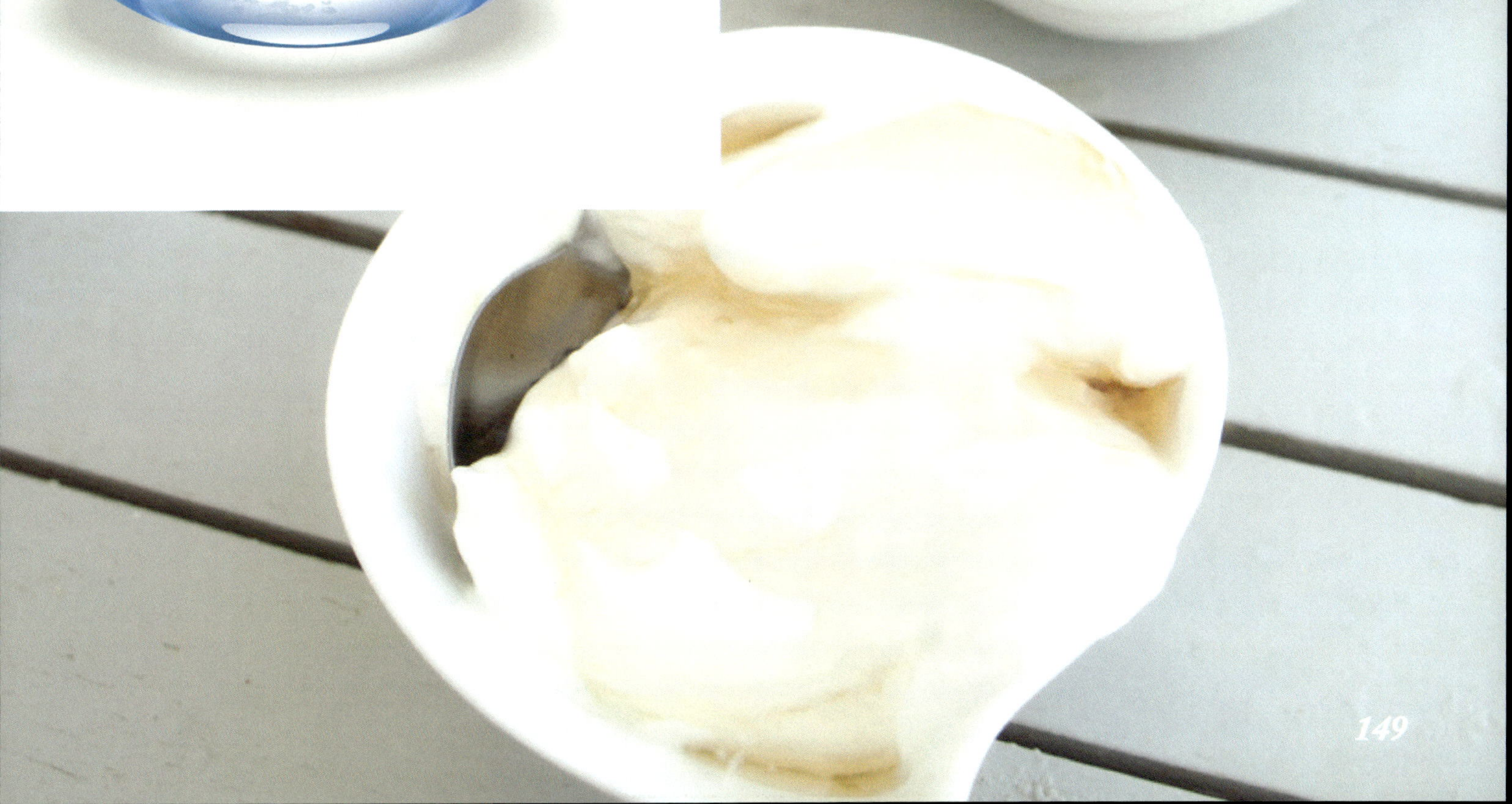

TONERS

ROSEWATER TONER

Rosewater has anti-inflammatory properties that can help reduce the redness of irritated skin and reduce acne, dermatitis and eczema. It is a great cleanser and aids in removing oil and dirt accumulated in clogged pores, Ideal for acne.

5 Cups rose petals (free of chemicals and pesticides)
Distilled Water
Enamel or stainless steel pot (any size)
Food-safe plate approximately 1-inch smaller in diameter than your cooking pot

Pick roses in the morning, after the morning dew has evaporated, and gently wash to remove any bugs or dirt. Fill the bottom of the pot with rose petals a few inches deep. Place the plate on top to weigh them down and pour distilled water over the petals until they are just covered. Heat the water over medium heat to be steaming hot, but do not boil. Let the water steam until the water has taken on the color of the rose petals, has become a bit thick and oily, and you see rose oil forming on the surface. This will take approximately 60 minutes. Strain the water into a glass bowl and squeeze as much liquid as you can from the petals. Place in a glass jar immediately or store in the refrigerator. You can use once cool. Use like any toner, after cleansing your skin morning and the evening.

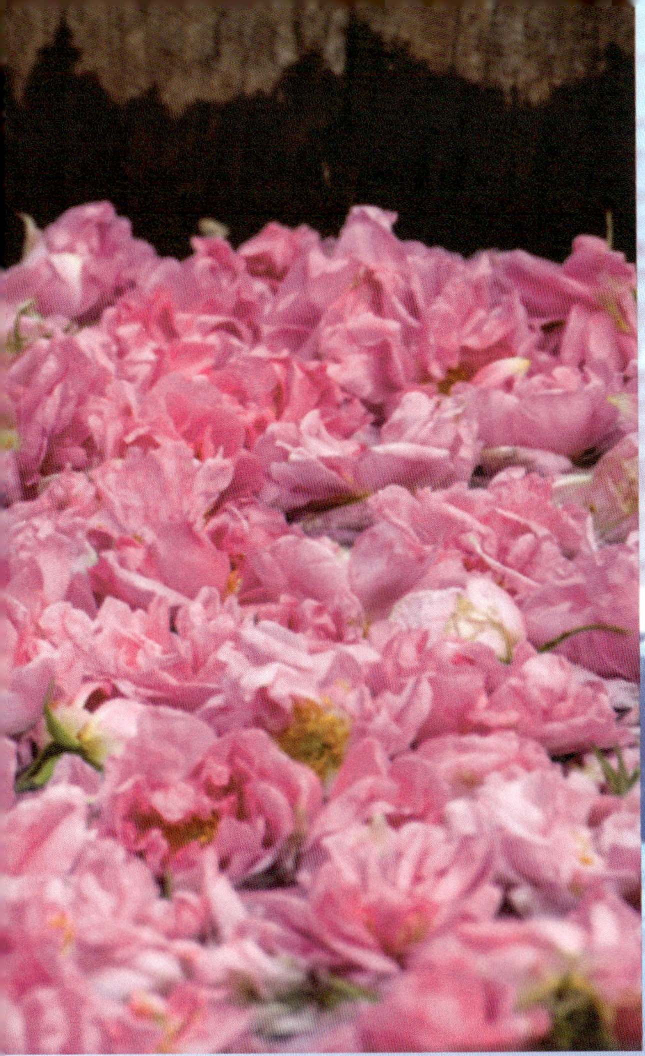
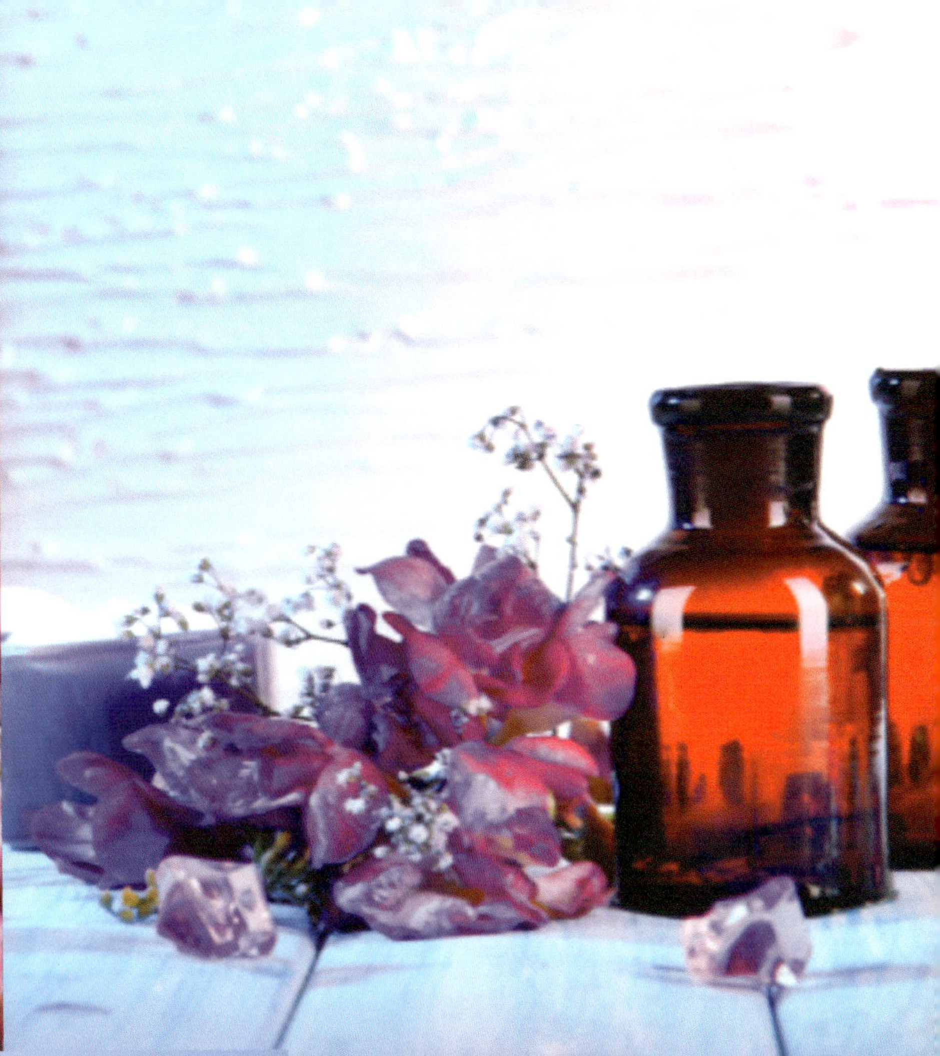
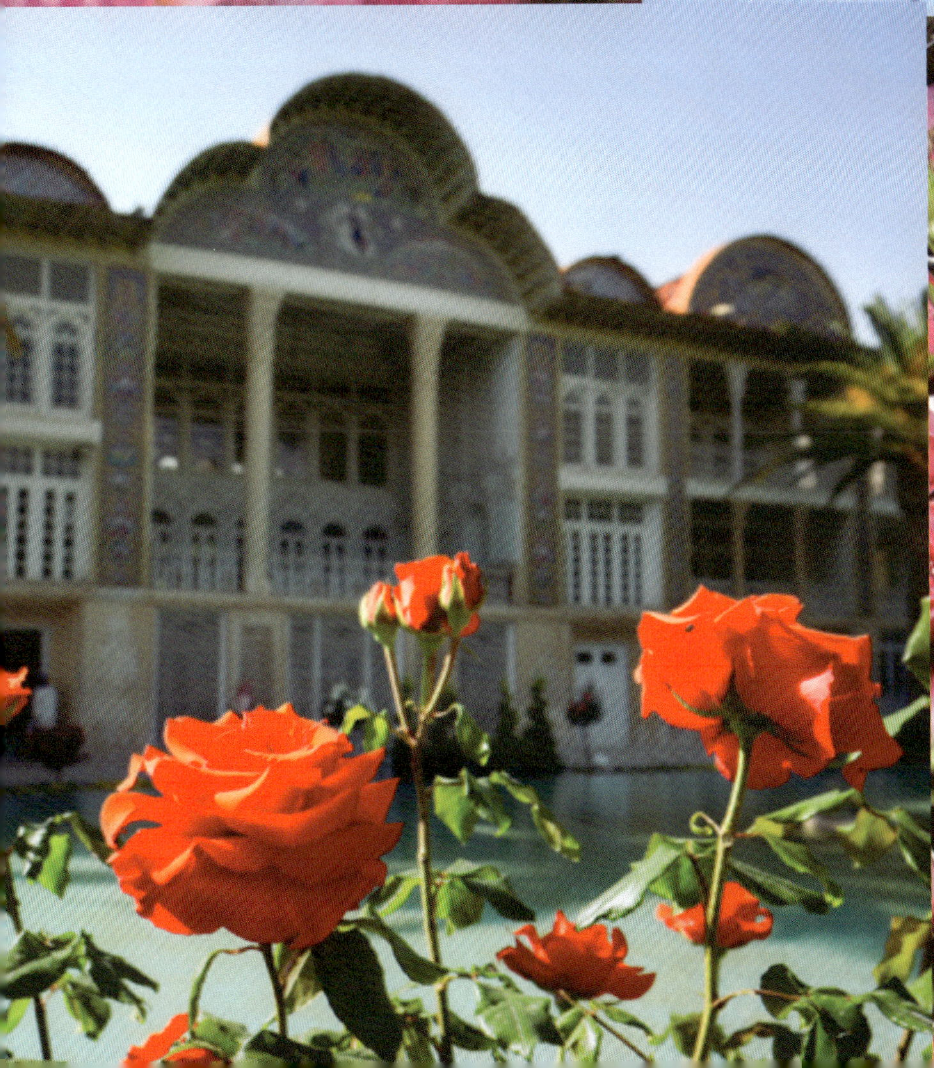
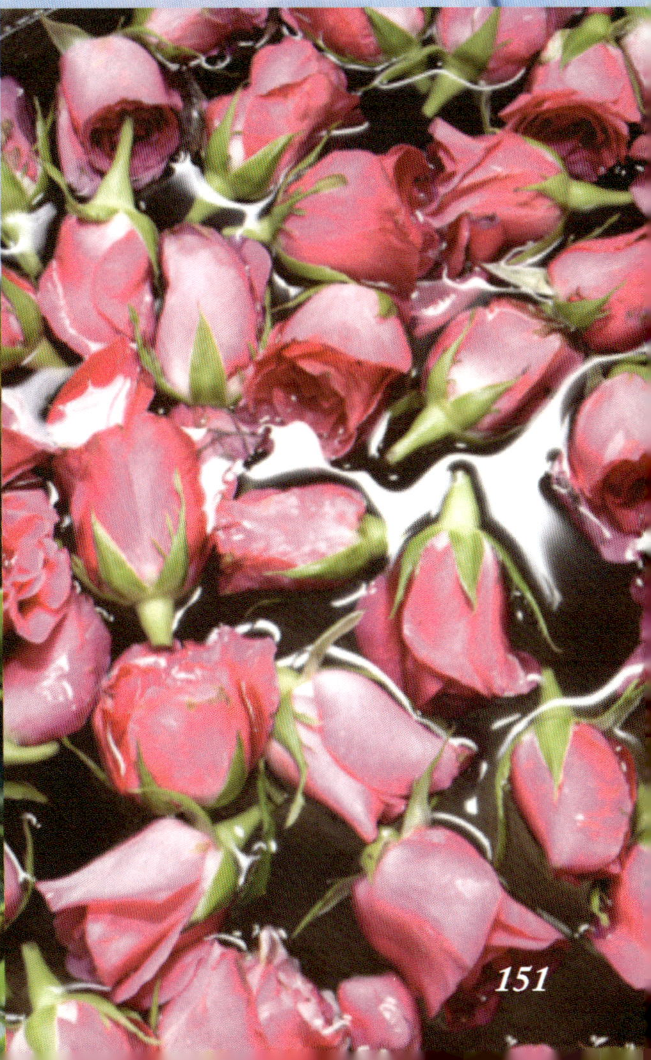

APPLE TONER

For acne and greasy skin

1 Tablespoon organic apple cider vinegar (Braggs)
3 Drops chamomile oil
Distilled or acid water

Mix the ingredients and pour into blue or amber glass jar and use as is.

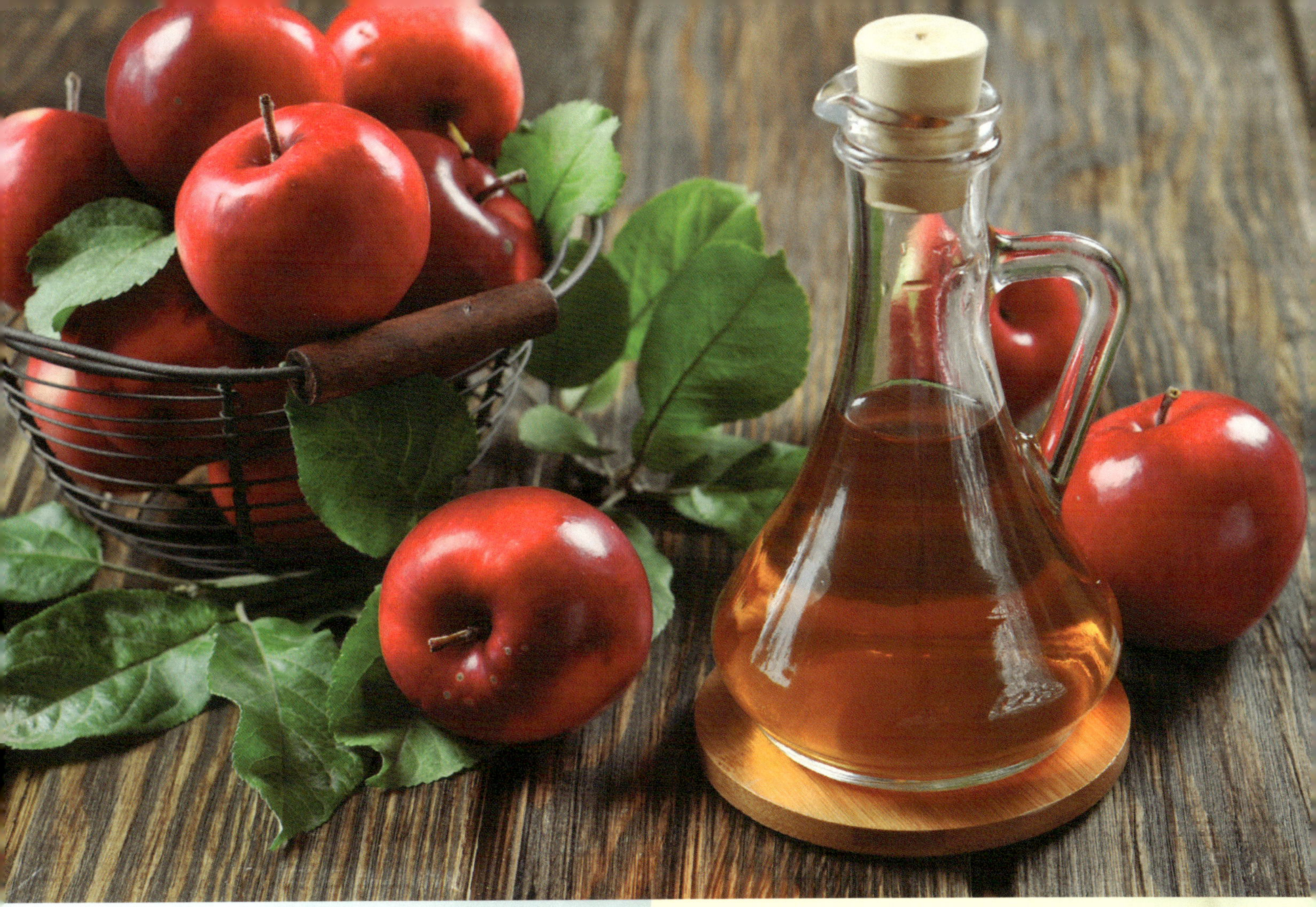

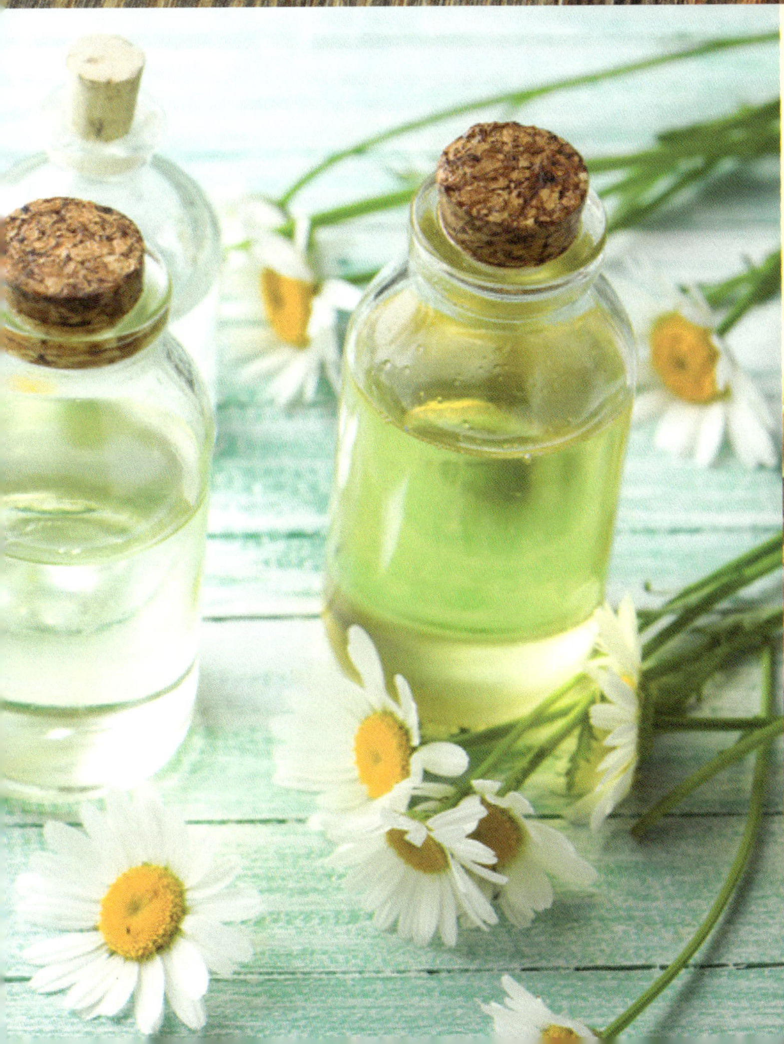

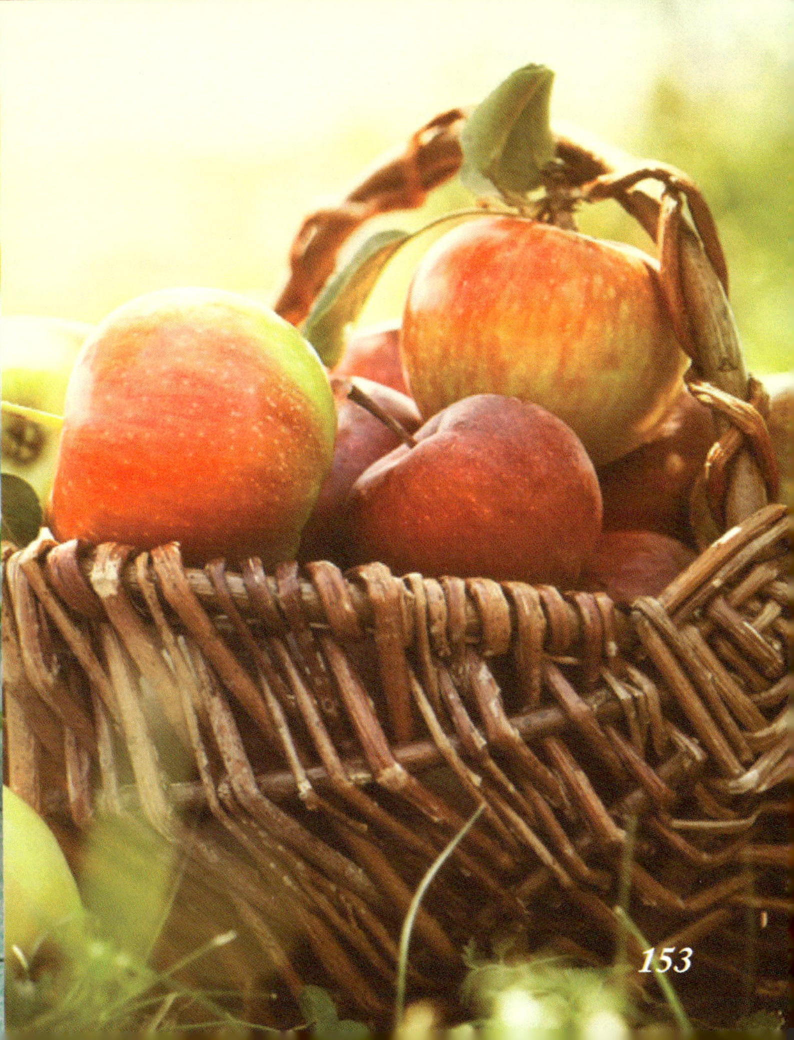

CUCUMBER TONER

For normal skin

2 Medium organic cucumbers
1/2 Tablespoon apple cider vinegar (Braggs)
3 Drops juniper essential oil

Mix the ingredients and pour into blue or amber glass jar. Shake before use.

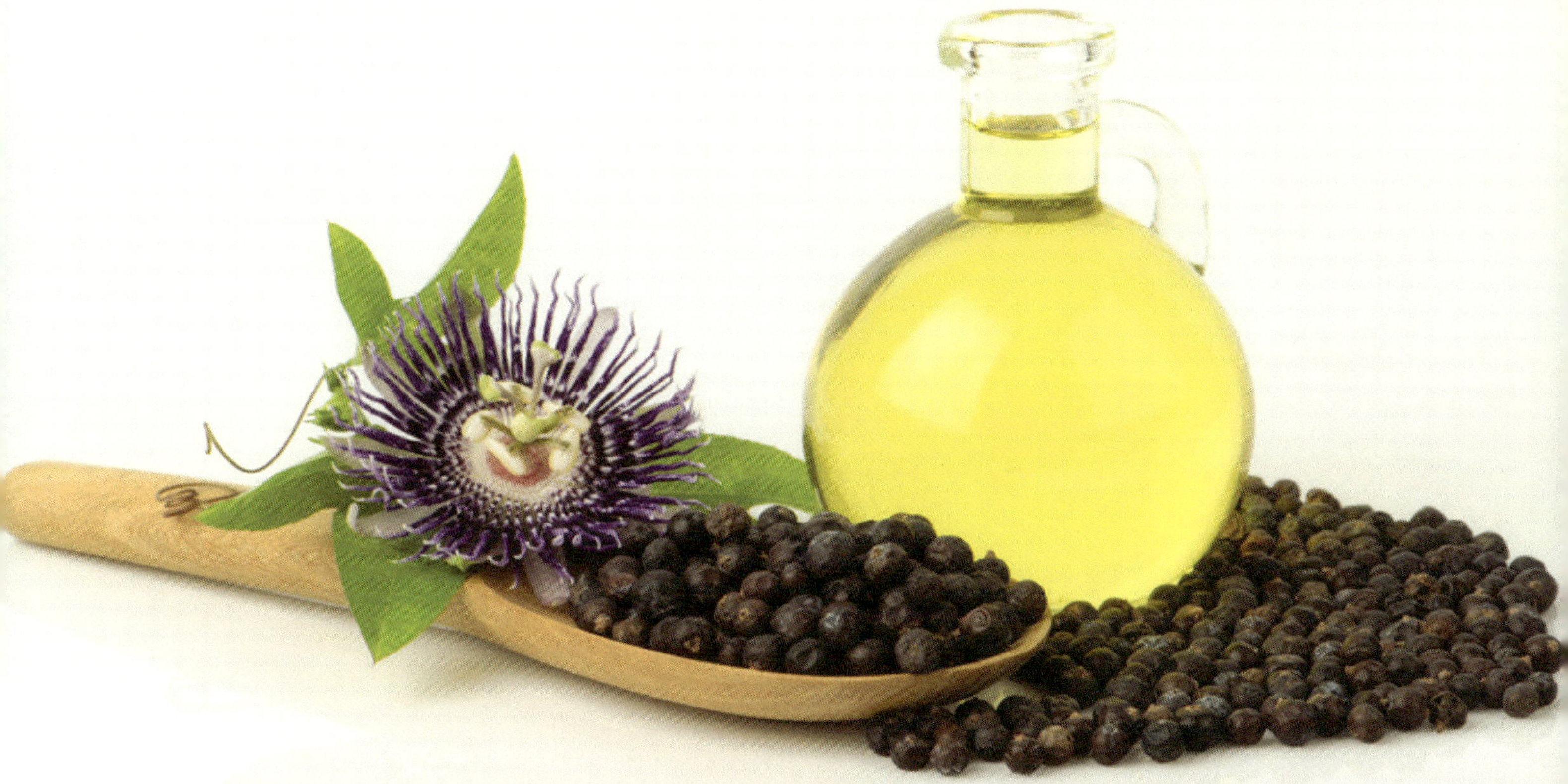

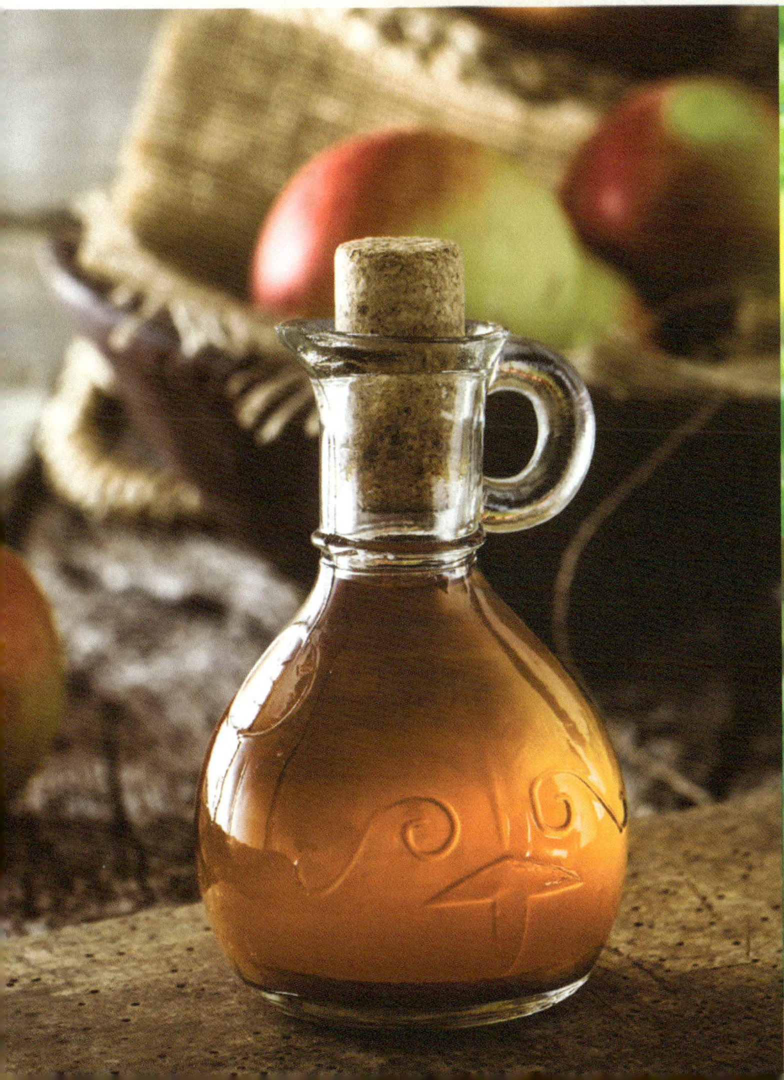

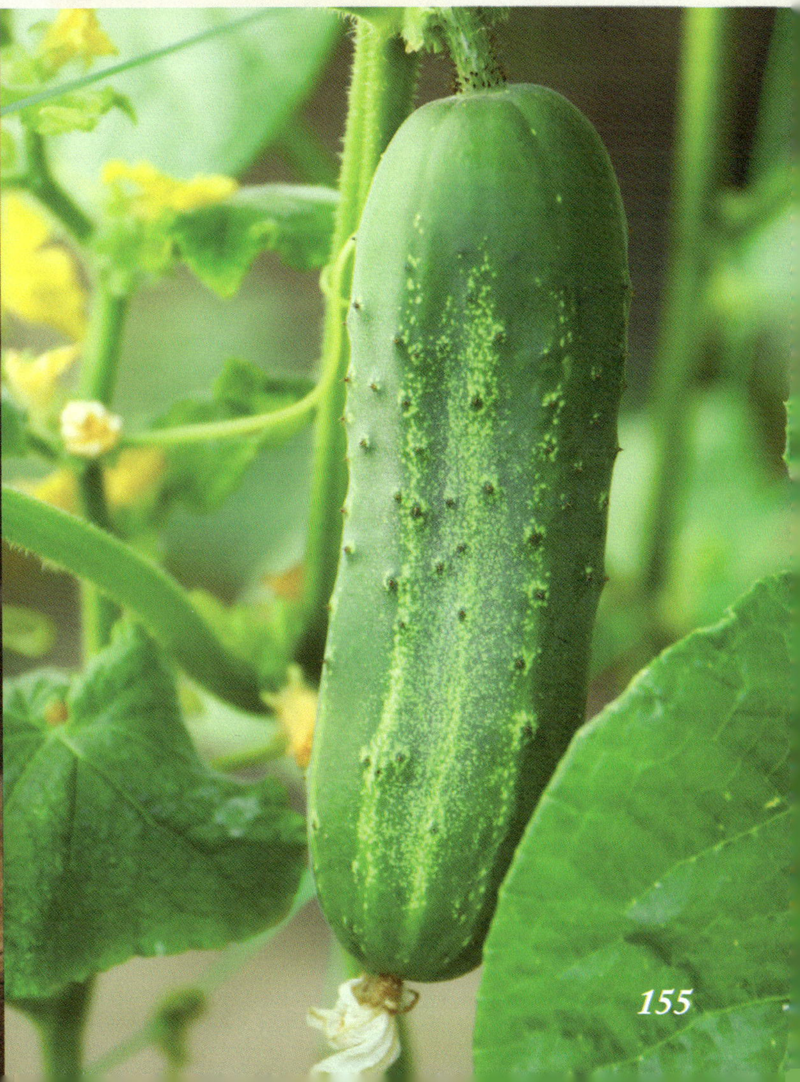

WATERMELON TONER

For all skin types

2 Tablespoons fresh watermelon juice
2 Tablespoons distilled water
1 Tablespoon vodka
2 Teaspoons organic rosewater (can be purchased at your local health food store)

Watermelon is food for your skin because it has significant levels of vitamins A, B6 and C, lycopene, antioxidants and amino acids. There's even a modest amount of potassium.

Extract the watermelon juice by placing it in your blender. Strain. If you want it absolutely pulp-free, strain it again through a fine cheesecloth. Stir the watermelon juice into the water and add vodka. Pour into a small glass bottle and store in a cool place, preferably the refrigerator.

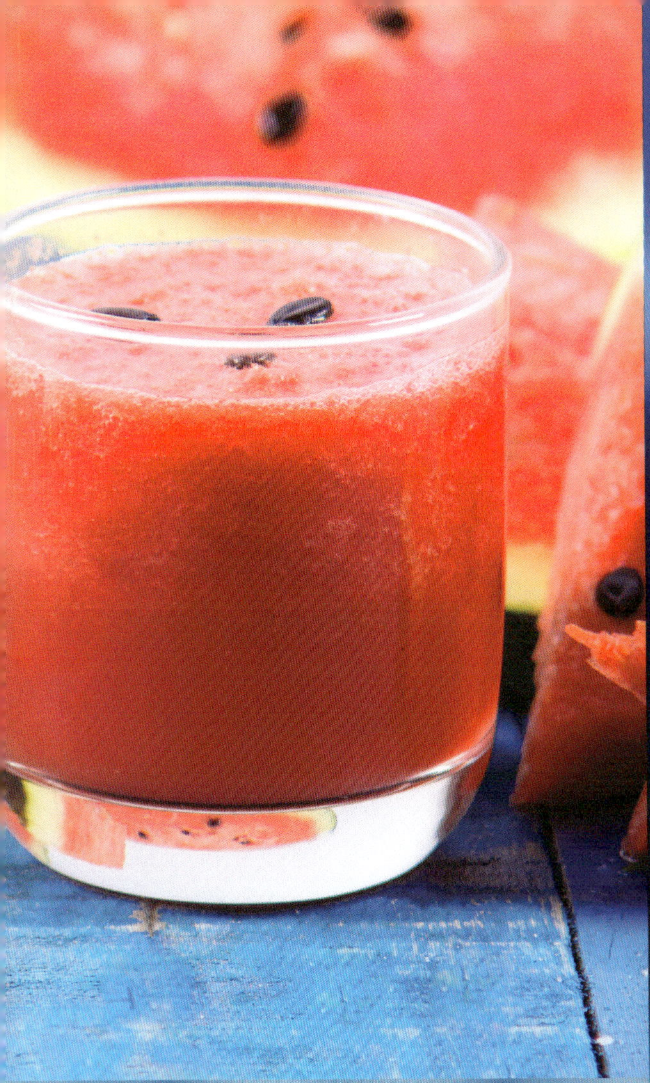
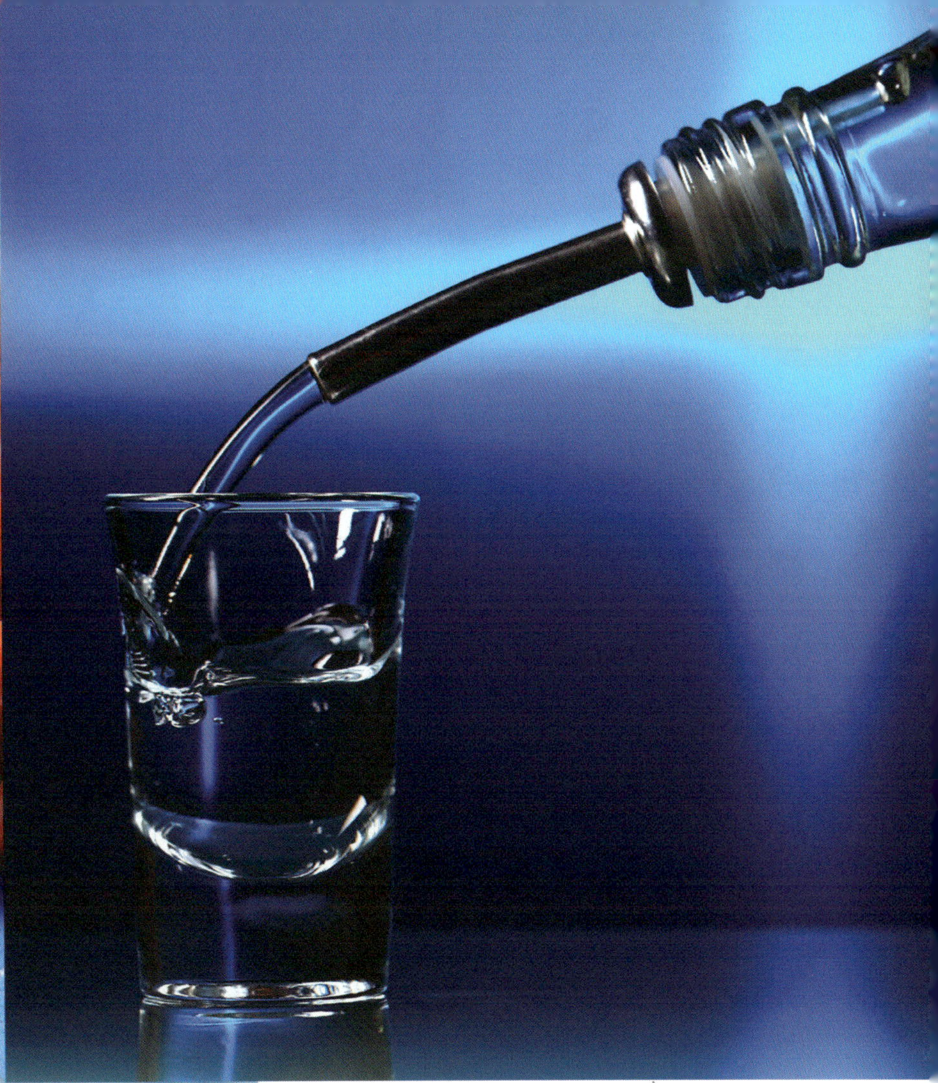
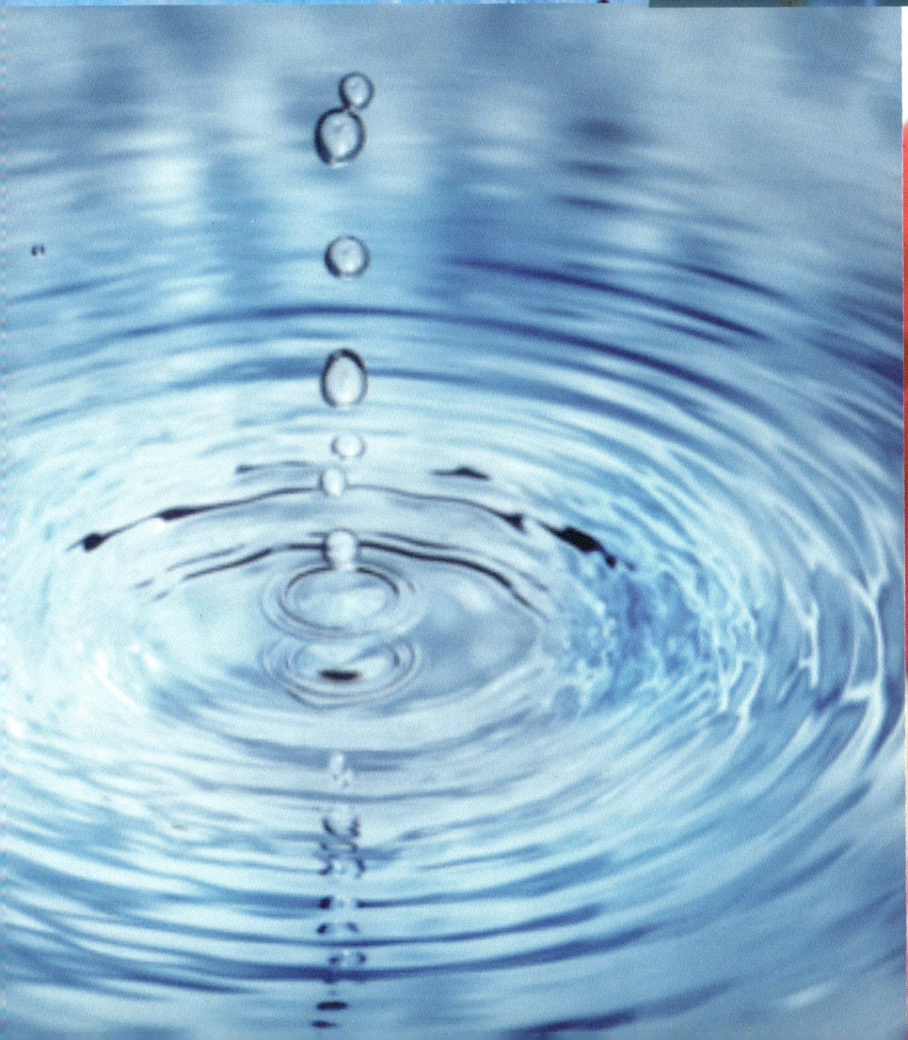
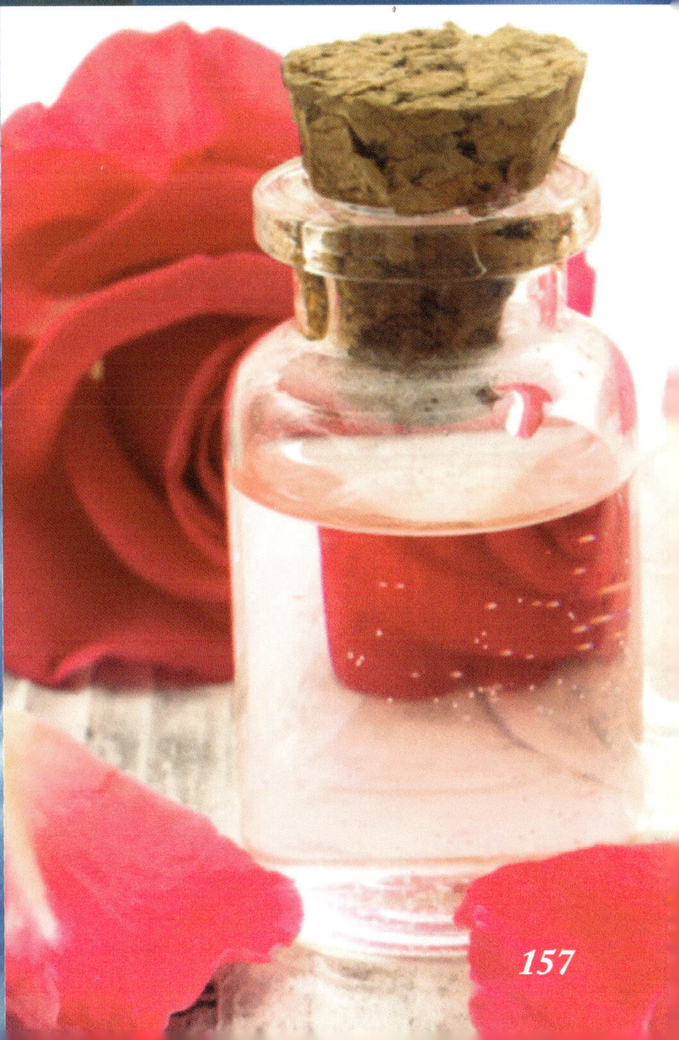

TOMATO TONER

For older pigmented skin

1 Organic tomato
2 Tablespoons distilled or acid water
2 Tablespoons white sparkling wine
4 Large organic strawberries

Place all ingredients in your blender. Strain. If you want it absolutely pulp-free, strain it again through a fine cheesecloth. Pour into a dark glass bottle and store in a cool place, preferably the refrigerator.

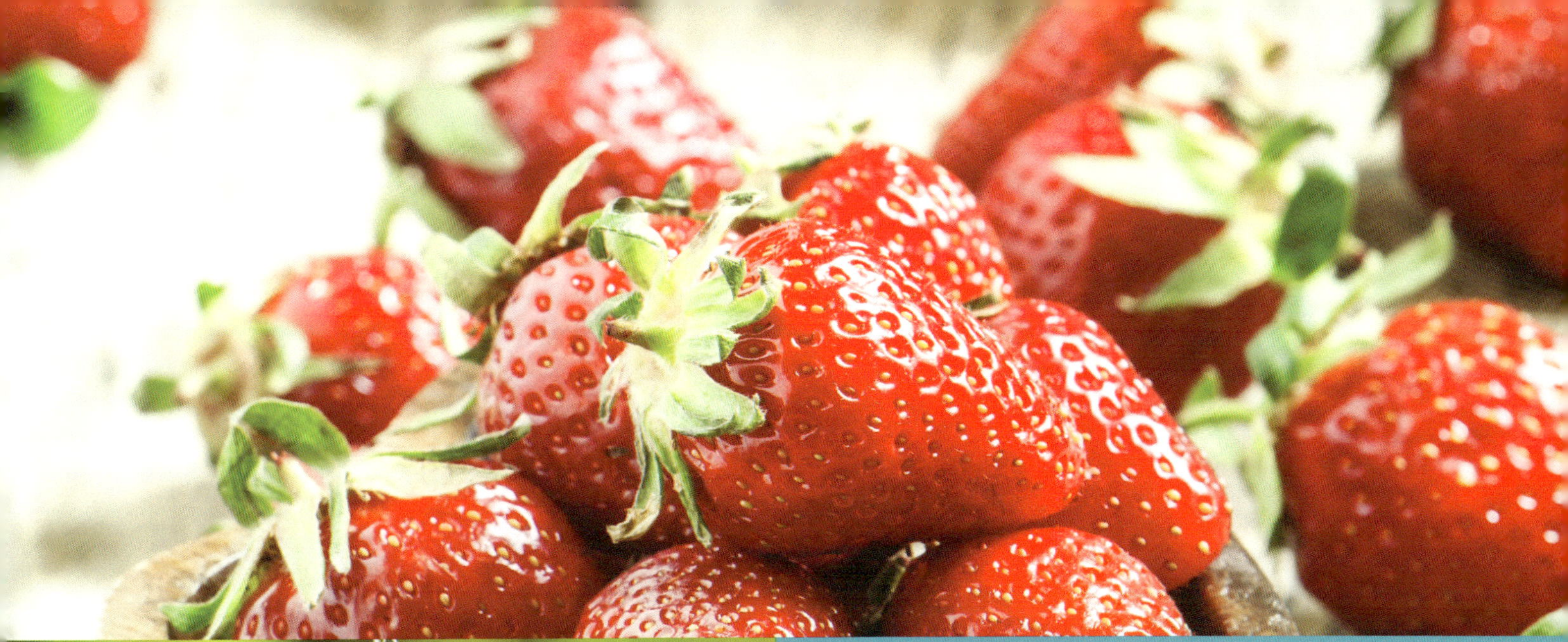

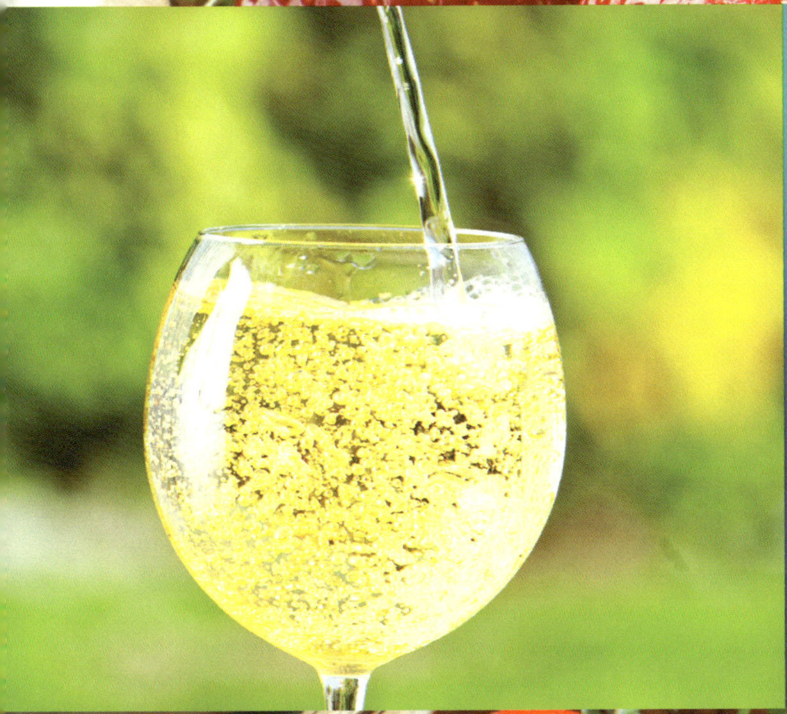

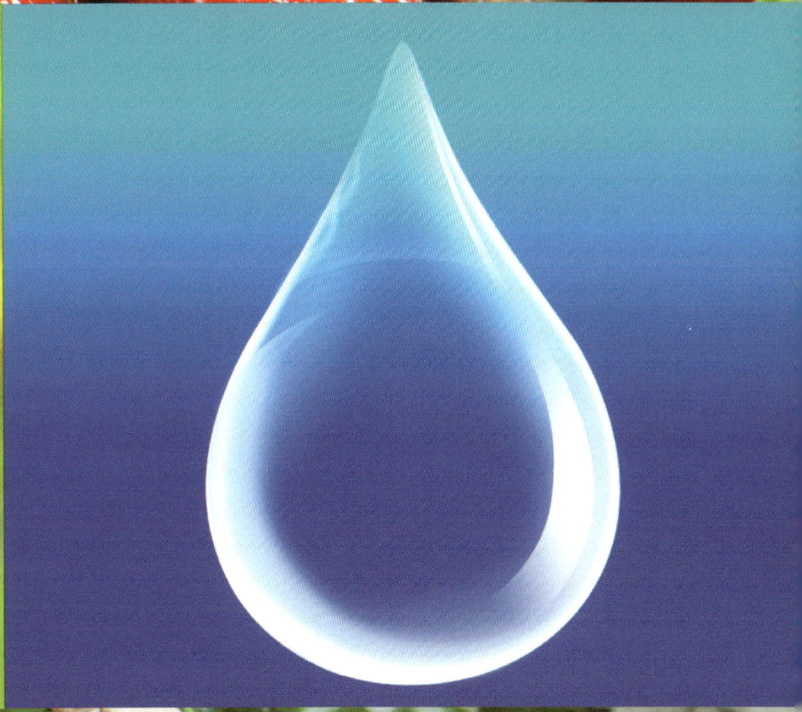

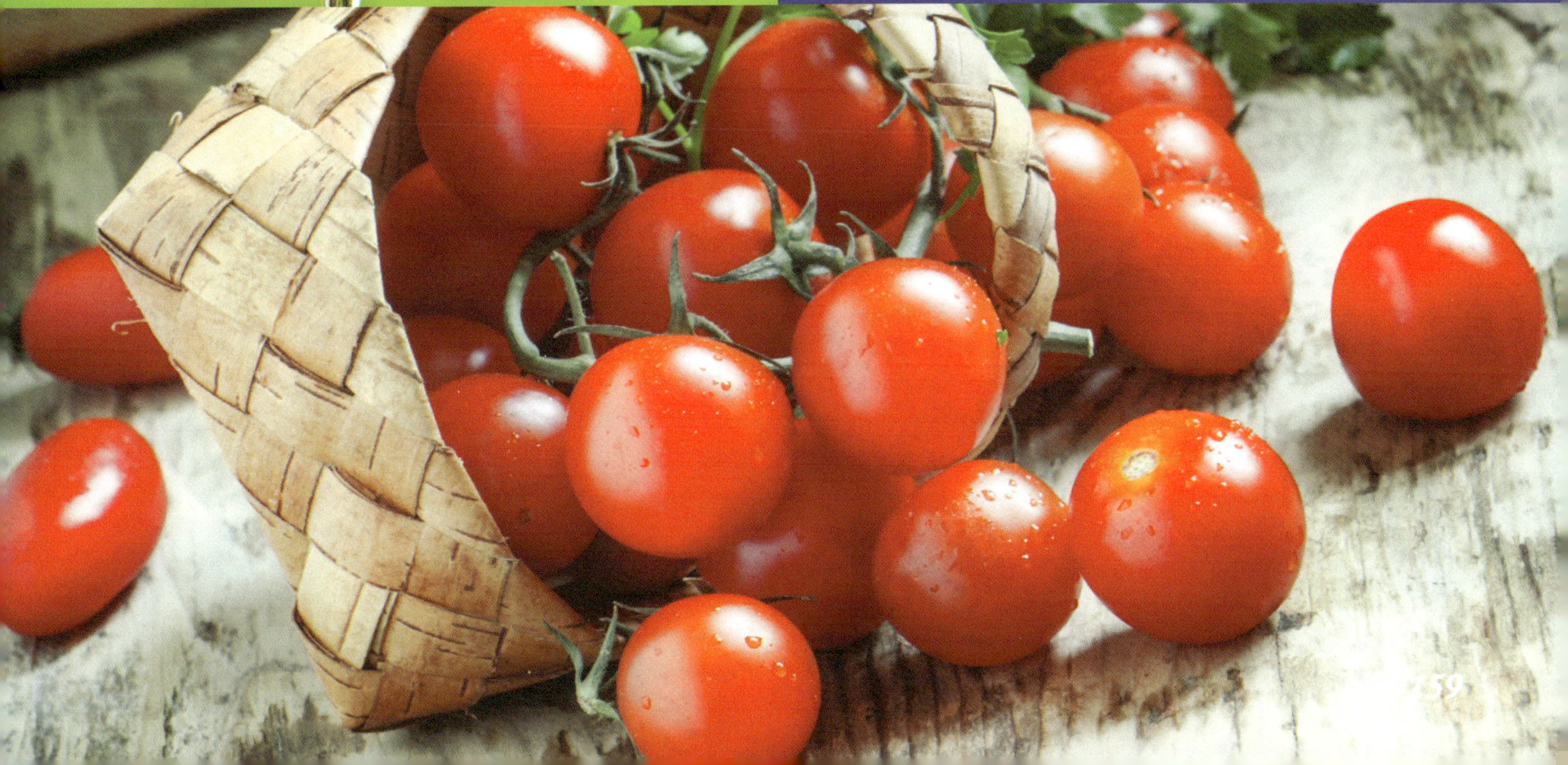

CUCUMBER-GREEN TEA TONER

4 Tablespoons cucumber juice (approximately 1 medium cucumber)
4 Tablespoons steeped green tea
1 Tablespoon vodka (optional)

Mix all ingredients well. Pour into a small glass bottle and store in a cool place, preferably the refrigerator.

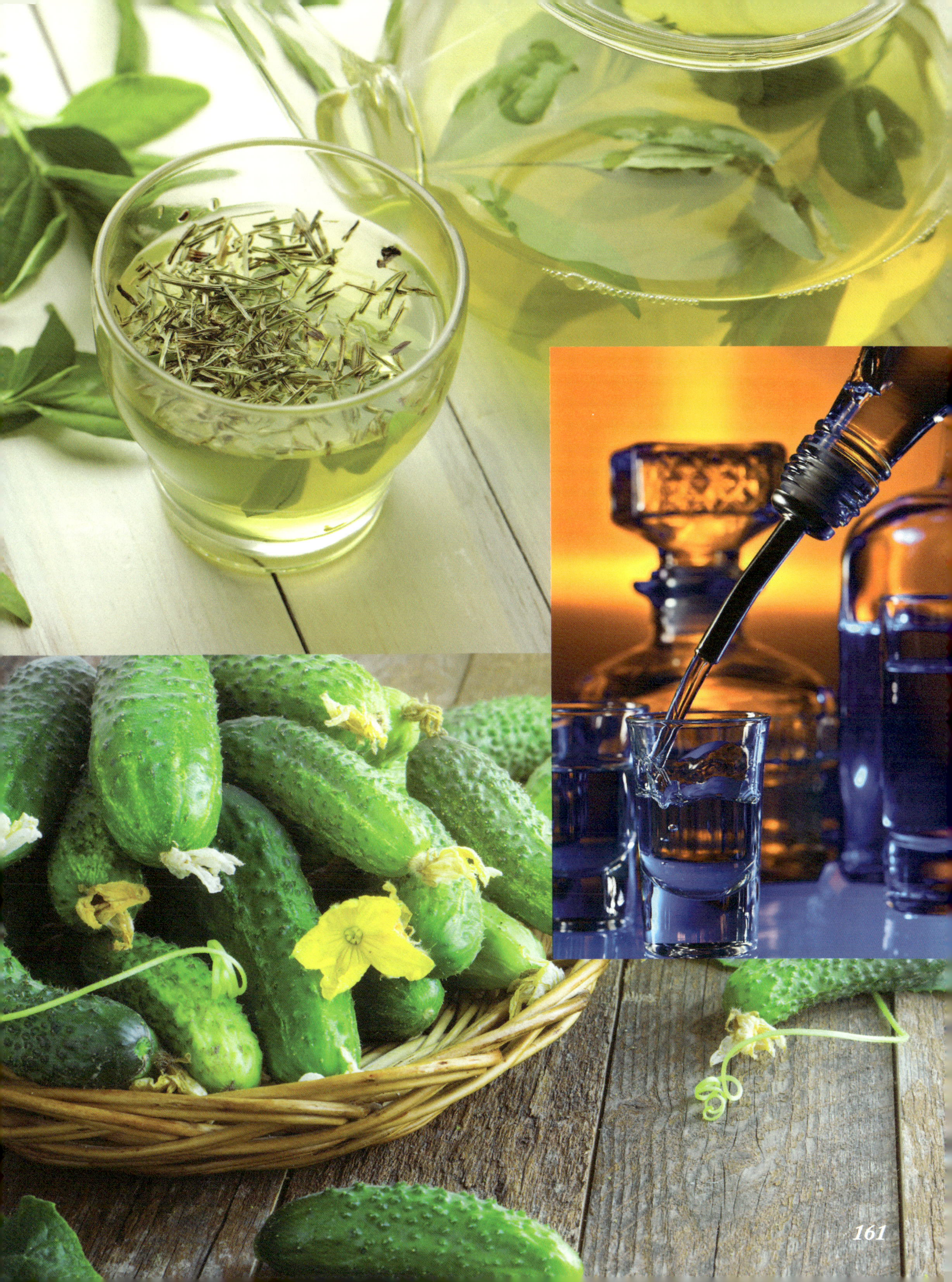

APPLE-MINT TONER

3-4 Teaspoons chopped fresh mint
2 Tablespoons raw apple cider vinegar (Braggs)
1 1/4 cups distilled or filtered water

Place the mint and apple cider vinegar in a small Mason jar or other glass jar with a screw-top lid. Let sit at room temperature for 1 week. The mint will infuse the vinegar and give it a lovely scent. Strain the mixture into a large measuring cup. Add the water. Stir well and pour into a clean glass bottle or jar and store in a cool place.

Apply to the face as a cleanser once a day or splash on your face as cool refreshment on a hot day.

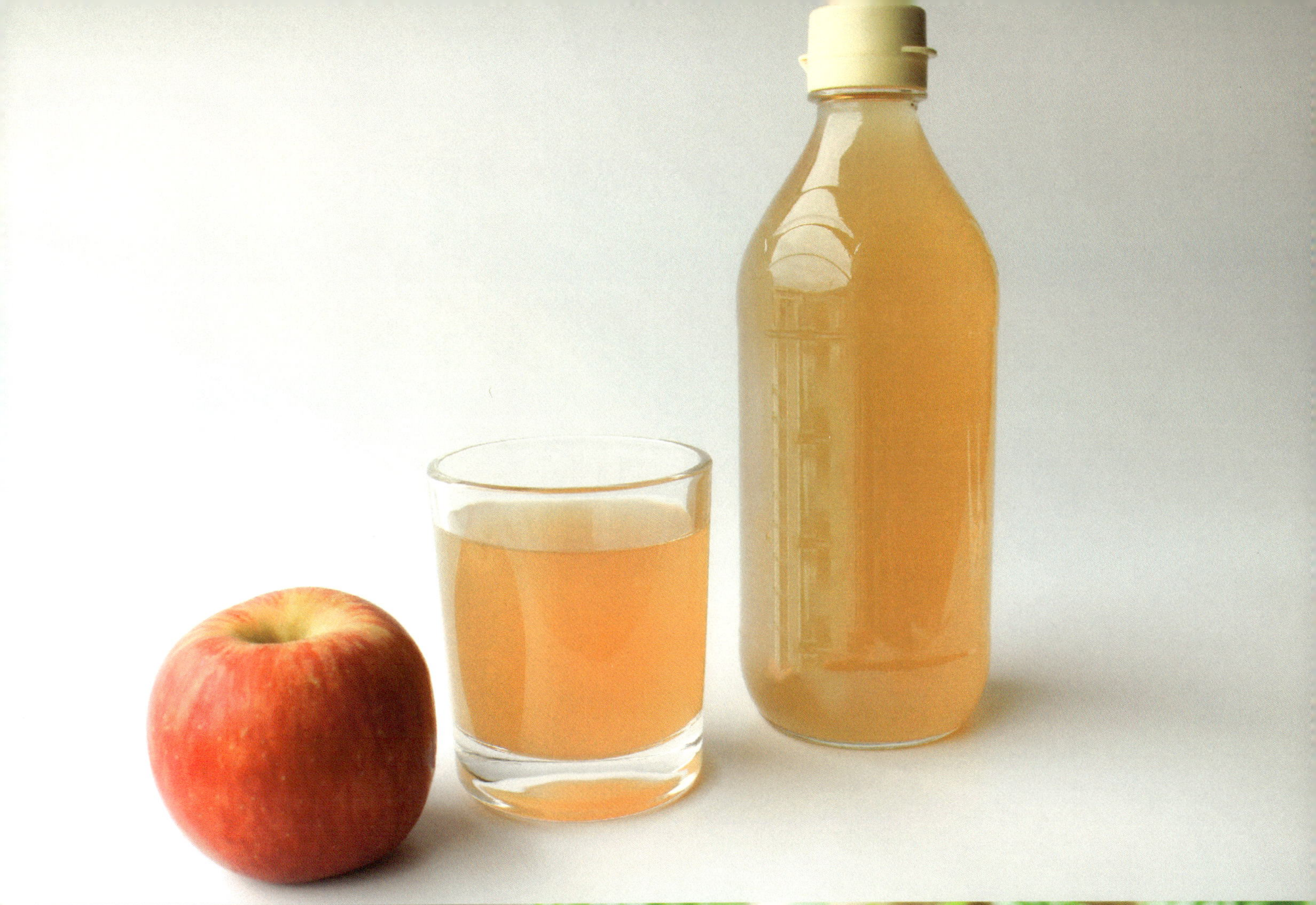

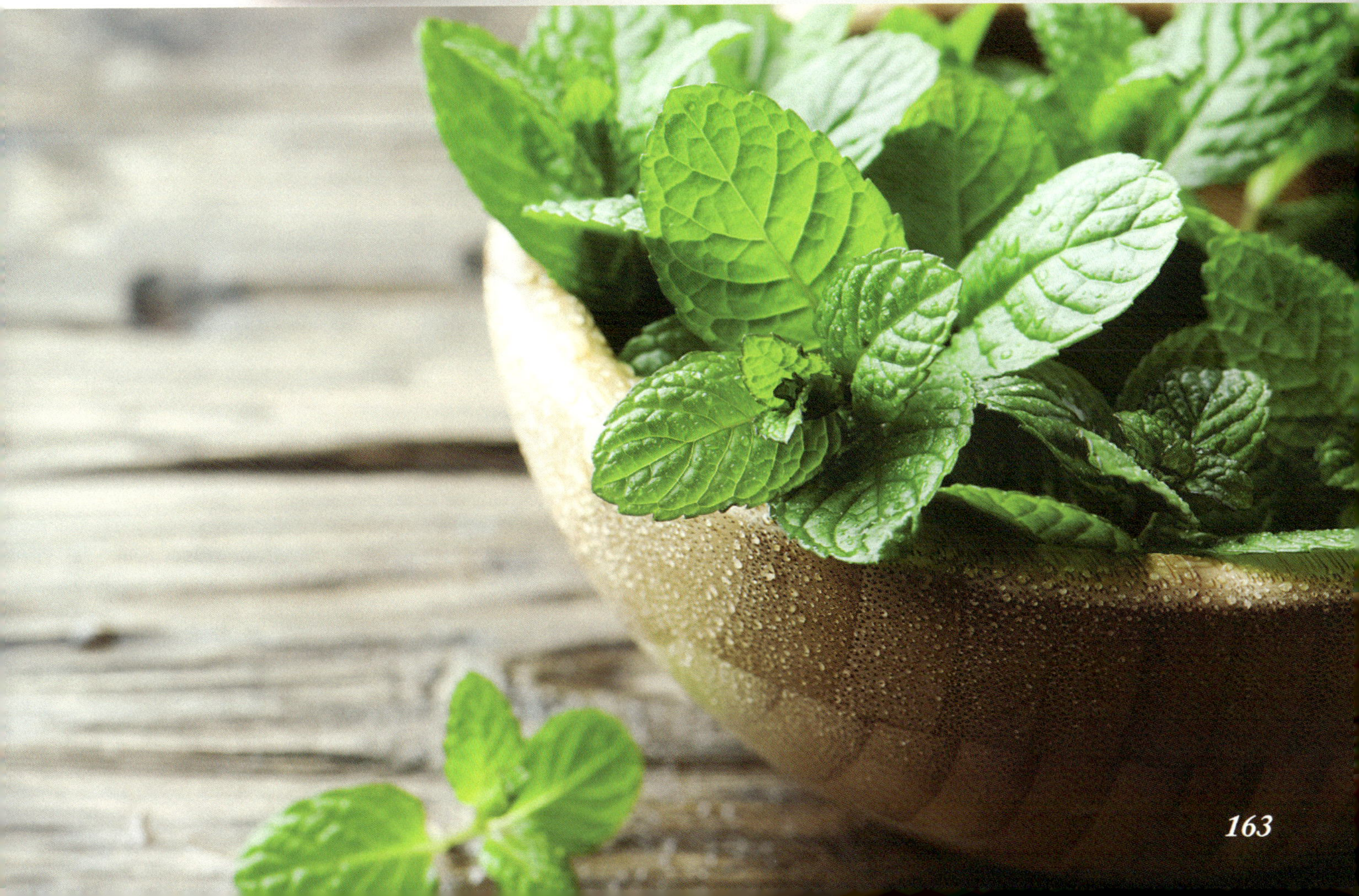

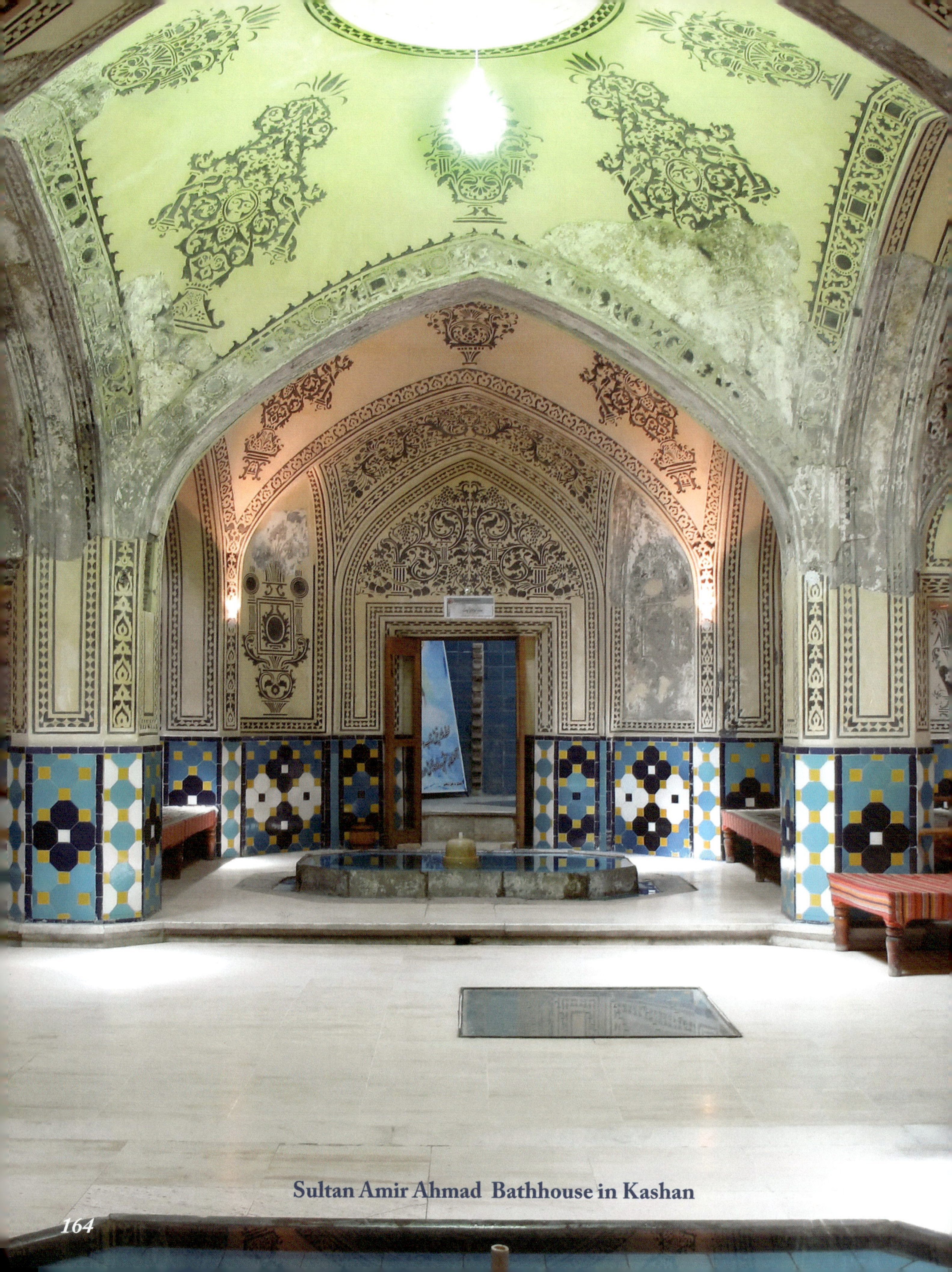

Sultan Amir Ahmad Bathhouse in Kashan

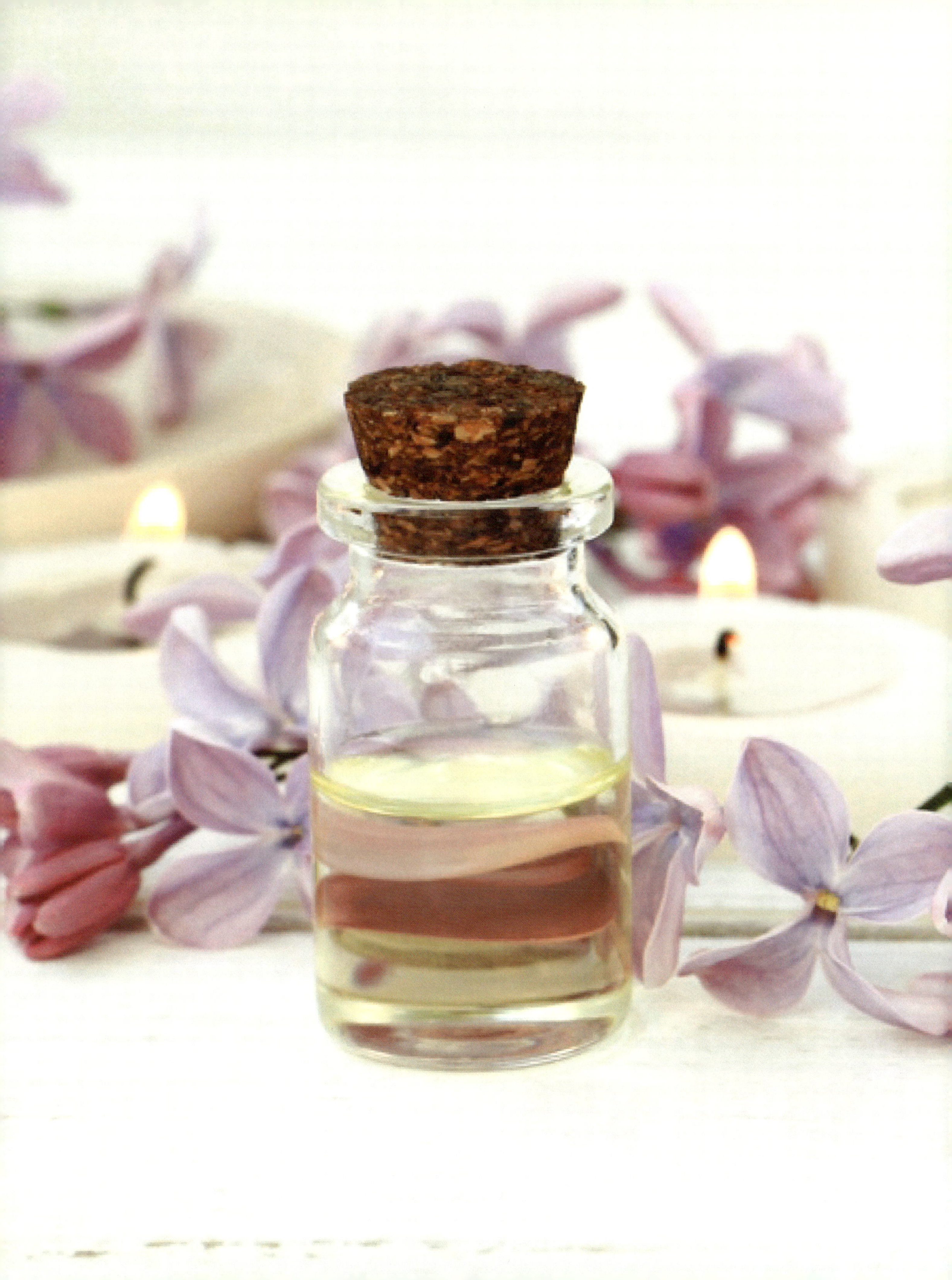

ROSE OIL

1 Cup rose petals
1 Cup jojoba, almond or grapeseed oil (a light olive oil will work in a pinch.)

Bring a few inches of water to a boil in a saucepan, then remove from heat. Pour oil in a glass jar. Crush, shred or "bruise" a cup of rose petals and place in the oil. Swirl the jar around to coat the petals, but don't shake.

Cover the jar and place into the hot water. Warming the oil will help release the scent from the rose petals. When the water cools, you can move the jar to a warm area like a sunny windowsill. Leave for at least 24 hours. Strain the oil through a cheesecloth, pressing the petals to extract as much oil as you can. (If you want a stronger-smelling oil, you can repeat steps 1-6 with fresh petals.) You may need to repeat the process 5 or 6 times to get the desired level of scent.) Pour clear oil into a dark bottle with a lid (dark glass will help block out sunlight and keep the oil more stable.)

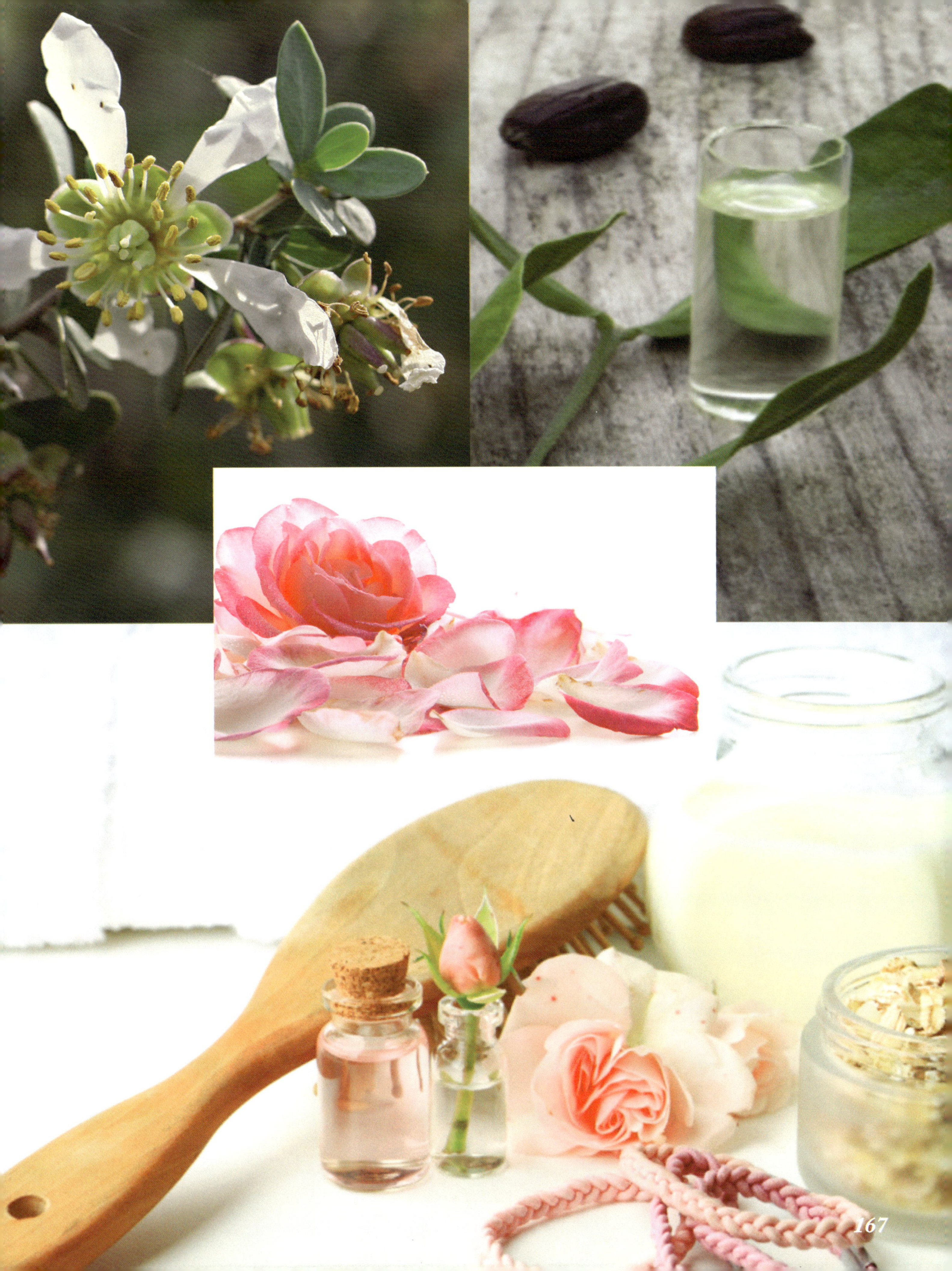

TURMERIC MASSAGE OIL

2 Tablespoons turmeric paste (recipe on page)
1 Cup virgin organic coconut oil

Heat coconut oil on low heat, add the turmeric paste, the oil will start sizzling. Remove the oil, and let it cool. Make sure not to burn the turmeric paste. Once completely cool, strain and store in glass bottles.

For diaper rash, skin infection, reduces colic pain, relieves constipation.

Massaging helps babies to sleep peacefully. Massage gently all over the body and then give baby a warm bath. Use this oil twice weekly for best results.

Warning: Be careful. Turmeric stains.

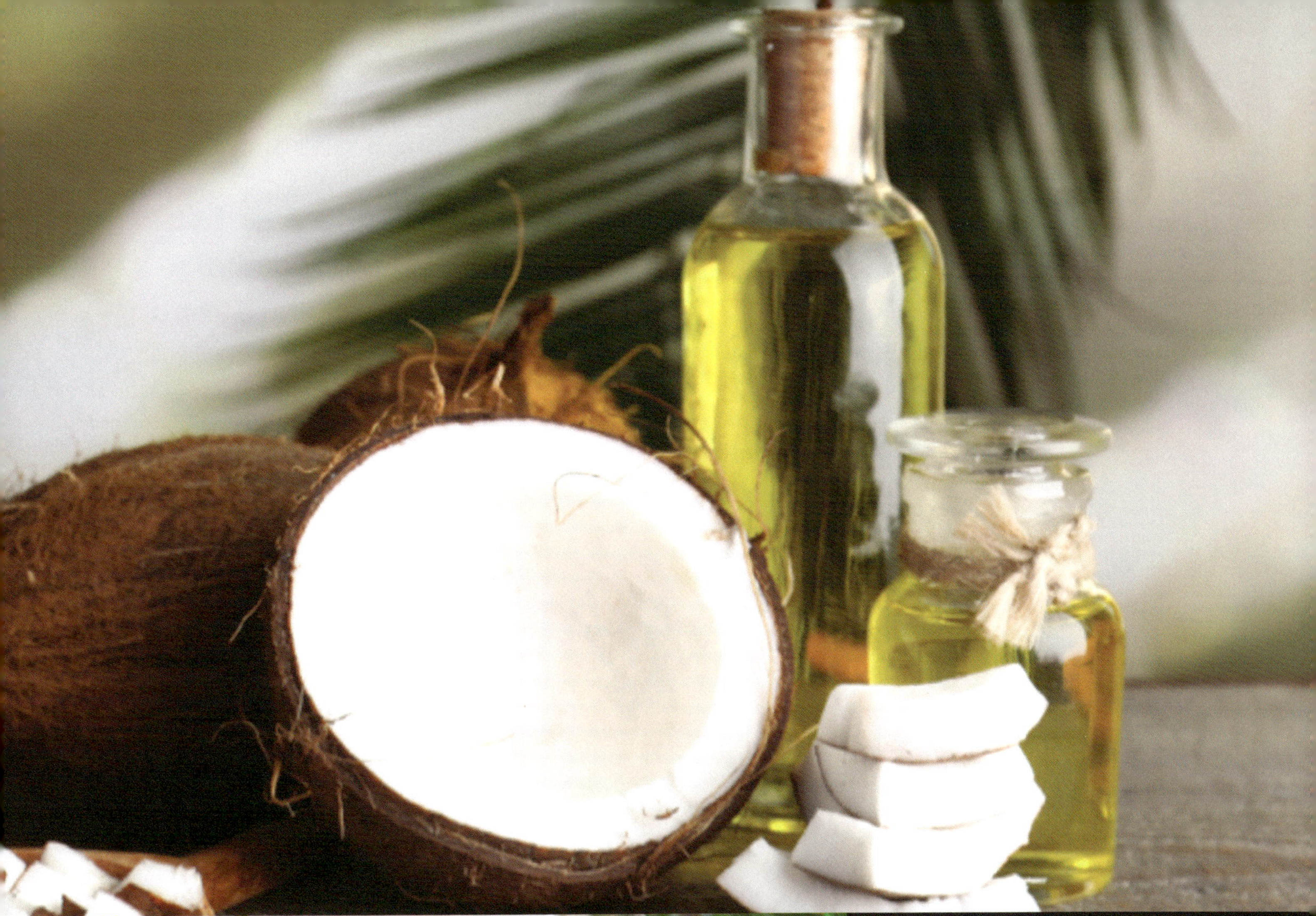

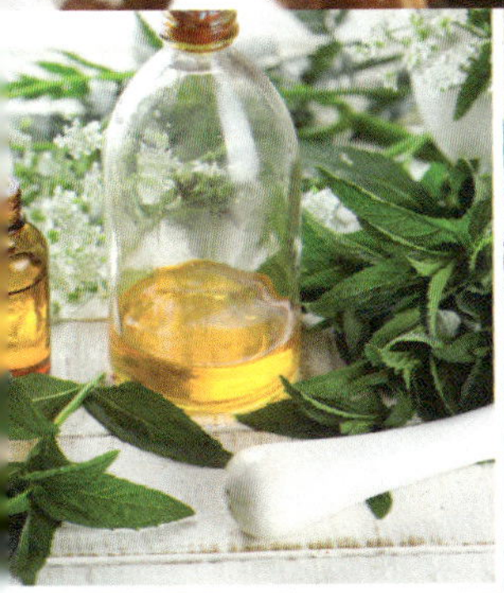

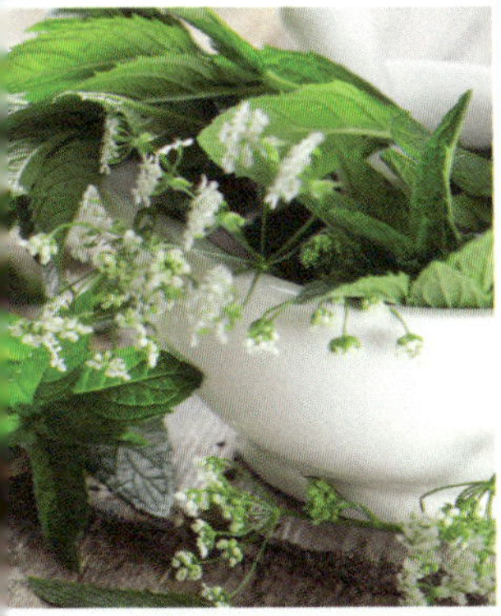

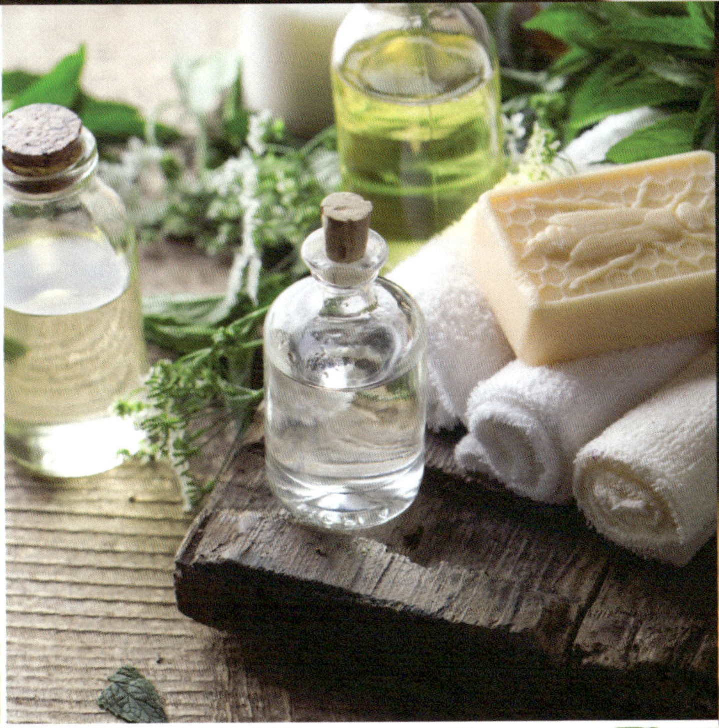

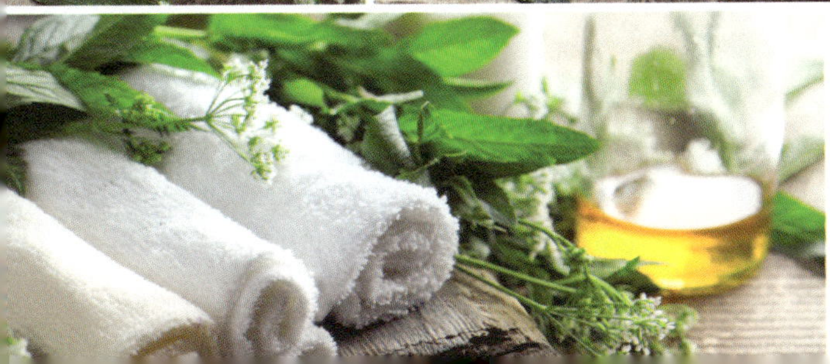

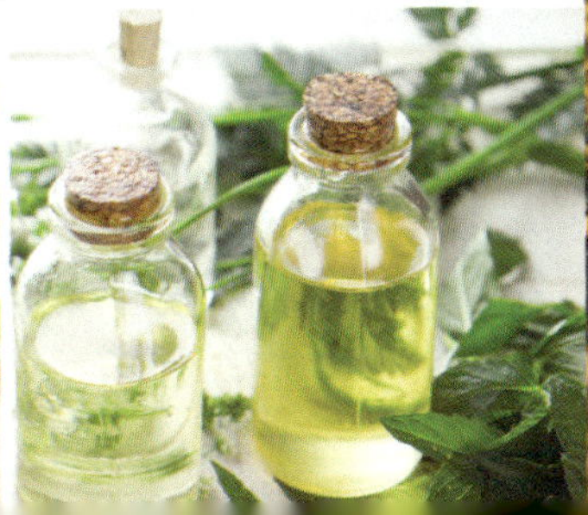

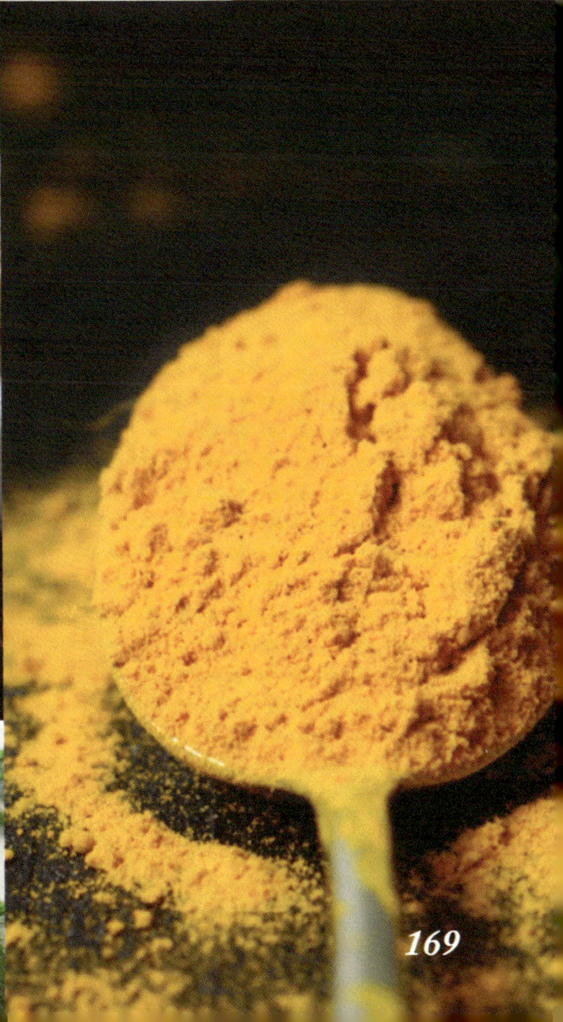

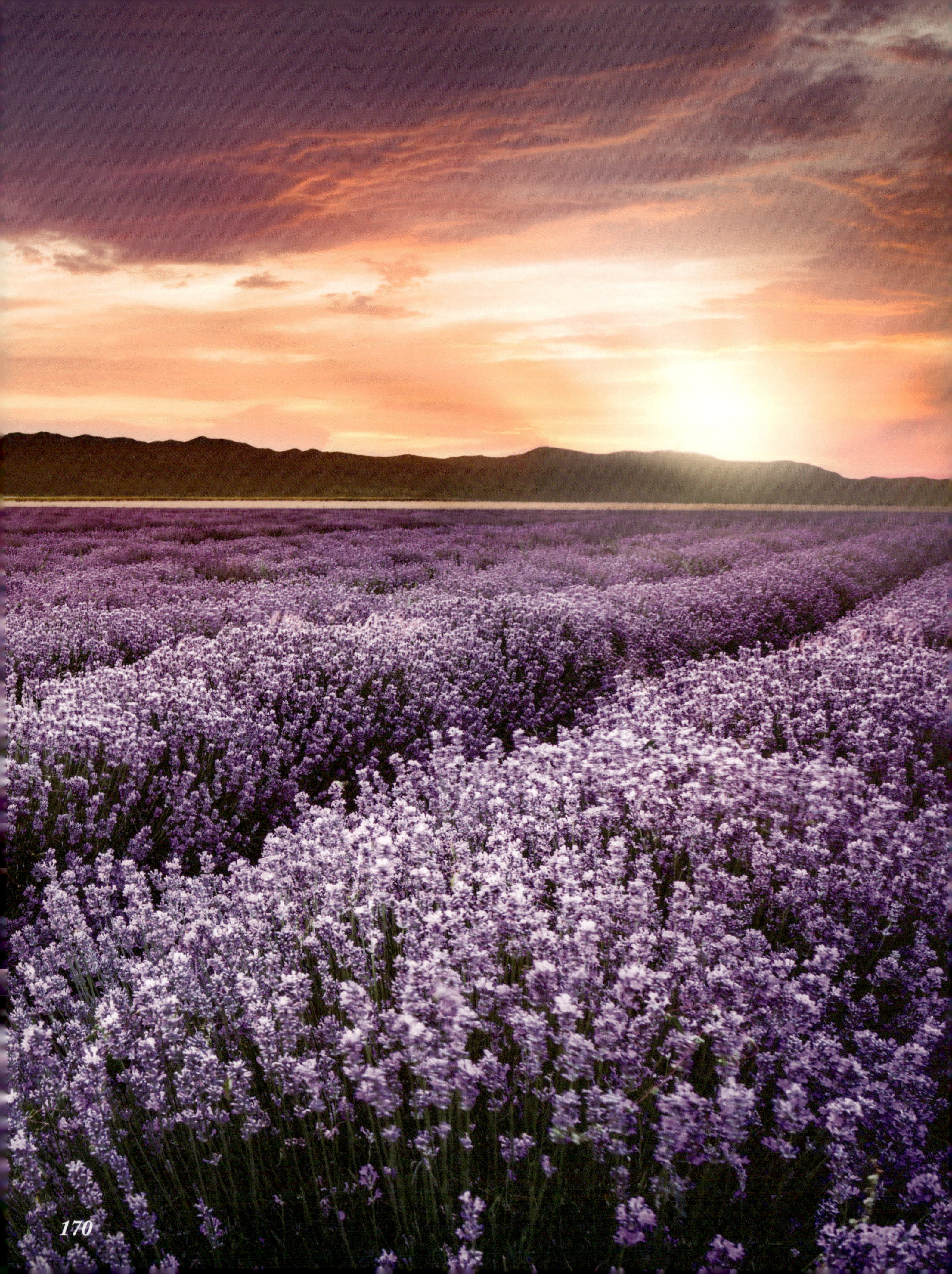

LAVENDER OIL

Soothes aching muscles, reduces anxiety, diminishes stress and so much more!

Linalol

Lavender oil contains up to 50% of the alcohol linalol. Linalol helps to kill bacteria and viruses. It also helps to heal burns, wounds and sores.

Ketones

Ketones are compounds that help to relieve pain, build new tissues and reduce inflammation. They are also known to have a sleep-inducing effect. Ketones can be toxic, so lavender that contains above 35% should be avoided.

Esters

Esters are compounds that are known to ease swelling and soreness, prevent muscle spasms, fight fungal infections and prevent scarring. They also help to regulate your mood, alleviating depression and hysteria.

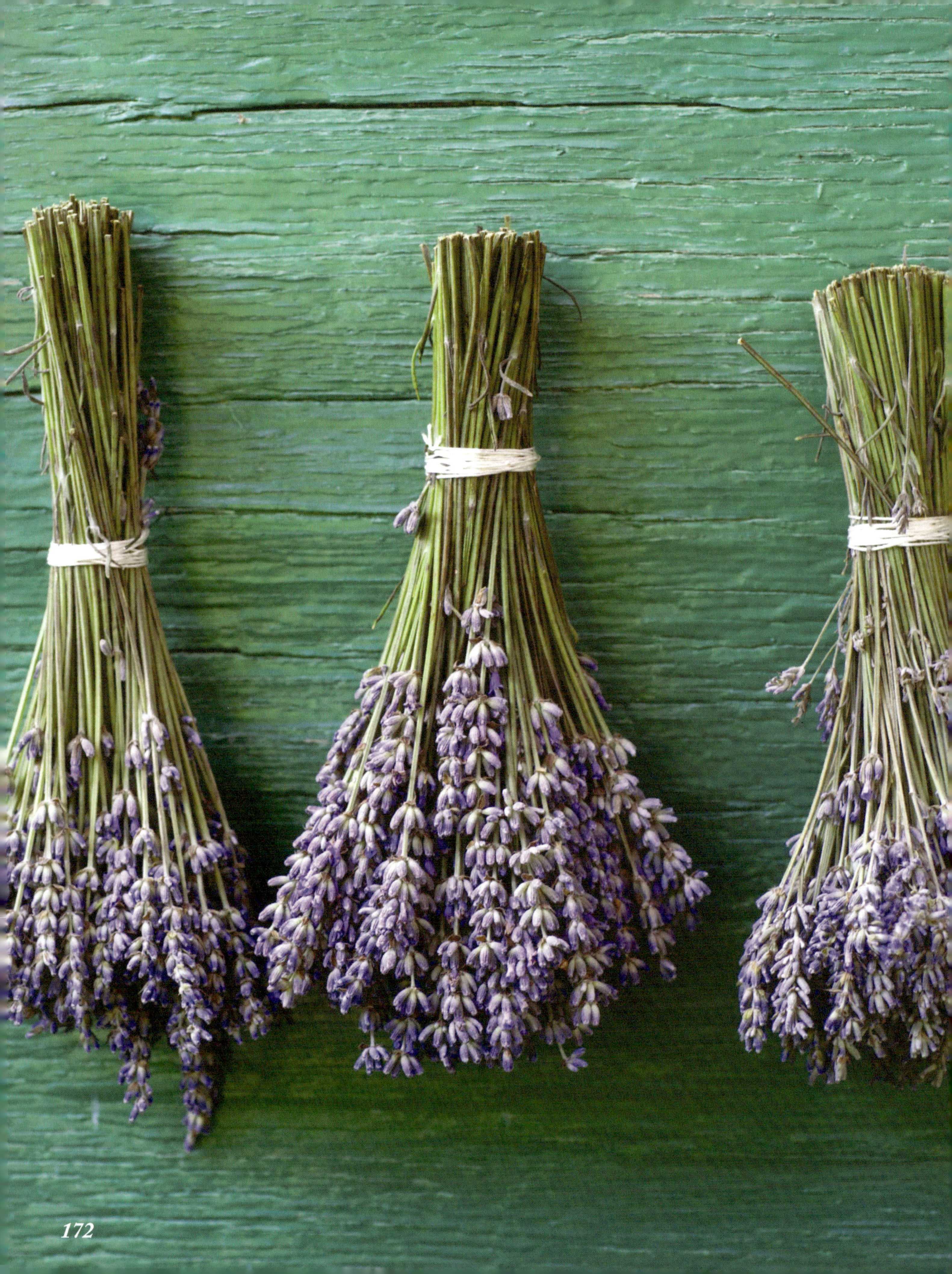

LAVENDER OIL

Dry lavender stalks
Castor oil (only the kind at health food stores)

First, make sure to use dry lavender to enhance its aroma and minimize the chance of the oil becoming rancid. If you have fresh lavender, dry it first by tying your sprig with a rubber band or string and let it hang upside down in a dry, warm area. Exposing it to sunlight will dry the lavender out much faster, but could break down some of its aromatic oils. Fresh-cut lavender may take two weeks to dry fully. Dehydrators take only one to three days to dry it.

Room Temp Method

Cut lavender stems into 6-inch segments. (The leaves, new stems, buds and flowers can be used, but not the woody stems near the base.) Lightly crush with your fingers or bruise it slightly with any clean, heavy object to expose its fragrance. If using buds, open them up with a knife or fingers and place in a jar. Pour oil into the jar to cover the lavender, leaving an inch or so at top to allow for expansion.

You can substitute almond oil, olive oil, or safflower oil. Steep in sunlight for about 48 hours. Can last several months in a dry dark location. For a noticeable scent leave it out for three to six weeks. If you do not have enough sunlight or time to use this method, continue to the next step . . .

Heated Method

Heat the oil and lavender mixture in a double boiler or crock pot for 2–5 hours, keeping it at a steady temperature between 100–120°F. This is only recommended if you have a cooking thermometer and a well-controlled, low temperature heat source, as too much heat can affect the aroma and the shelf life of the oil.

Lay a piece of muslin or cheesecloth over a bowl and pour the oil and herb mix over it. Discard the flowers and other lavender pieces. Store in a dark bottle or jar. The shelf life depends on the type and freshness of oil used, but lasts for months if kept in a dry, dark location.

Warning: Diabetics, epileptics and pregnant women should avoid lavender oil completely.

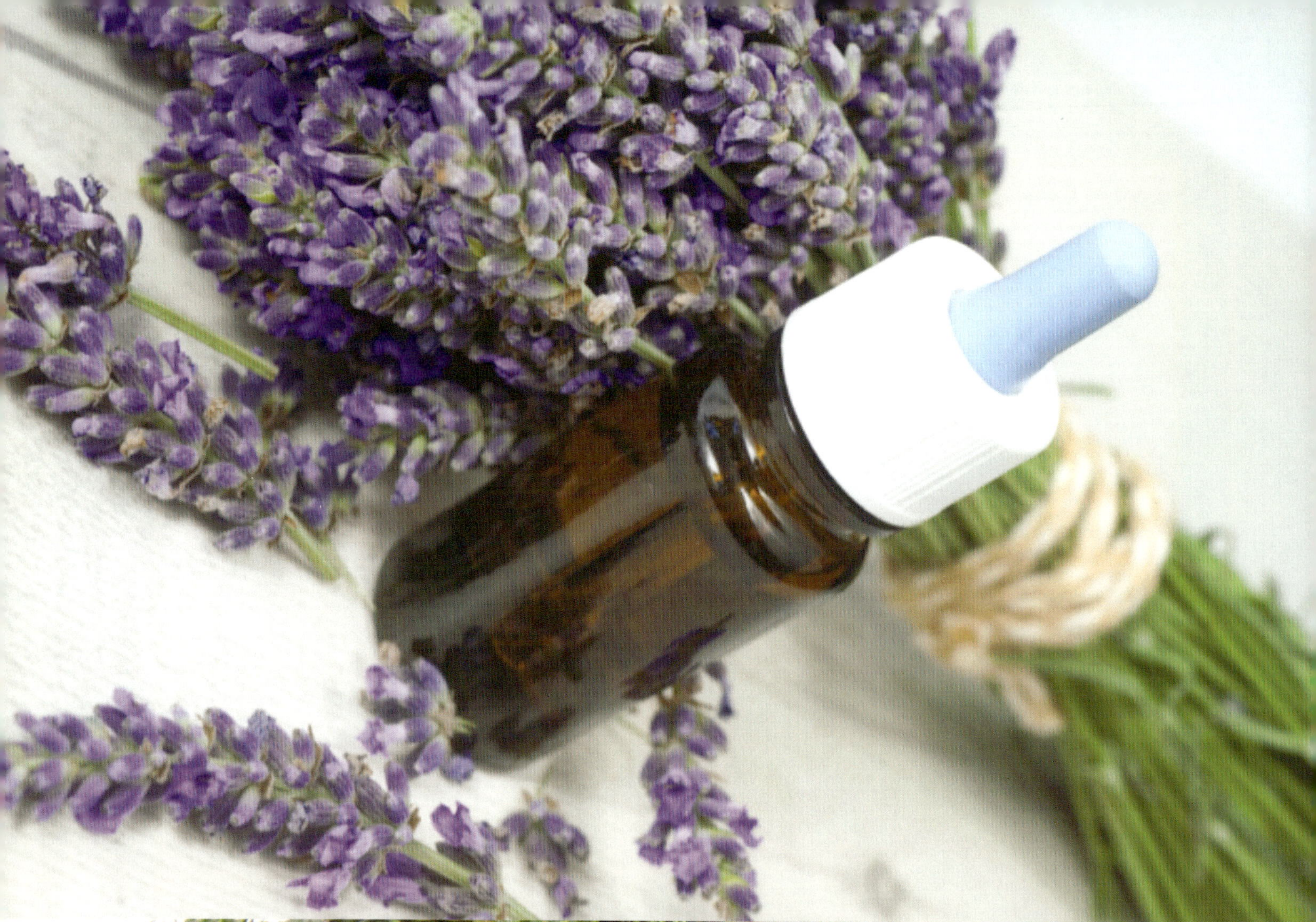

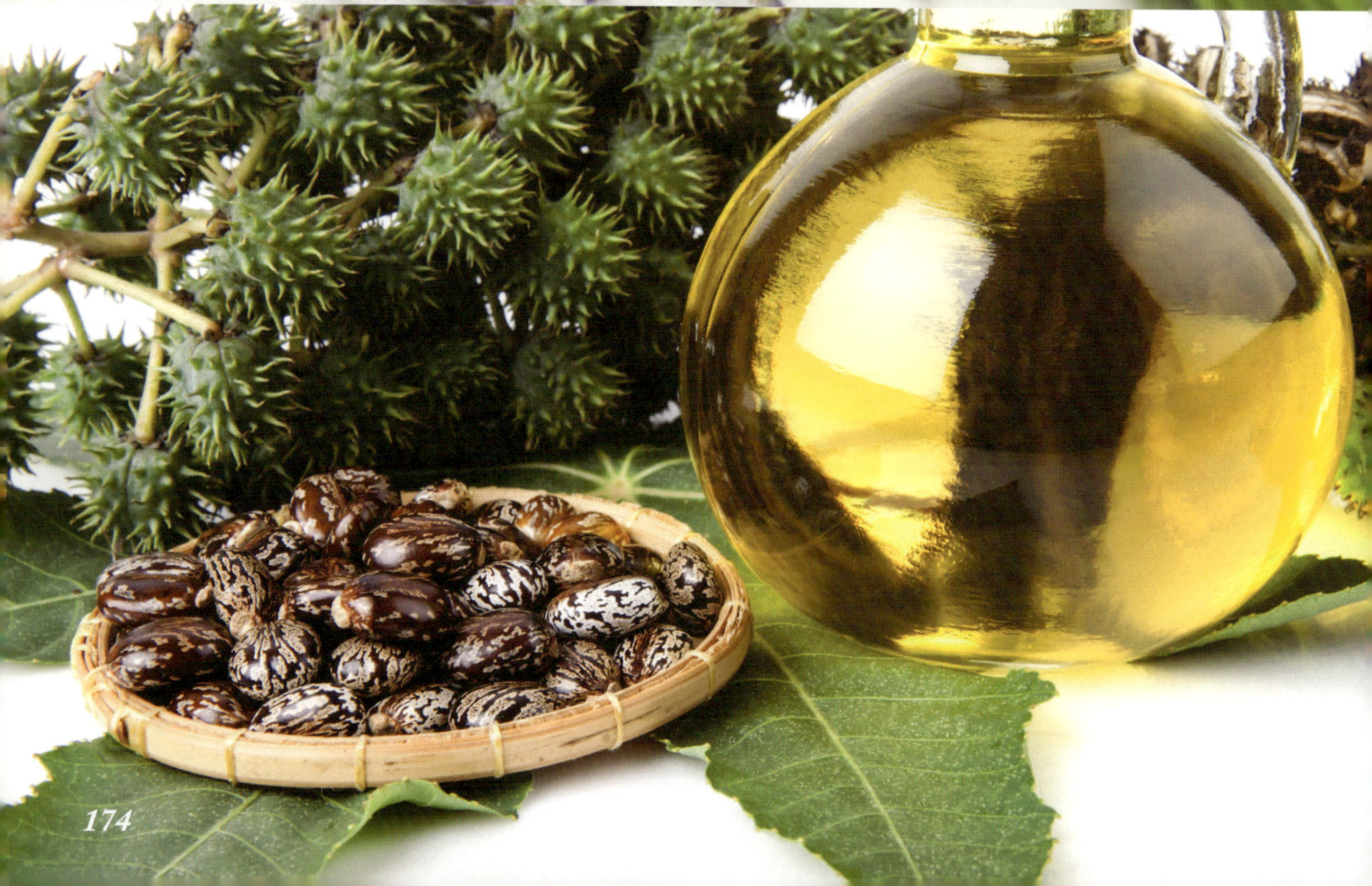

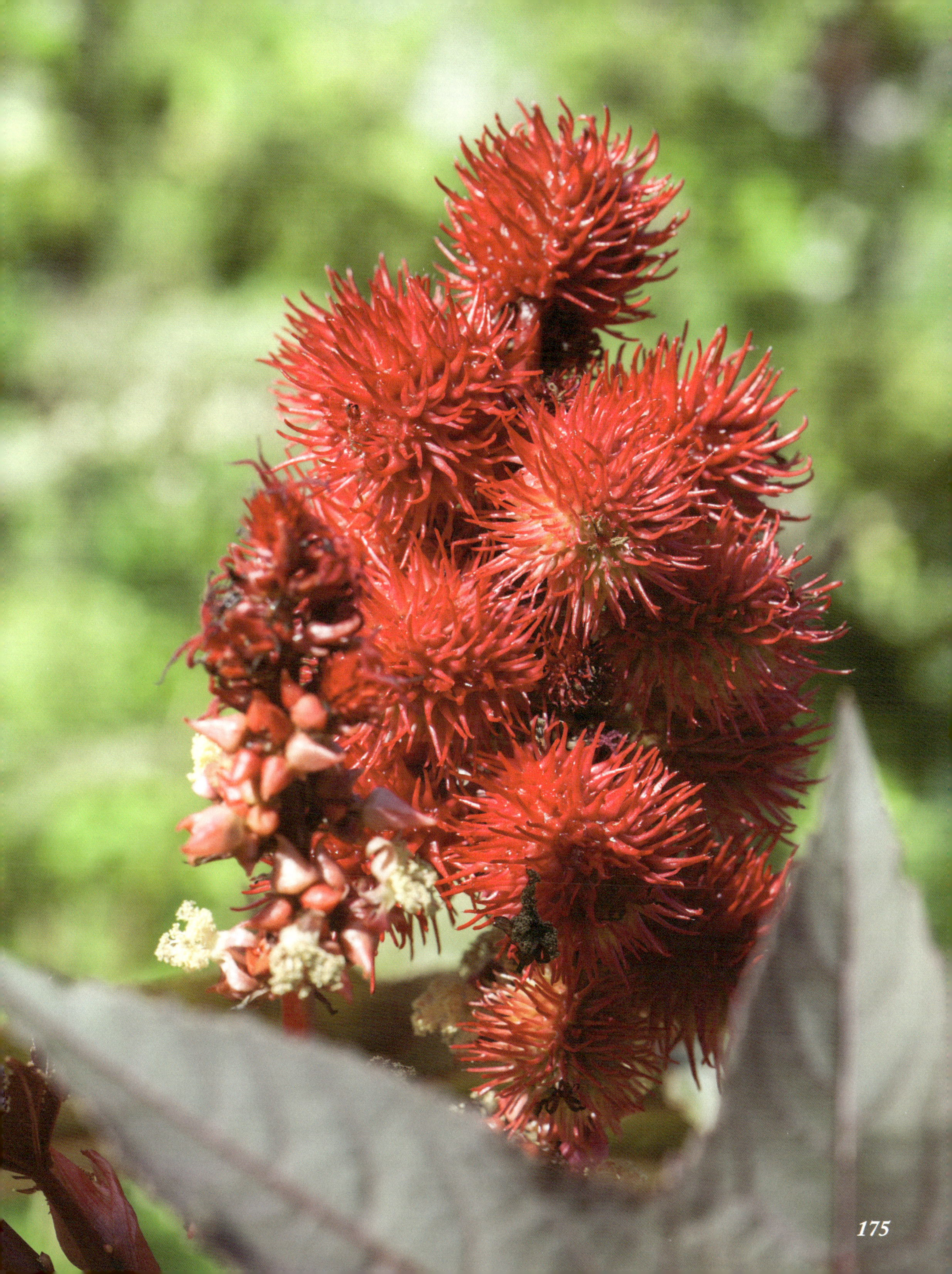

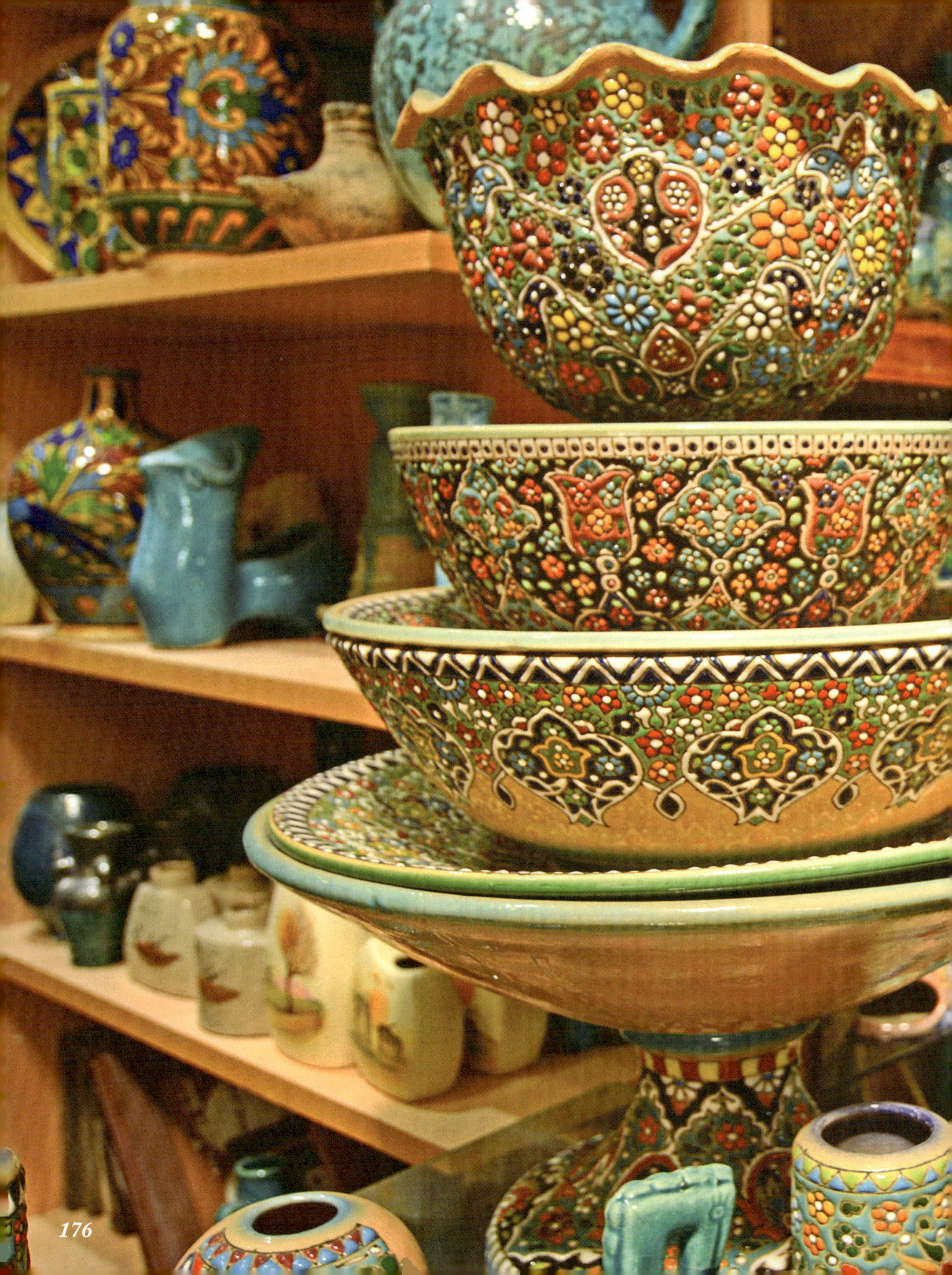

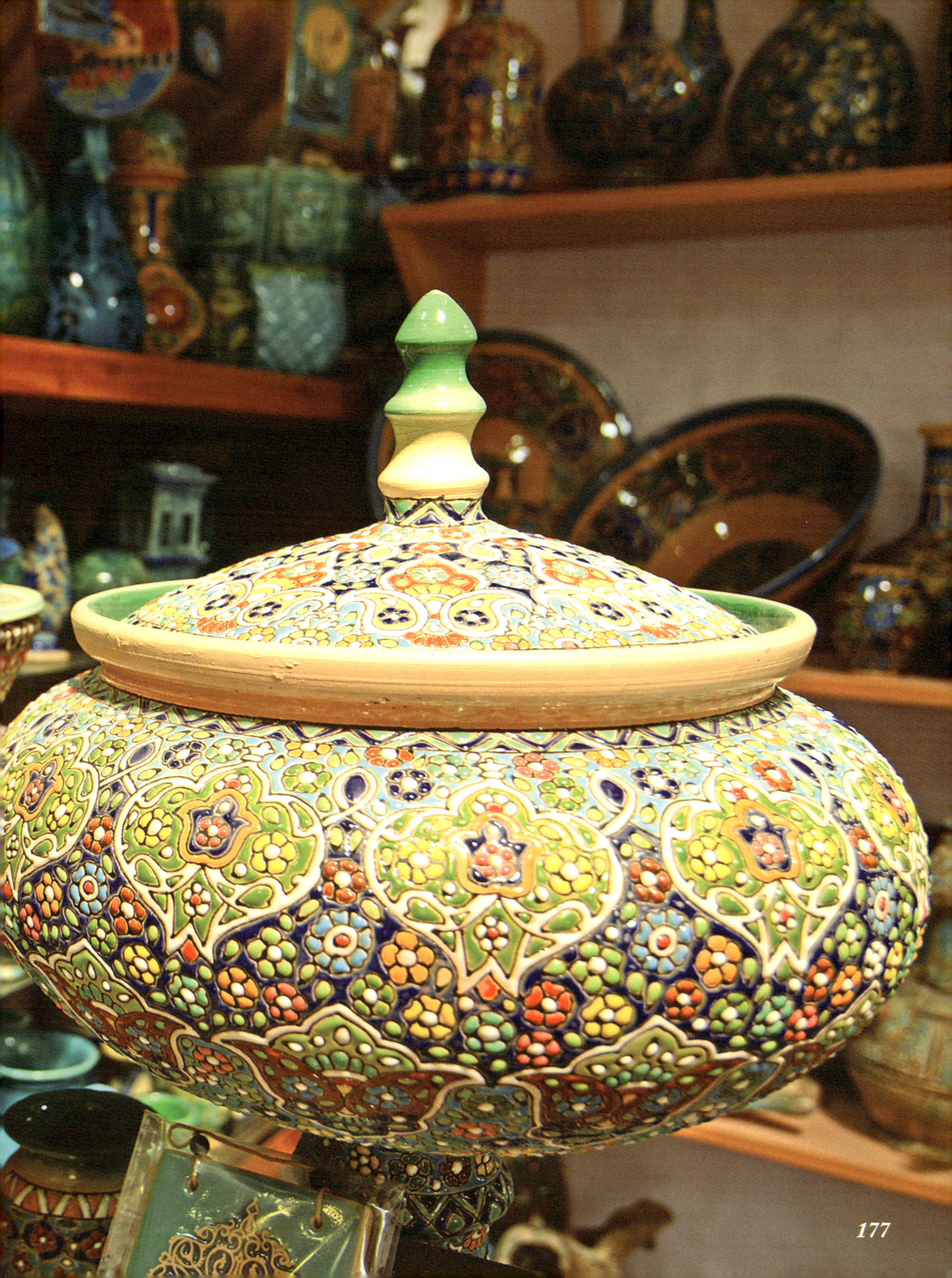

SEFIDAB ("WHITE WATER")

Sefidab is an ancient Persian mineral product that means white water in Farsi. Traditionally it combined zeolite, a volcanic mineral substance, and animal fats that were dried into a white rock. These days this fat has been replaced by vegetable oil for health concerns regarding animal diseases.

Sefidab has been used for thousands of years as a skin exfoliant in hamams (Middle Eastern public baths). It is known for its cleansing and exfoliating effect. It detoxes the body, stimulates circulation and gives you a more even skintone.

The microporous cellular structure of zeolite is one of nature's few negatively charged minerals, giving it the ability to attract positively charged contaminants. Zeolite swaps its beneficial negatively charged minerals for any positively charged contaminants on or in your body. Sefidab is an excellent exfoliator, especially when used with a loofah, and peel for the entire body. While showering, rub some sefidab on to your scrubbing mitt and thoroughly scrub to remove dead skin.

SEFIDAB EXFOLIANT

To erase cellulite

1 cup – Coconut oil (virgin raw organic)
1 cup – Cacao butter (raw organic)
1 cup – Micronized zeolite (4ppm or smaller so that it's small enough to penetrate the skin)

Melt the coconut oil and cacao butter at very low heat in a double boiler. Add zeolite and pour into a sealed jar.

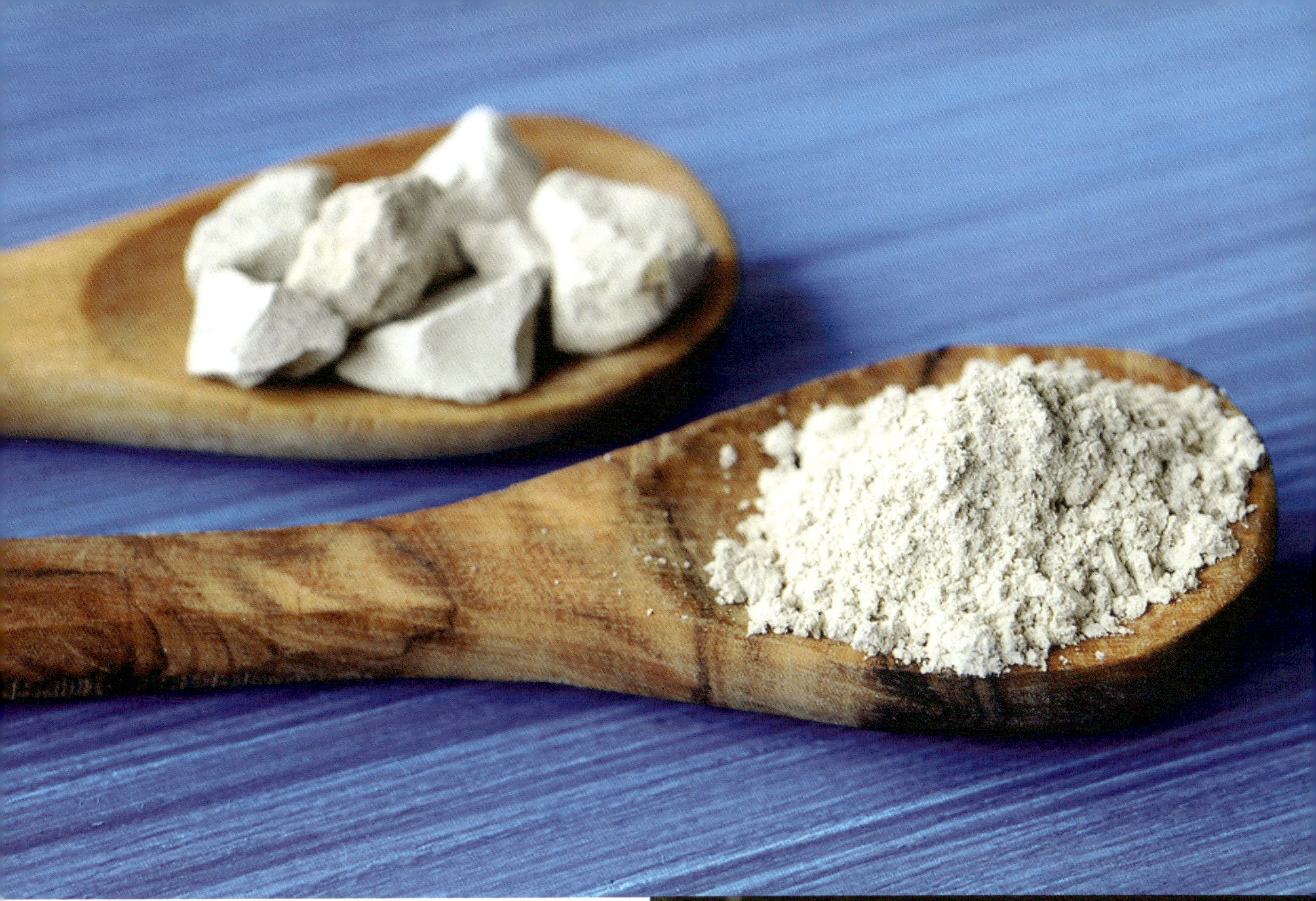

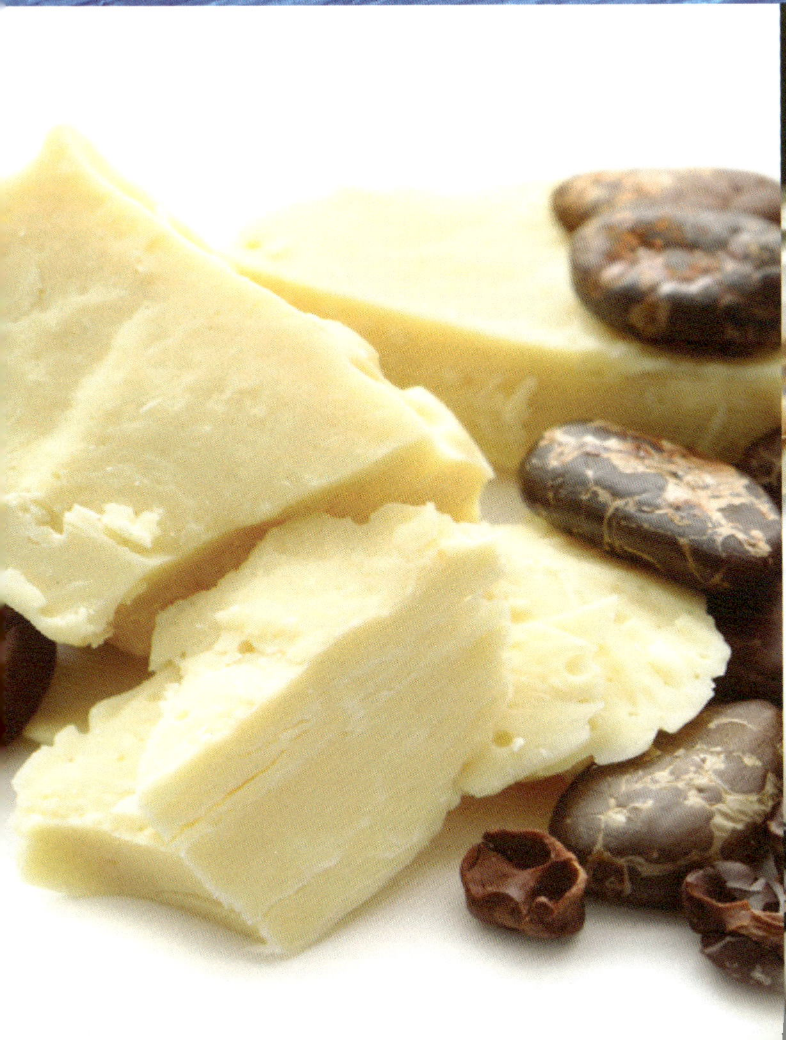

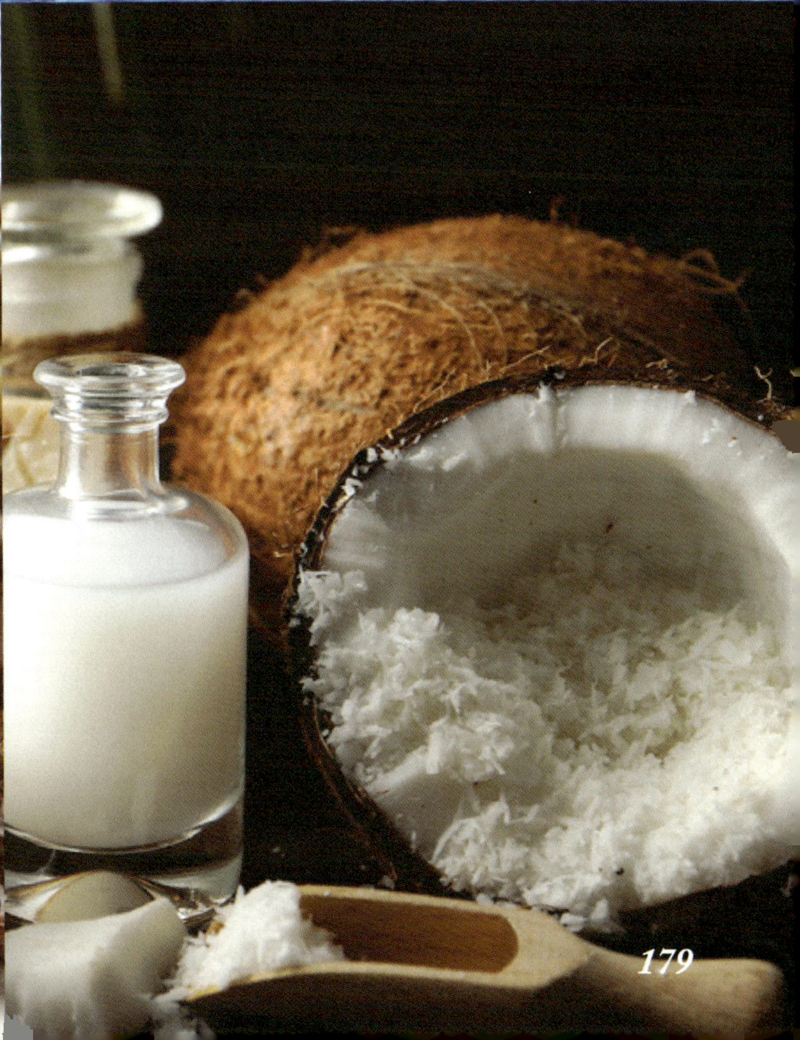

SWEET POTATO

Sweet potatoes are an incredibly nutritious food packed with antioxidants like beta carotene, vitamins C, E & D, and minerals such as manganese and iron. They are also high in potassium which helps to lower blood pressure by removing excess sodium and regulating fluid balance in the body. Sweet potatoes are an excellent anti-stress food and are known to help relax muscles, steady nerves, and balance cognitive function. They are also one of the best anti-cancer foods and can particularly help to prevent breast, colon, lung, skin, and oral cancers.

Sweet potatoes are known for being easy to digest and are very good for ulcers, inflamed colons, digestive disorders, and constipation. Sweet potatoes contain compounds called phytochelatins that can bind to heavy metals such as lead, mercury, copper, and cadmium and safely remove them through the body. Mothers have even given children who have accidentally swallowed a metallic object such as a coin, plenty of sweet potato so that it will stick to the object and allow it to pass through easier.

The health benefits of sweet potatoes are the most bioavailable when eaten raw, steamed, or baked. Try making a simple fat-free sweet potato soup by steaming sweet potatoes until soft and then placing in a blender or food processor and blend until creamy smooth. Spices such as cloves, cinnamon, ginger, chili pepper, or curry can be added for a flavor and nutritional boost. Baked sweet potatoes can be stored in the refrigerator and later sliced over a fresh green salad for a hearty lunch or dinner. Sweet potatoes are also delicious mashed with a drizzle of olive oil, coconut butter, or avocado. Sweet potatoes are a comforting, satisfying, and very healing food.

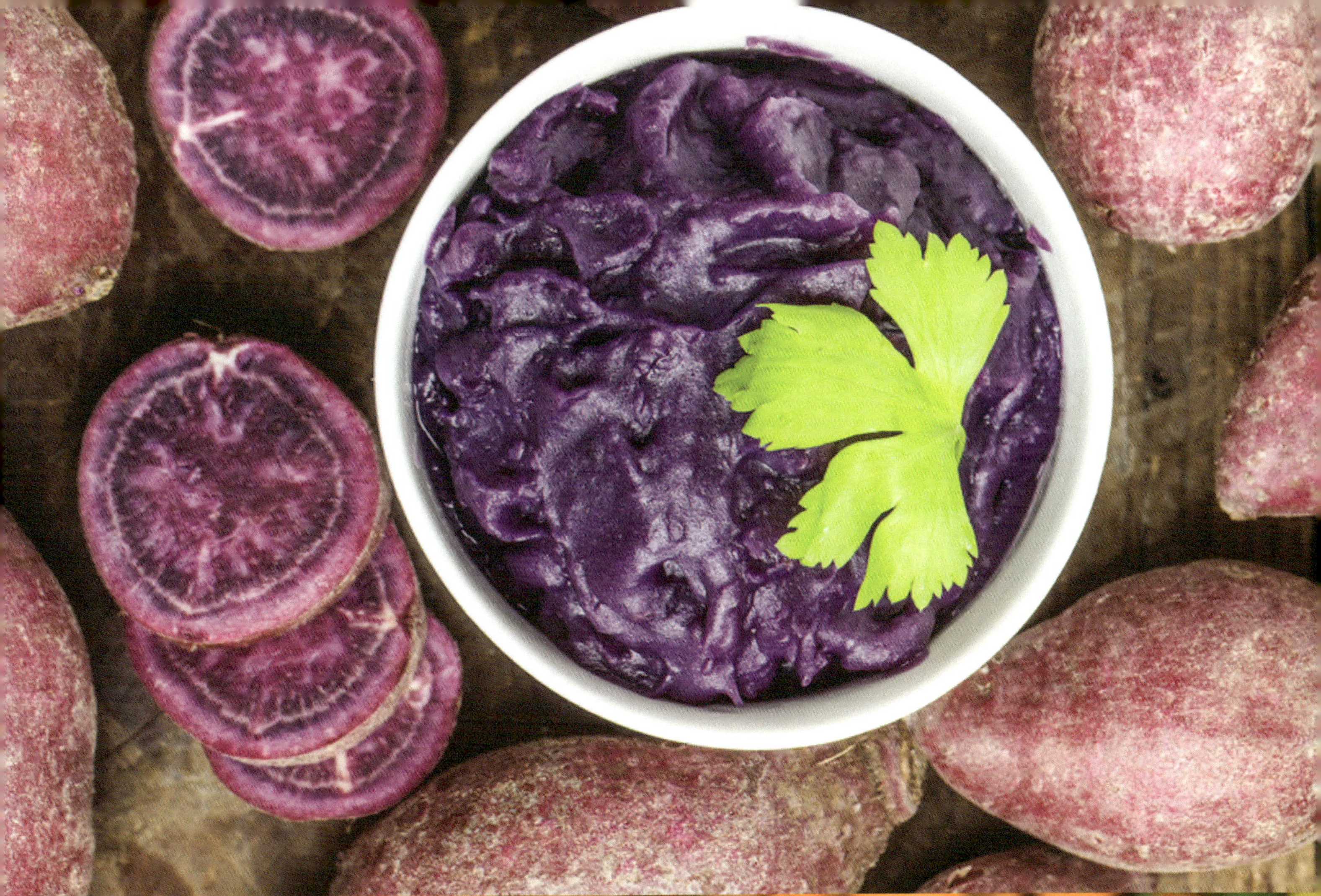

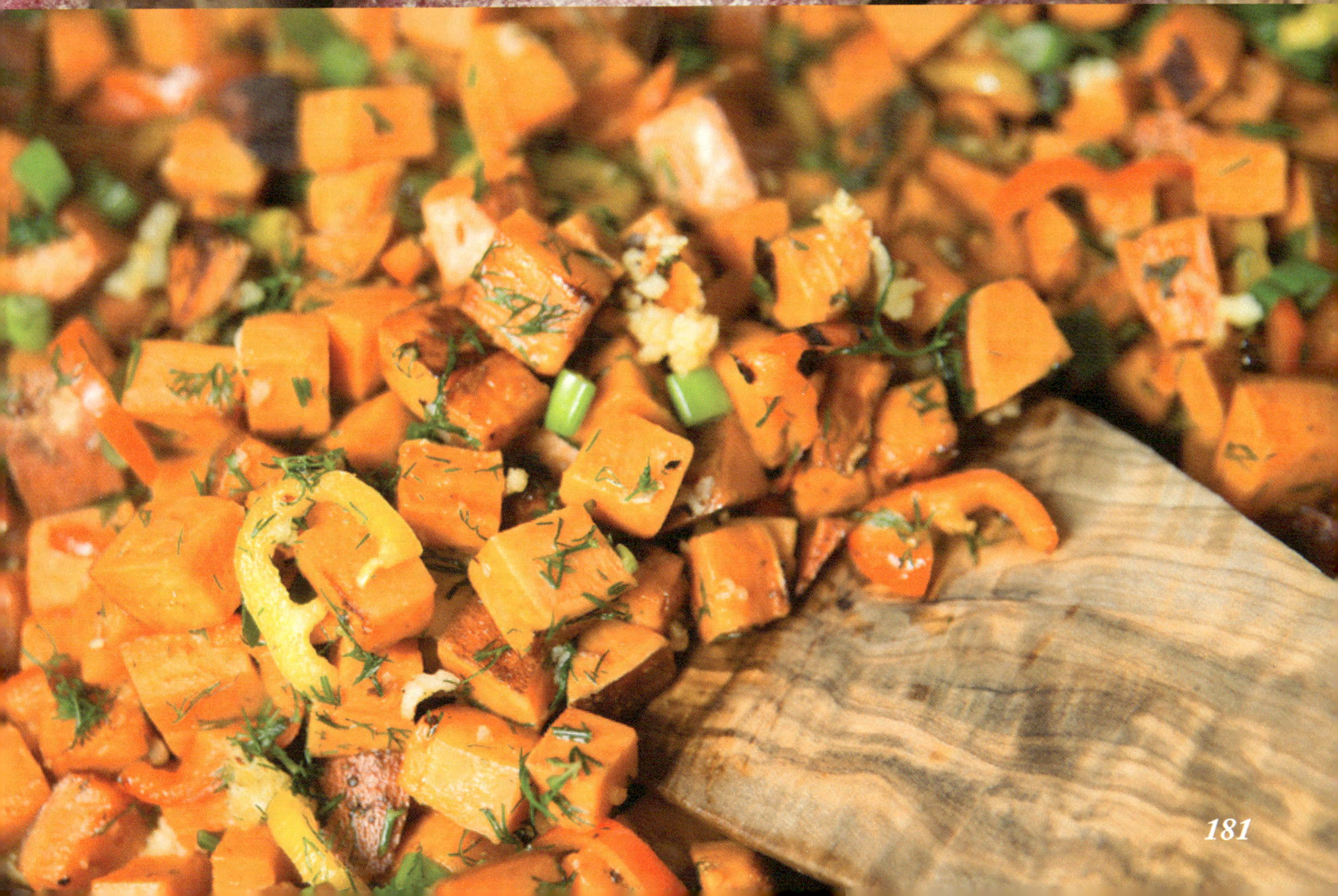

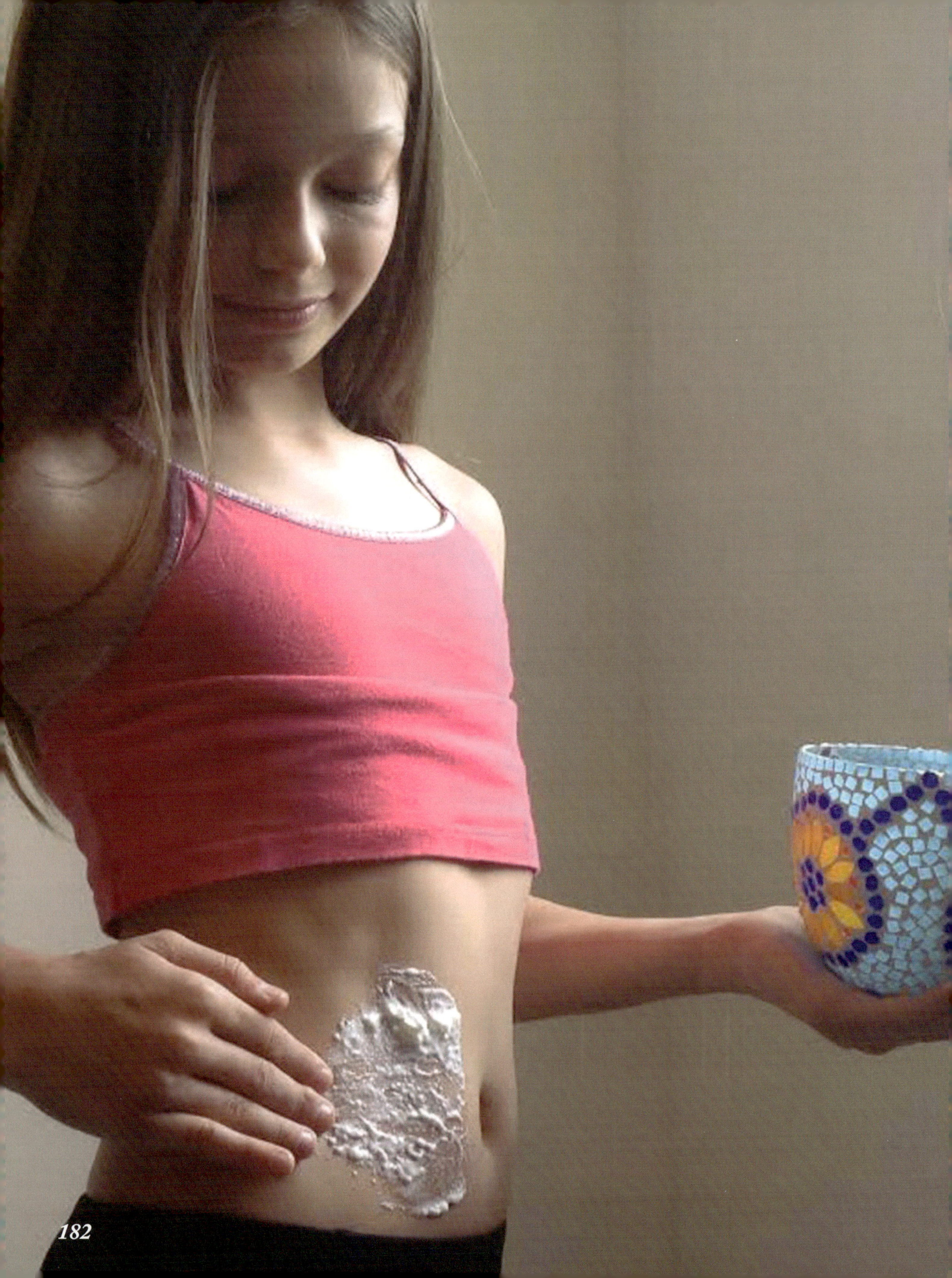

ERASE STRETCH MARKS

1 Medium yam peeled and chopped
2 Tablespoons coconut oil
1/4 Cup raw honey or Manuka honey

Place ingredients in a blender, until a paste. Rub on stretch marks and leave for 25 minutes. Wash off. Repeat daily until you see the stretch mark fade away.

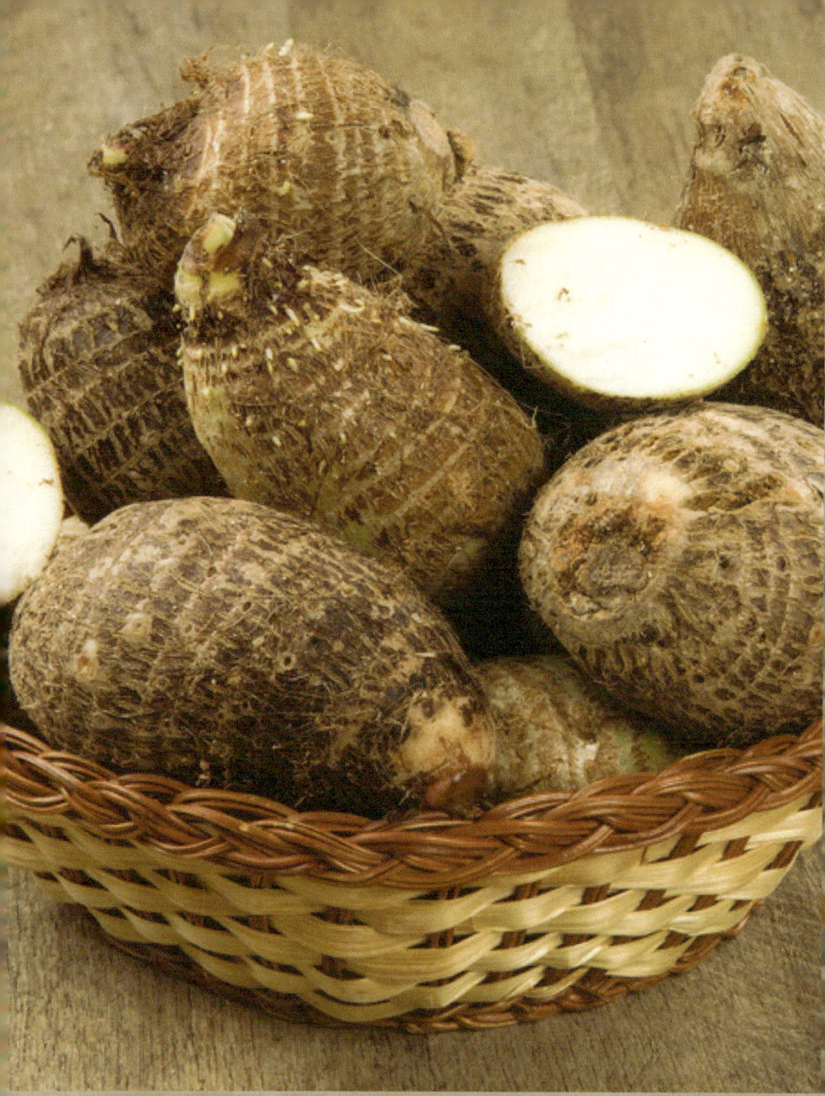

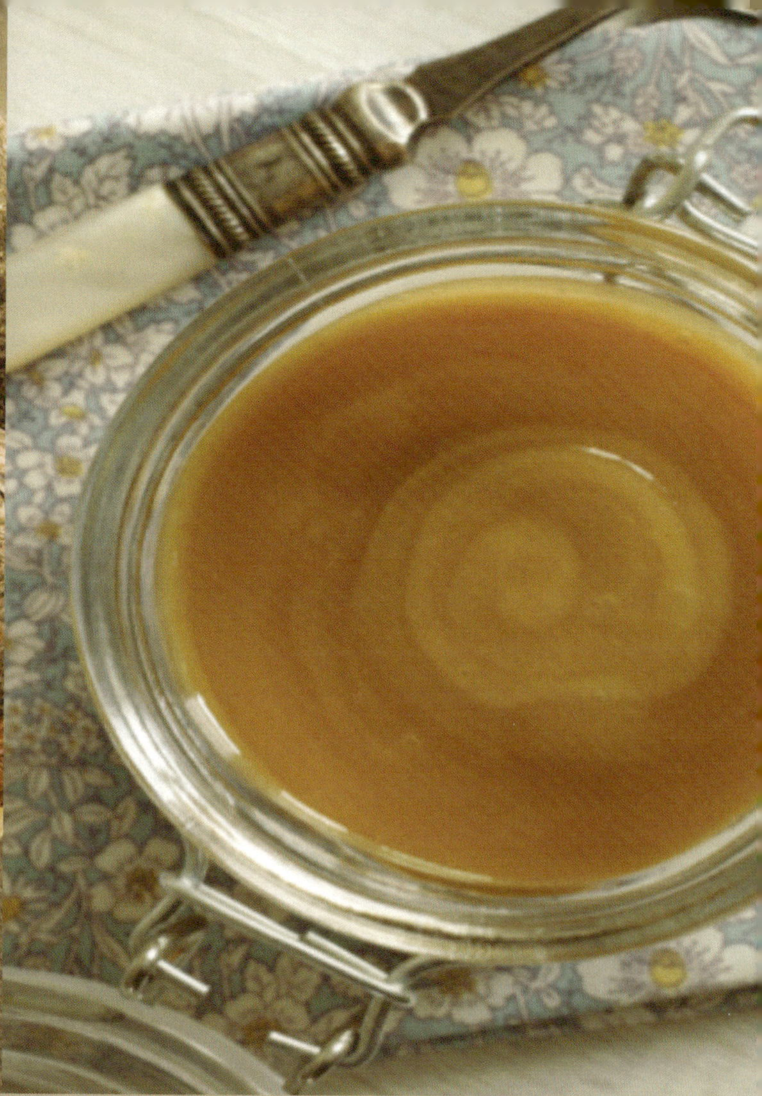

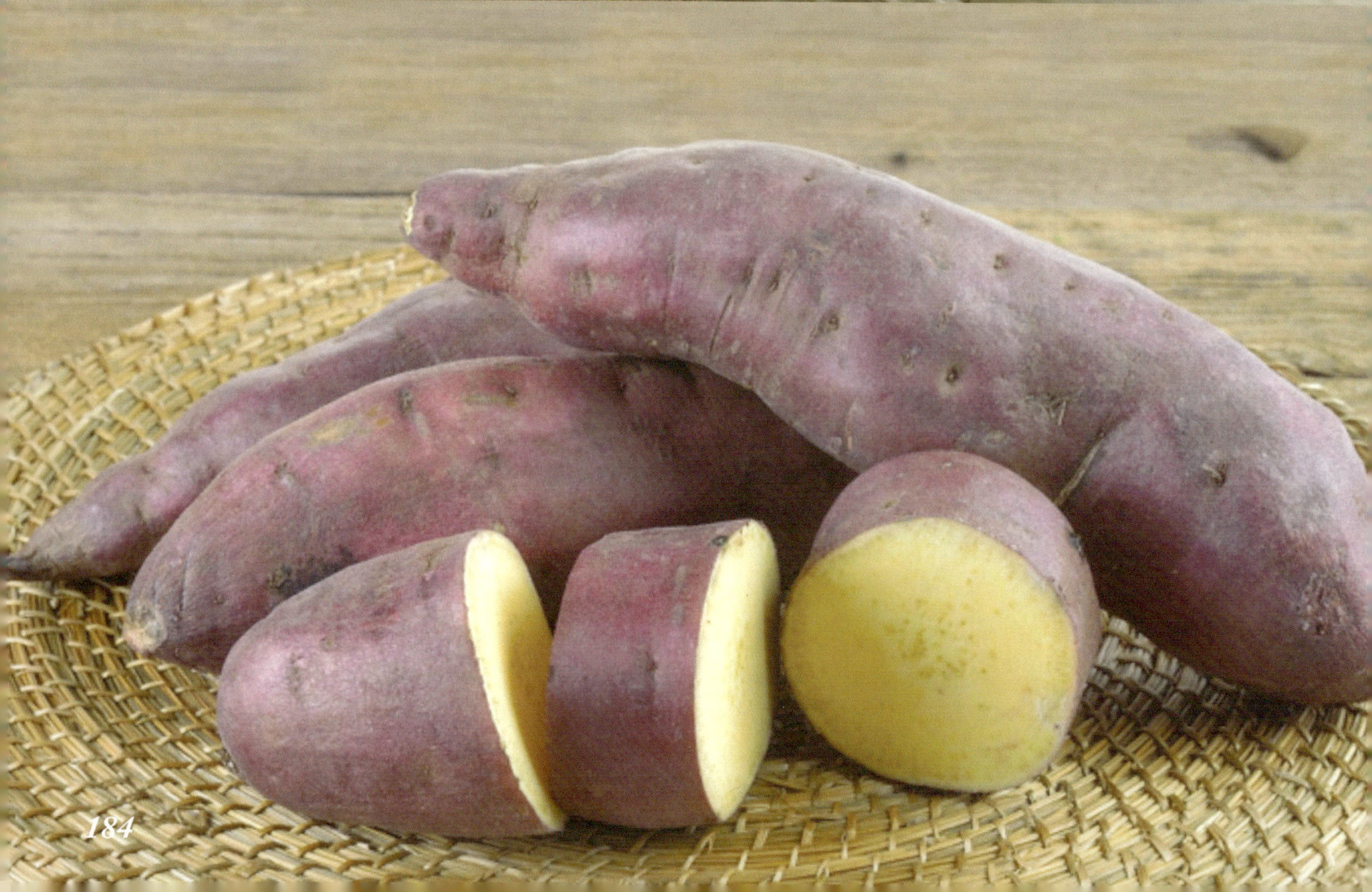

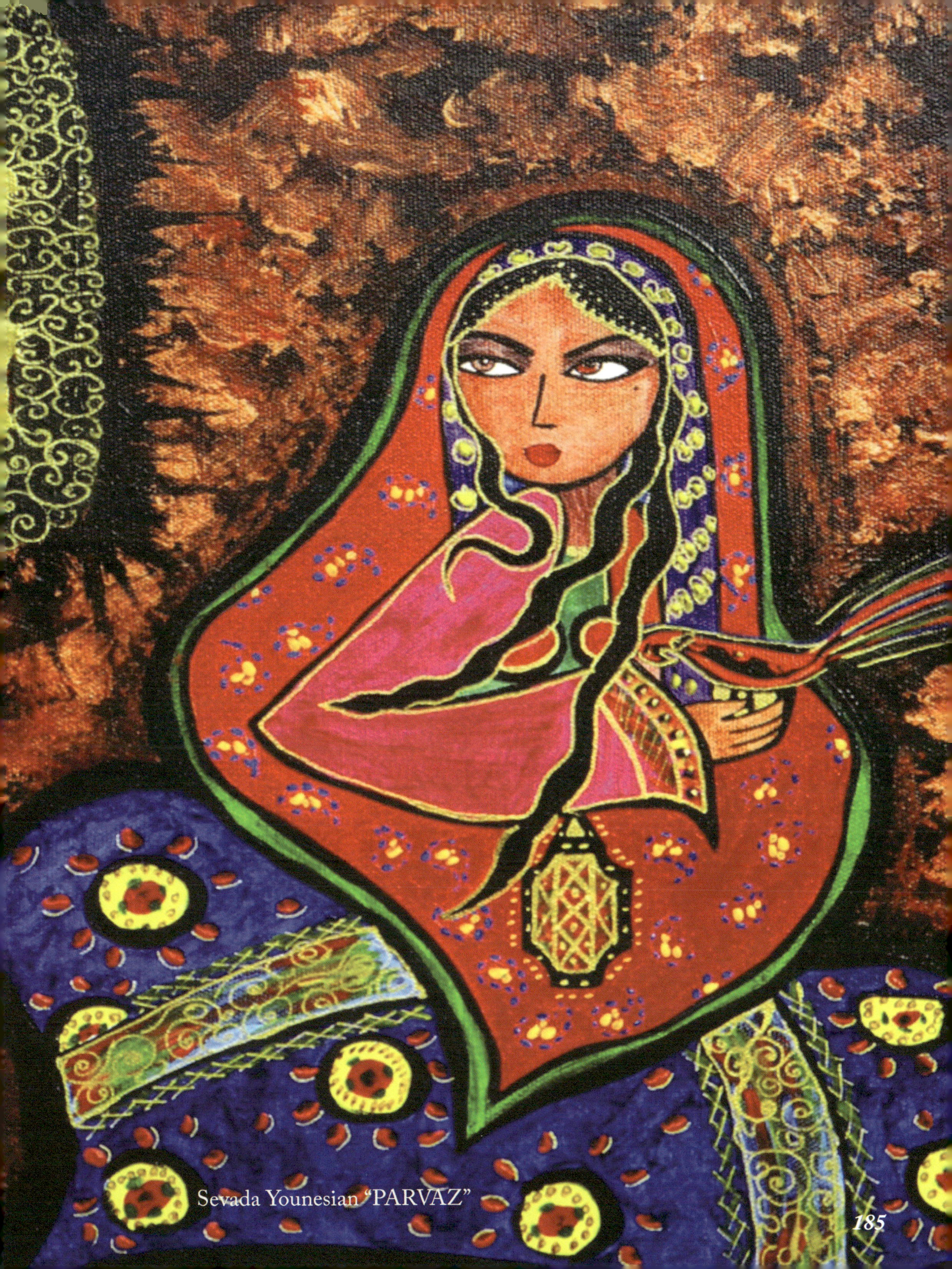

Sevada Younesian "PARVAZ"

BROKEN AND FRACTURED BONES

Turmeric works to reduce inflammation and heals both bone and muscle quickly. It's important to do the Turmeric Golden Milk every day too (page 36) so that you are also working from the inside out!

TURMERIC PASTE FOR HAIR FRACTURES

2 Tablespoons turmeric
1 Egg yolk

Mix turmeric and egg yolk well then paint on the inflamed area. Wrap with plastic wrap and cover with an Ace bandage for 2-day intervals. Reapply after each shower or bath. To heal the fracture continue for 4 to 5 weeks.

TURMERIC PASTE FOR SPRAINS

For ligament pain, inflammation, sprain.

2 Tablespoons turmeric
1/2 Teaspoon organic virgin coconut oil
1 Egg yolk (organic)

Mix well into a paste and apply all over the targeted area. (Make sure you put it on in the bathtub as turmeric stains.) Cover with plastic wrap, then Ace bandage. Leave on a day or two before reapplying.

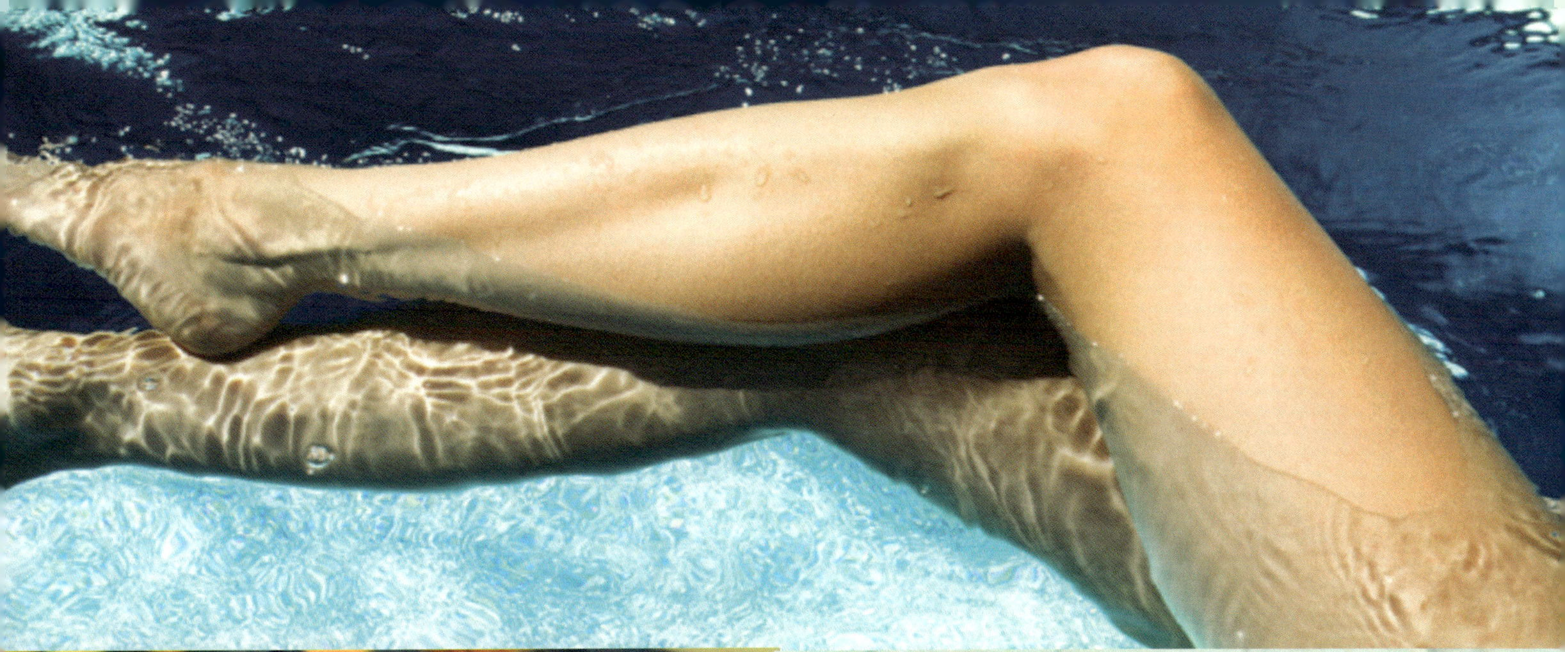

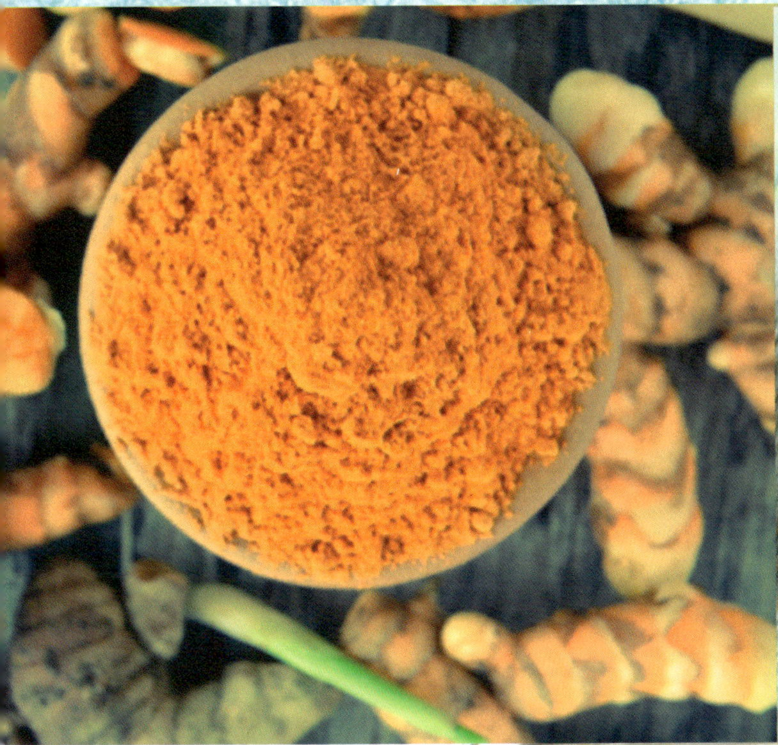

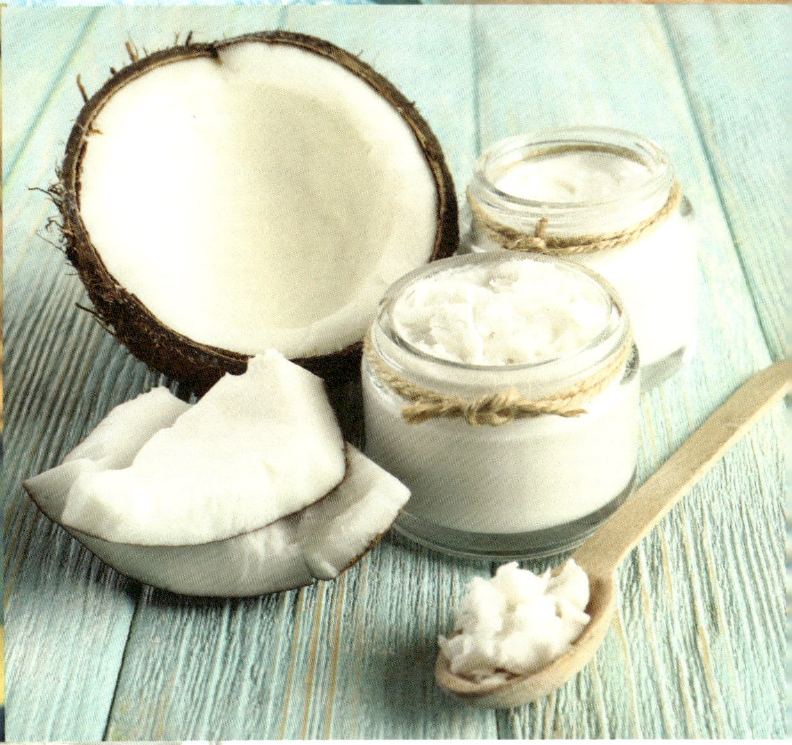

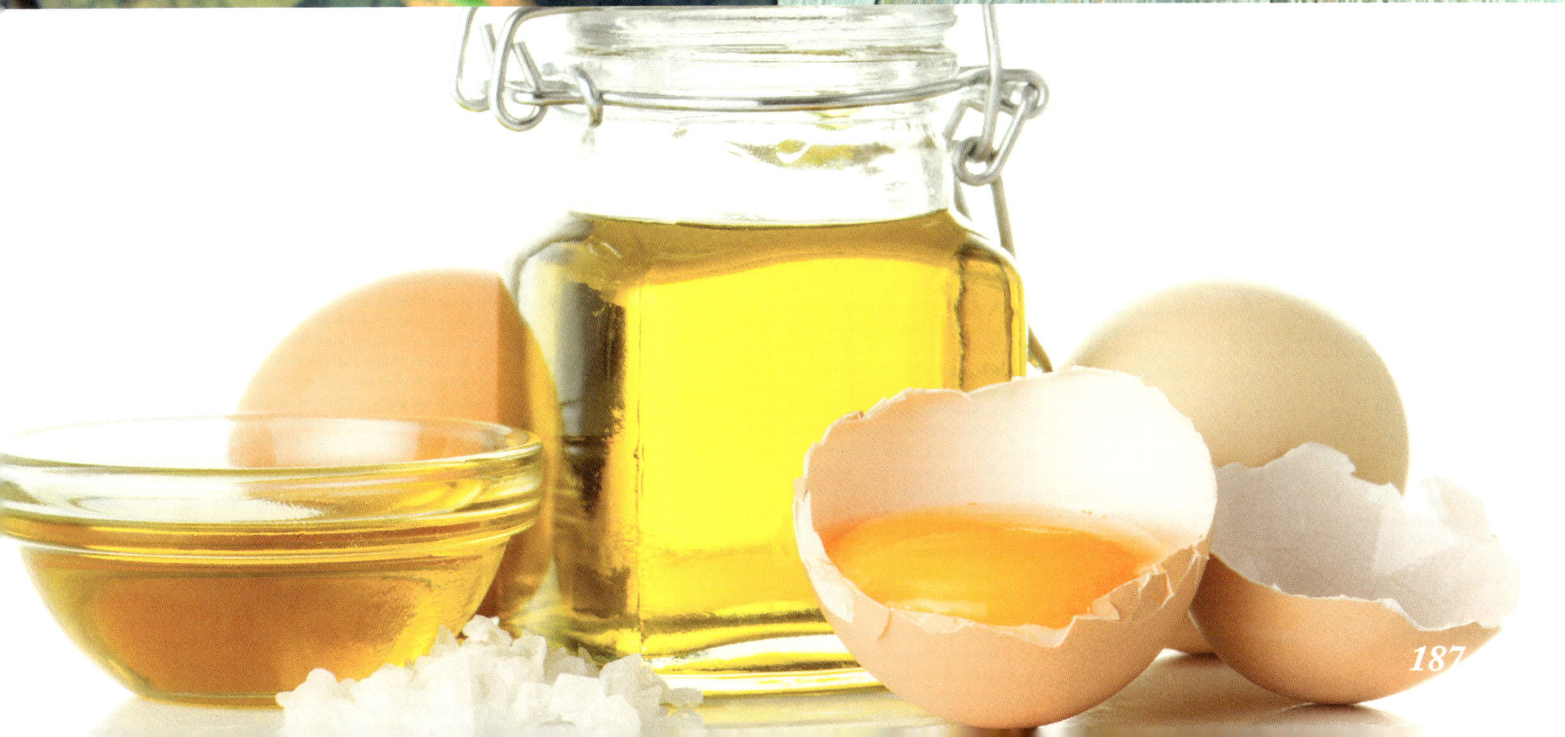

MEDICINAL HERBAL MOUTHWASH

This mouthwash is perfect during times when your gums need a little extra care. The antibacterial and astringent herbs in this recipe help disinfect, soothe inflammation and tighten tissue. I like to use this one as a medicinal preparation, rather than as a daily rinse.

Making your own herbal mouthwash is as easy as making tea, and allows you to avoid artificial colors, flavors, fluoride, sweeteners and other chemicals often found in commercial products. Using rose tea offers a wonderful astringent base to help tone your gums and keep them healthy, while the addition of tinctures lets you control and customize the medicinal potency you need, depending on your current oral health.

1 Cup organic rose bud or petal tea, brewed strong and cooled to room temperature
1 oz organic echinacea tincture
½ oz organic calendula tincture
¼ oz organic goldenseal tincture
¼ oz organic white oak bark tincture
¼ oz myrrh tincture

Mix together and store in a cool place. Swish in mouth for at least 3 minutes and spit out.

EVERYDAY HERBAL MOUTHWASH

This is a great recipe to use each day after you brush your teeth. The calendula, white oak bark, and myrrh are antibacterial, anti-inflammatory, and astringent to clean and protect.

1 Cup organic Rose bud or petal tea, brewed strong and cooled to room temperature
½ oz organic calendula tincture
¼ oz organic white oak bark tincture
¼ oz myrrh tincture

Mix all ingredients together in an amber bottle and store in the refrigerator for one to two weeks, unless it starts to get funky sooner. The alcohol and refrigeration should preserve it for quite a while, though I don't know for sure how long since I use a batch within a week. If your teeth are sensitive to cold, you can mix it with a little hot water to warm. Swish a mouthful or two each day for at least for 1minute and then spit out. For a fresher flavor, add a few drops of peppermint flavoring extract.

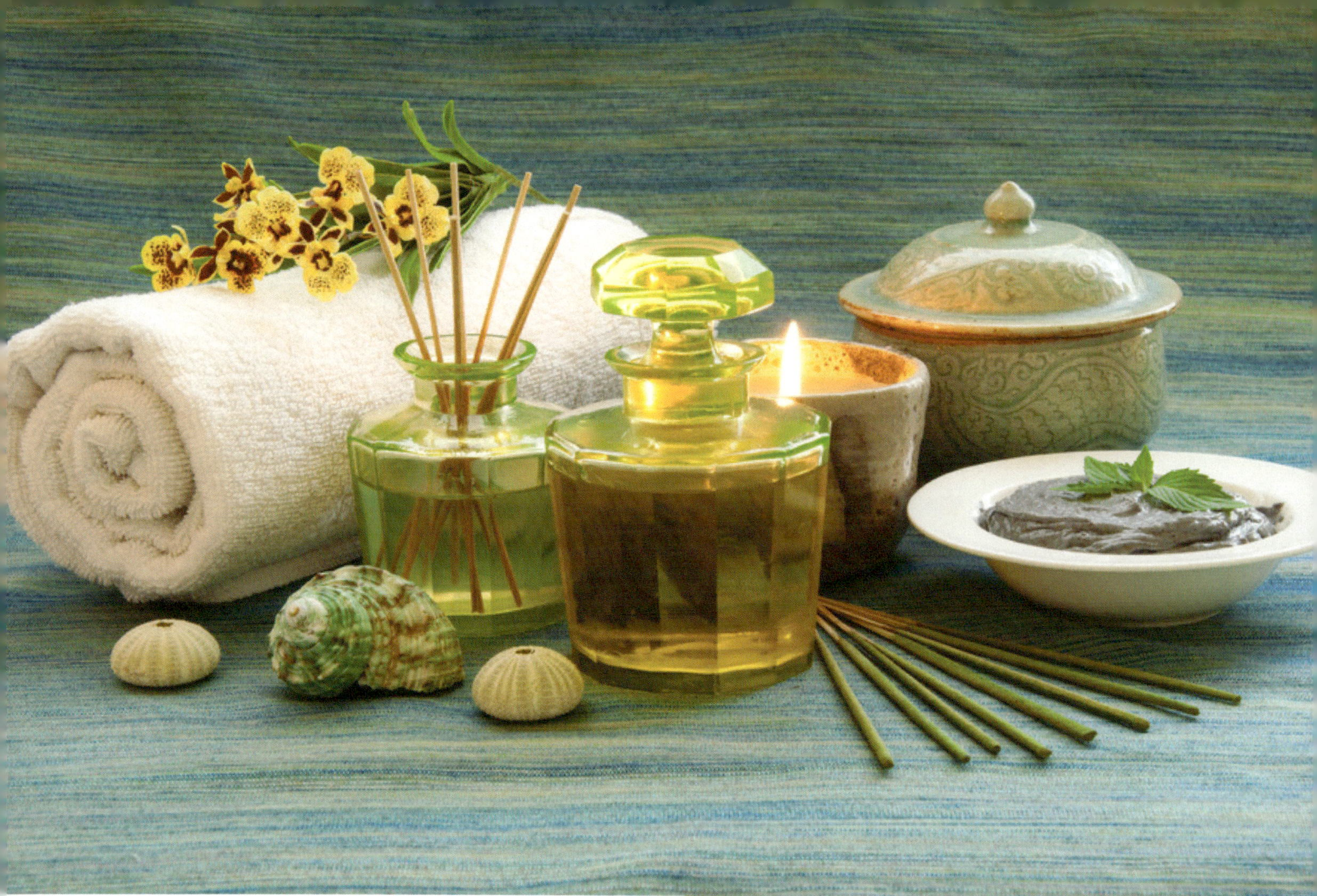

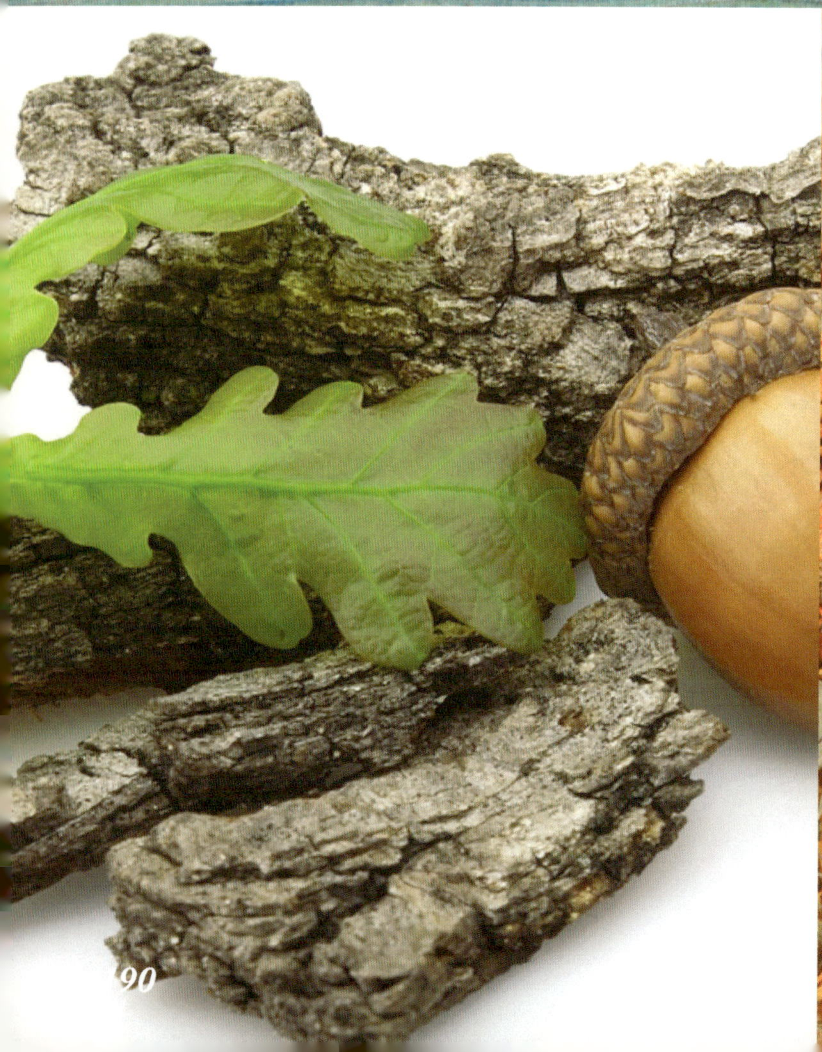

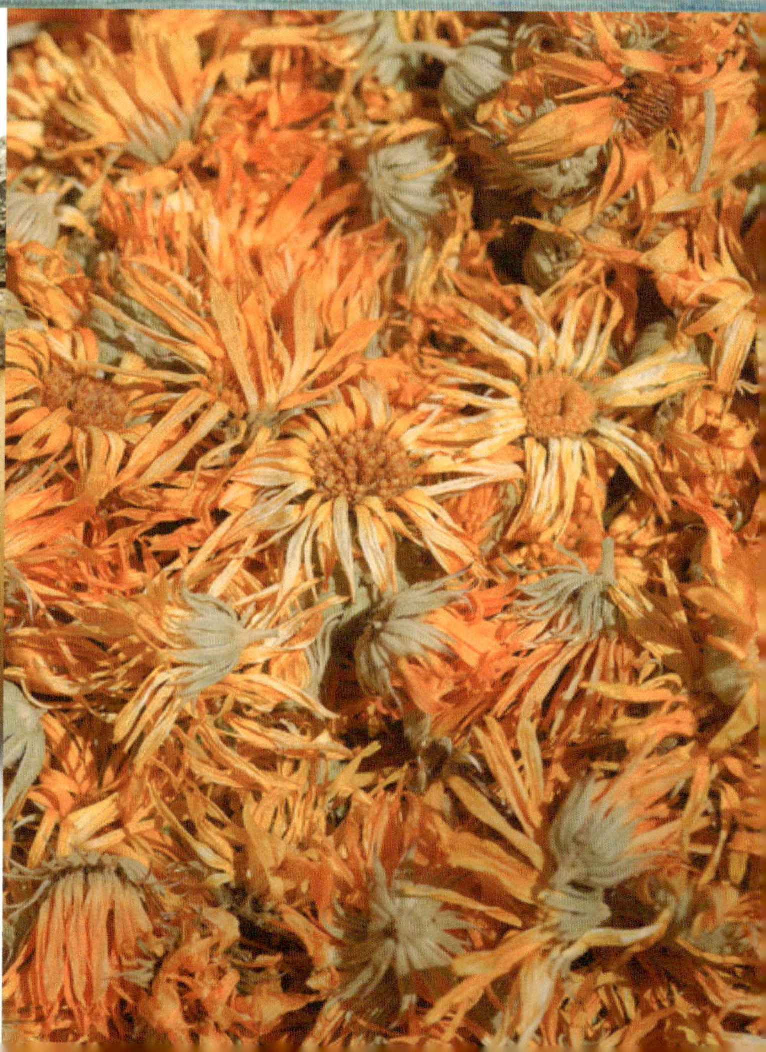

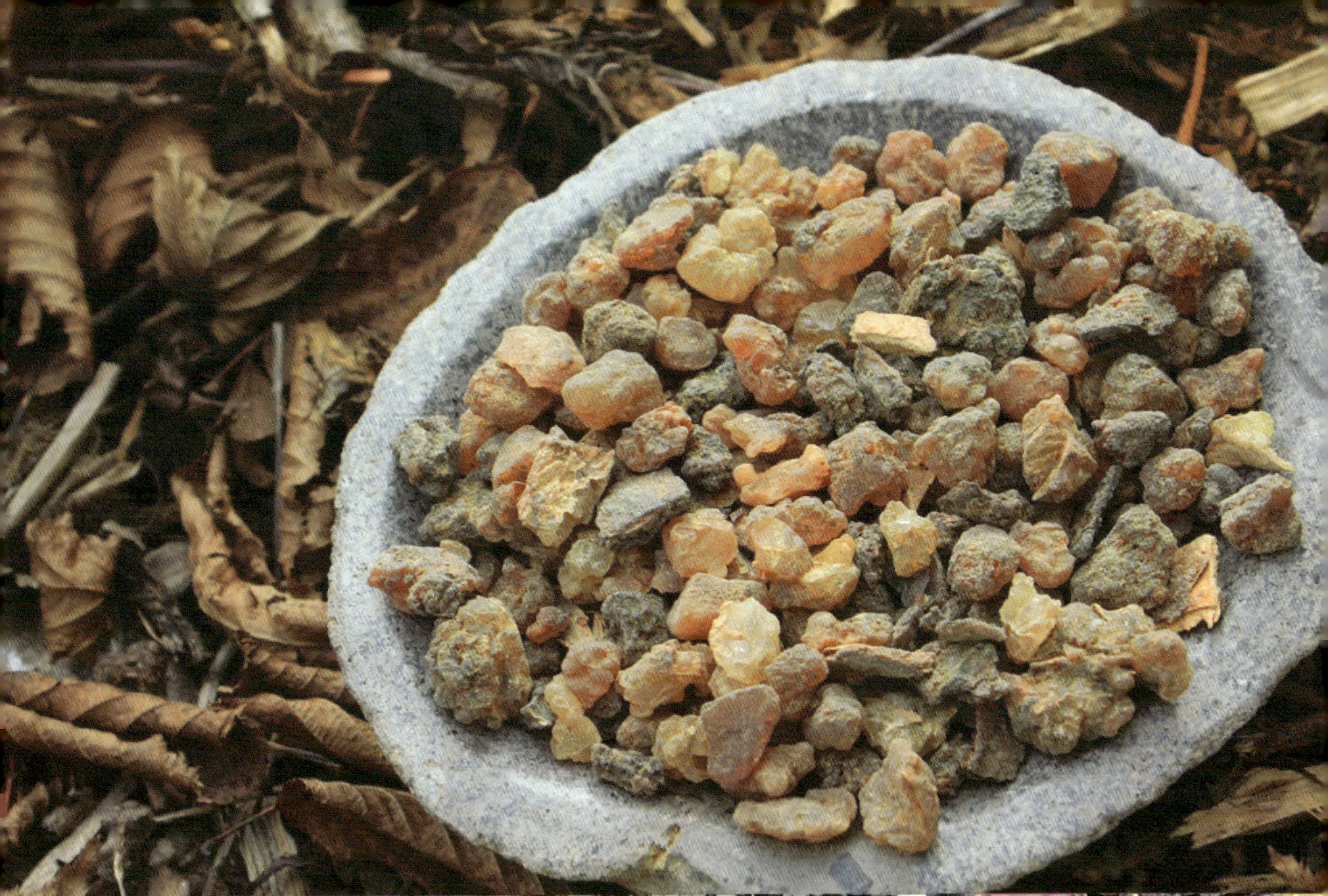

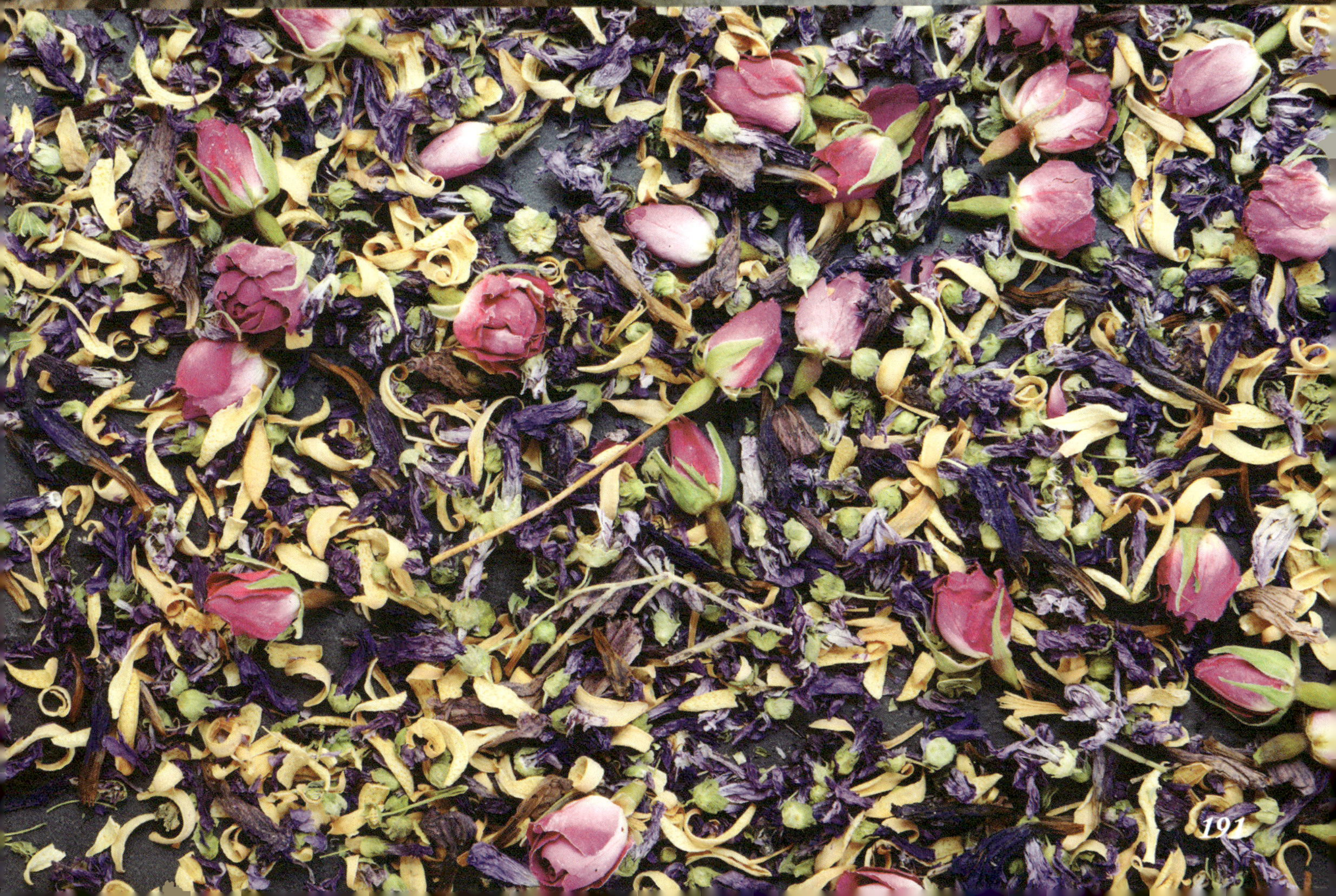

BAKING SODA

Baking soda has been used since ancient times by the Egyptians, 7,000 years ago, and in ancient Persia. In the old days they called it Soda Ash.

The ancient Egyptians used natural deposits of natron, a mixture consisting mostly of sodium carbonate decahydrate, and sodium bicarbonate. Like turmeric, baking soda has many diverse uses and applications. It alkalizes the body, purifies water, helps constipation, hangovers, headaches and is also known as a cancer cure in a special application.

CANCER CURE

Every morning upon rising and 45 minutes before breakfast drink a large glass of cold filtered water with one teaspoon of apple cider vinegar half a lemon and 1/4 teaspoon of baking soda (non GMO.)

TIRED FEET

1/2 Cup baking soda
1/4 Cup sea salt
Warm water
Soak your feet for 30 minutes or longer. It will sooth your feet, relax you and draw toxins out of your body.

SOOTHING BATH

1 Cup baking soda
1/2 Cup sea salt
Pour in your tub and soak for 30 minutes. Make sure you drink a large glass of water when you get out of the tub.

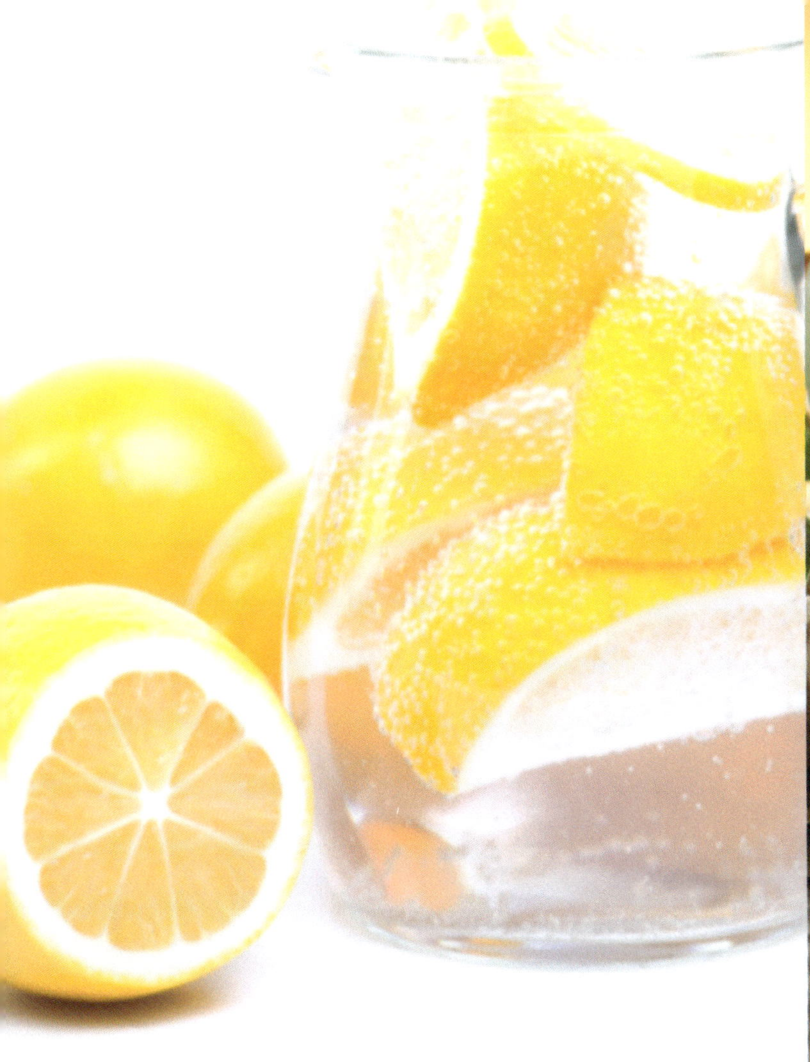
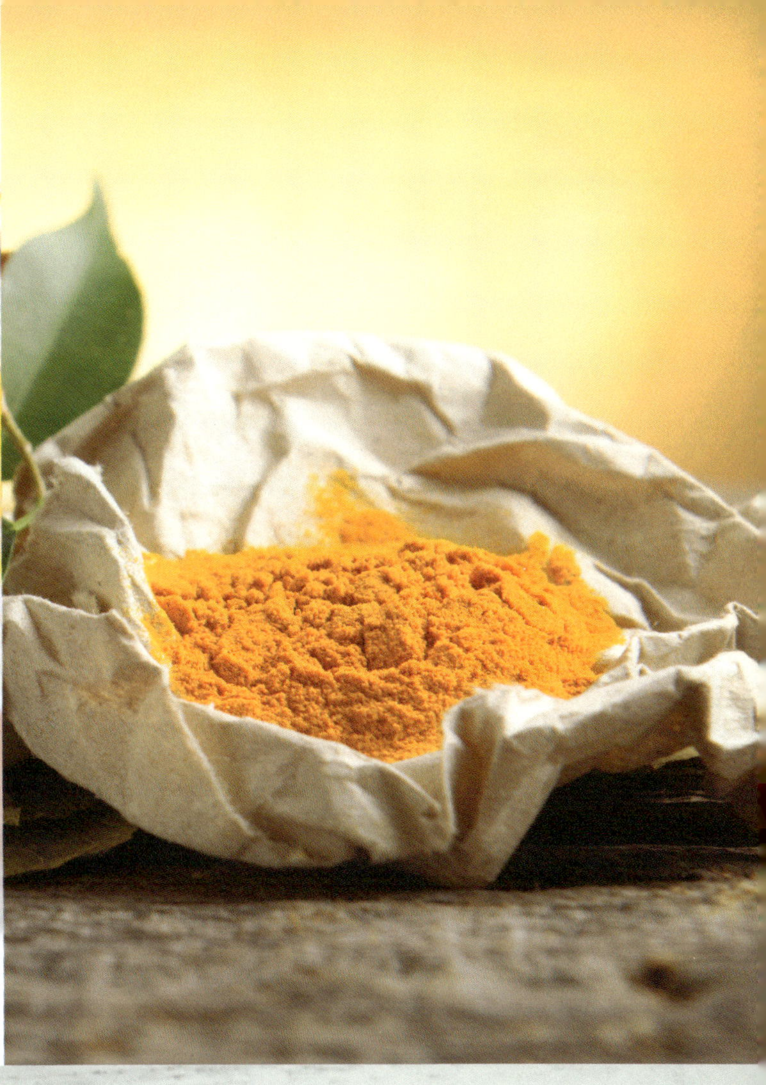
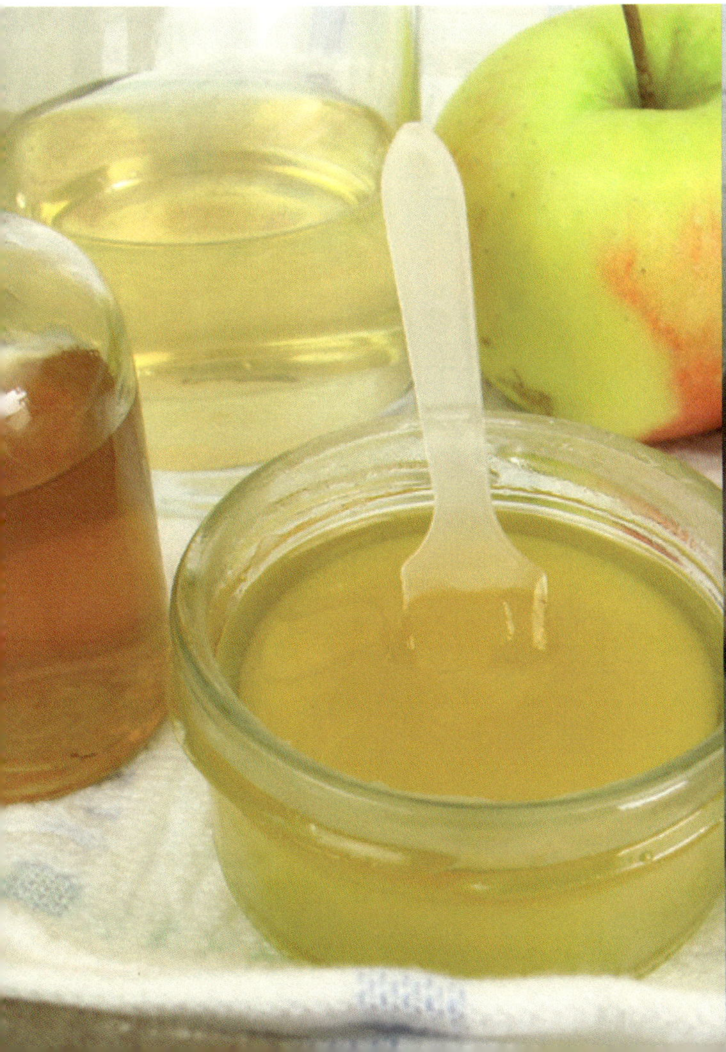
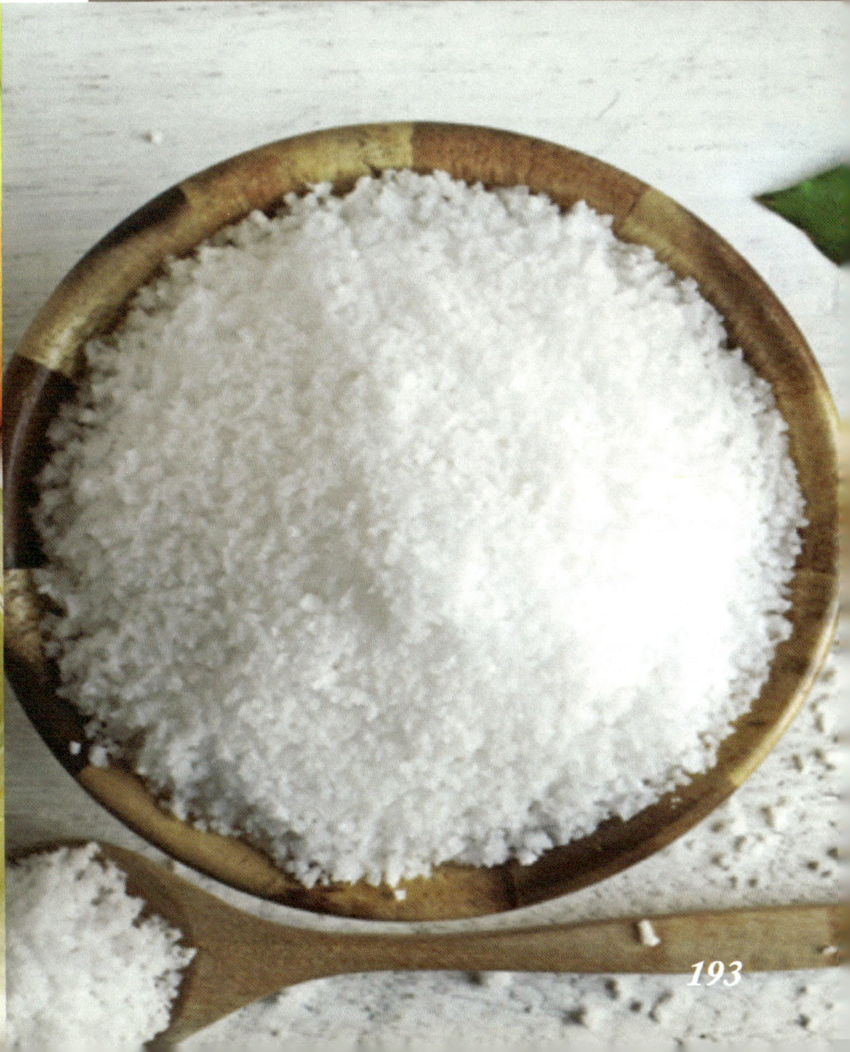

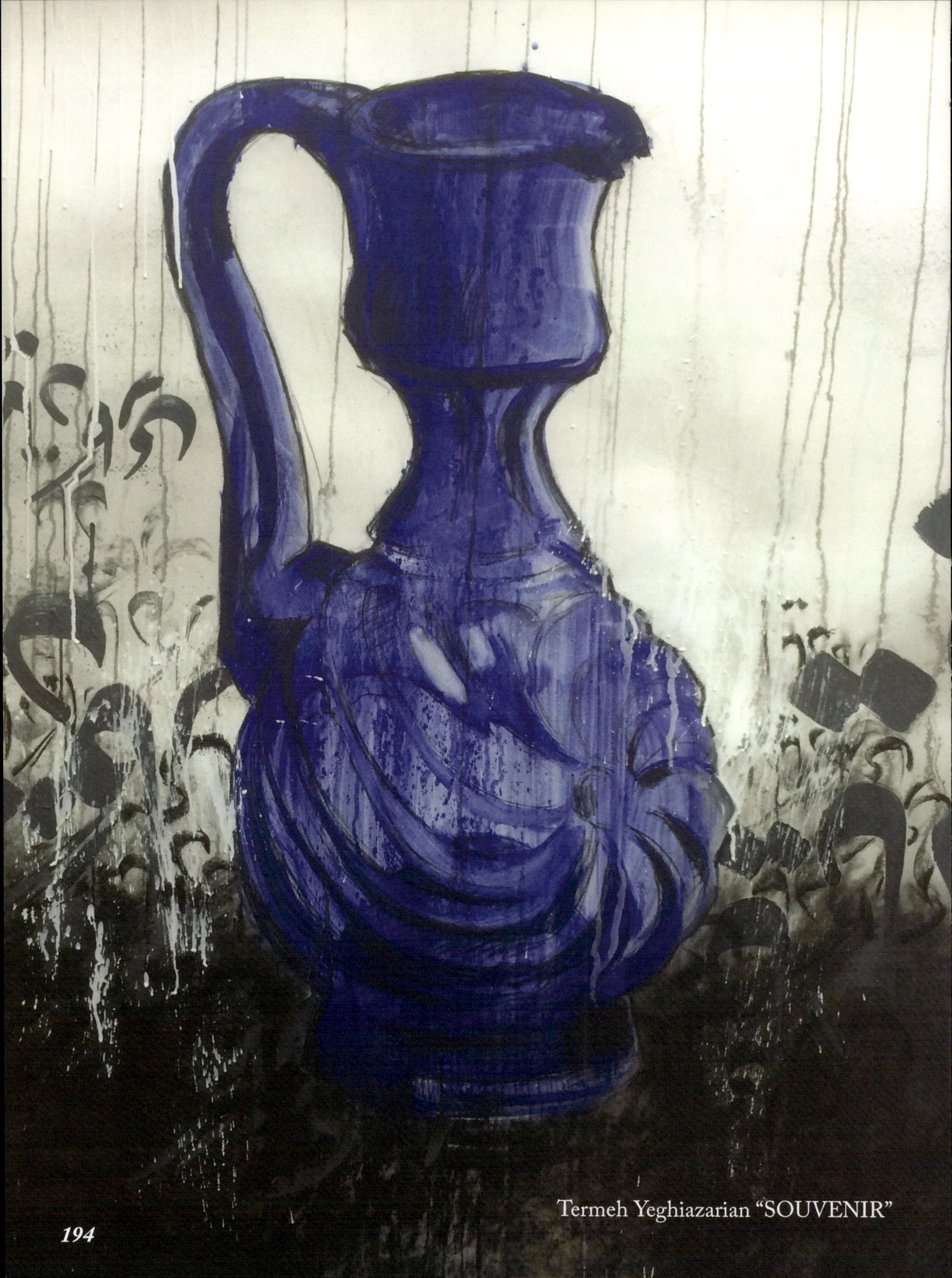

Termeh Yeghiazarian "SOUVENIR"

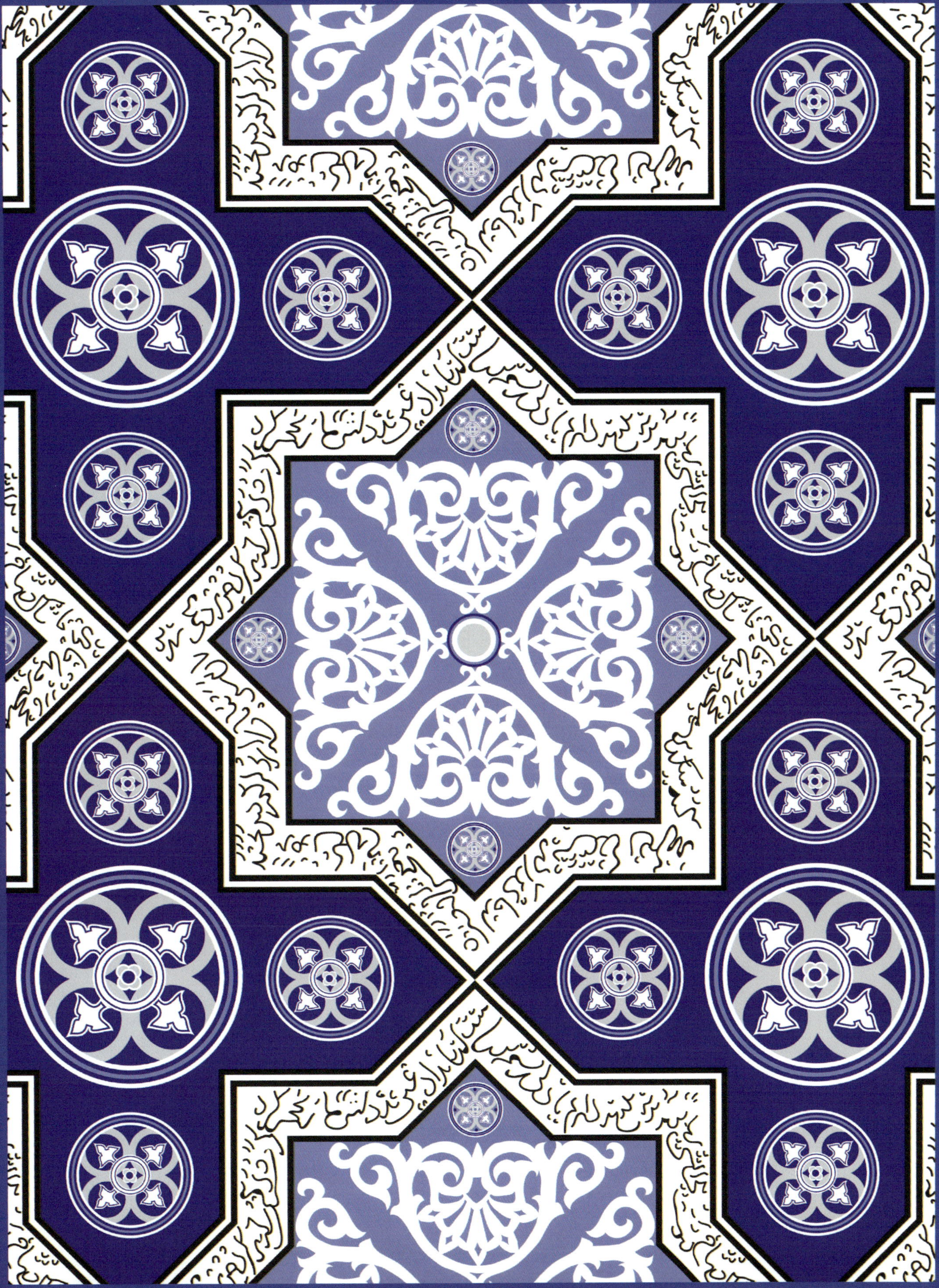

FACE MASK

Tightens the skin, shrinks pores and freshens the skin

2 Tablespoons full-fat (preferably raw) yogurt
1 Teaspoon baking soda

Mix well. When it starts to fizz brush evenly on your décolleté neck and face. Lay down and relax for 30 minutes. You will feel your skin tighten and tingle. Remove with lukewarm water followed with cold water.

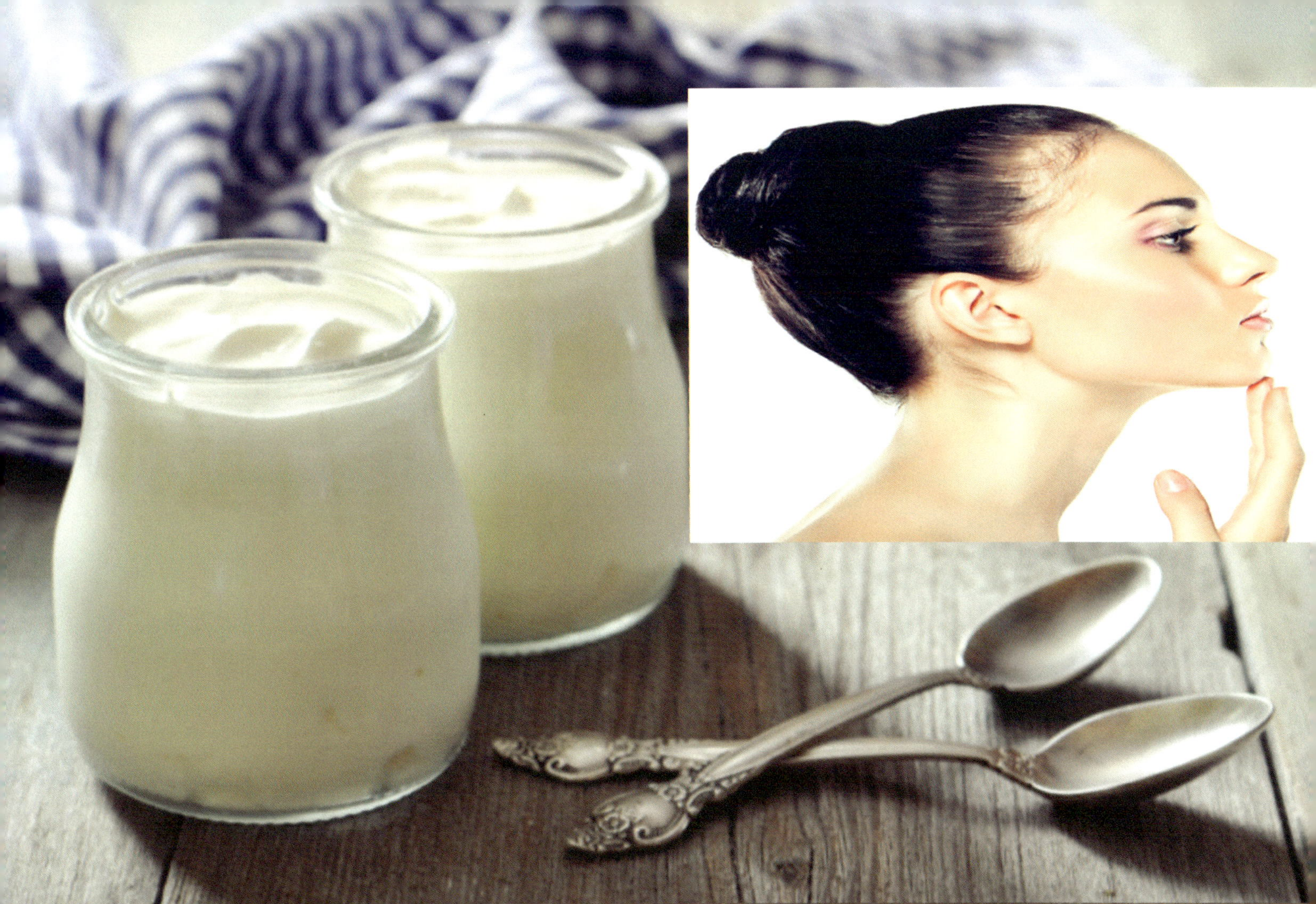

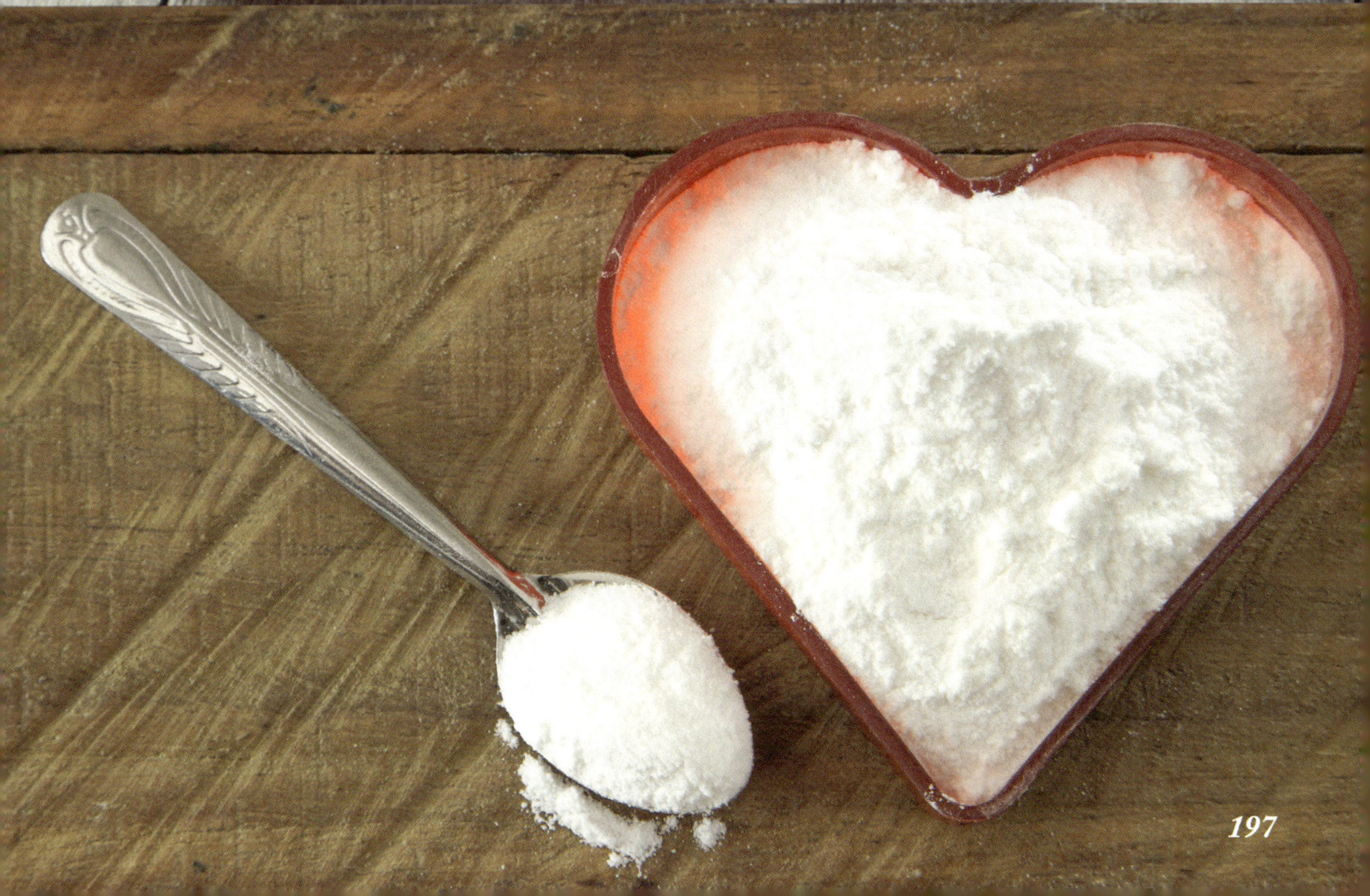

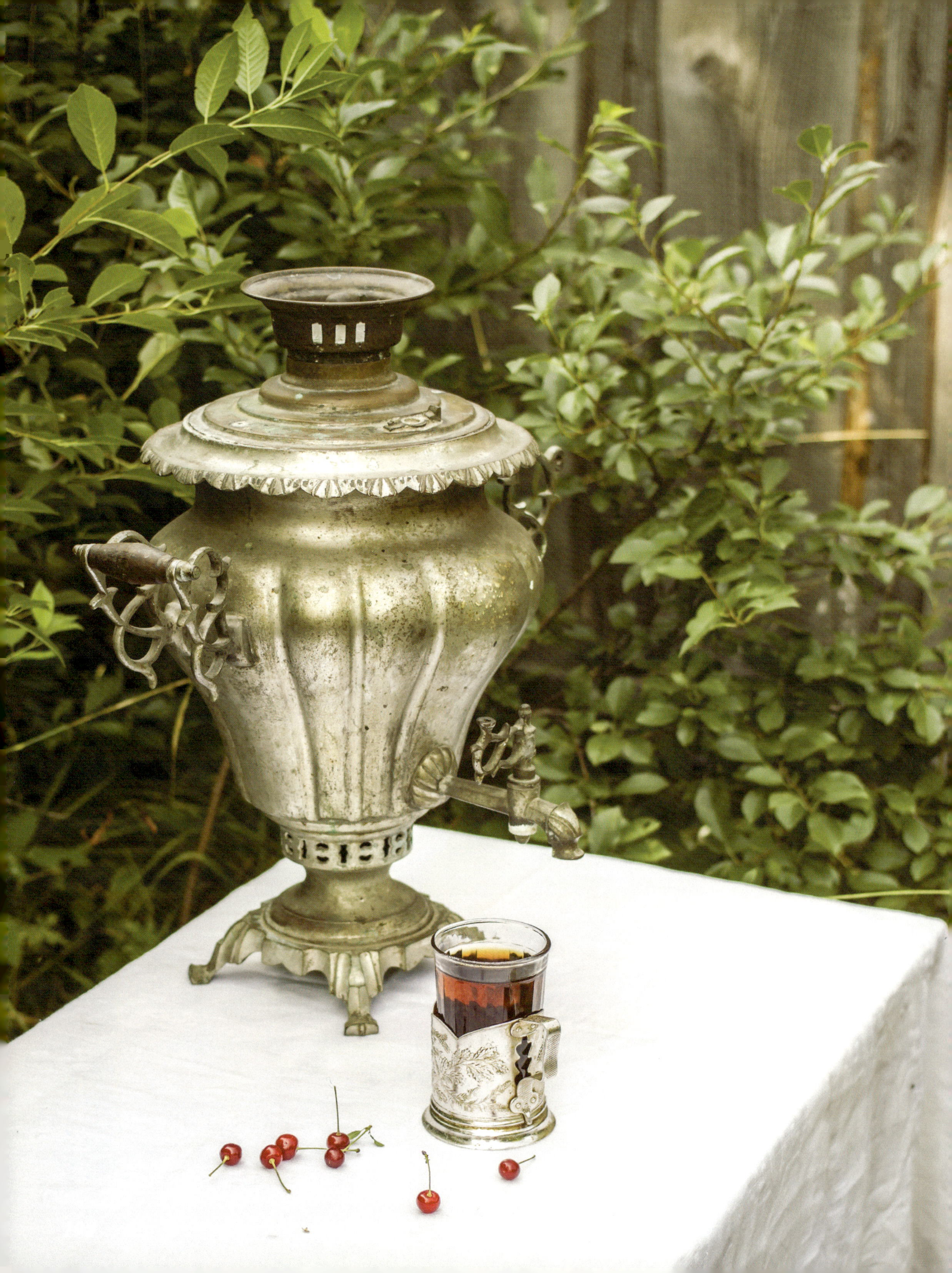

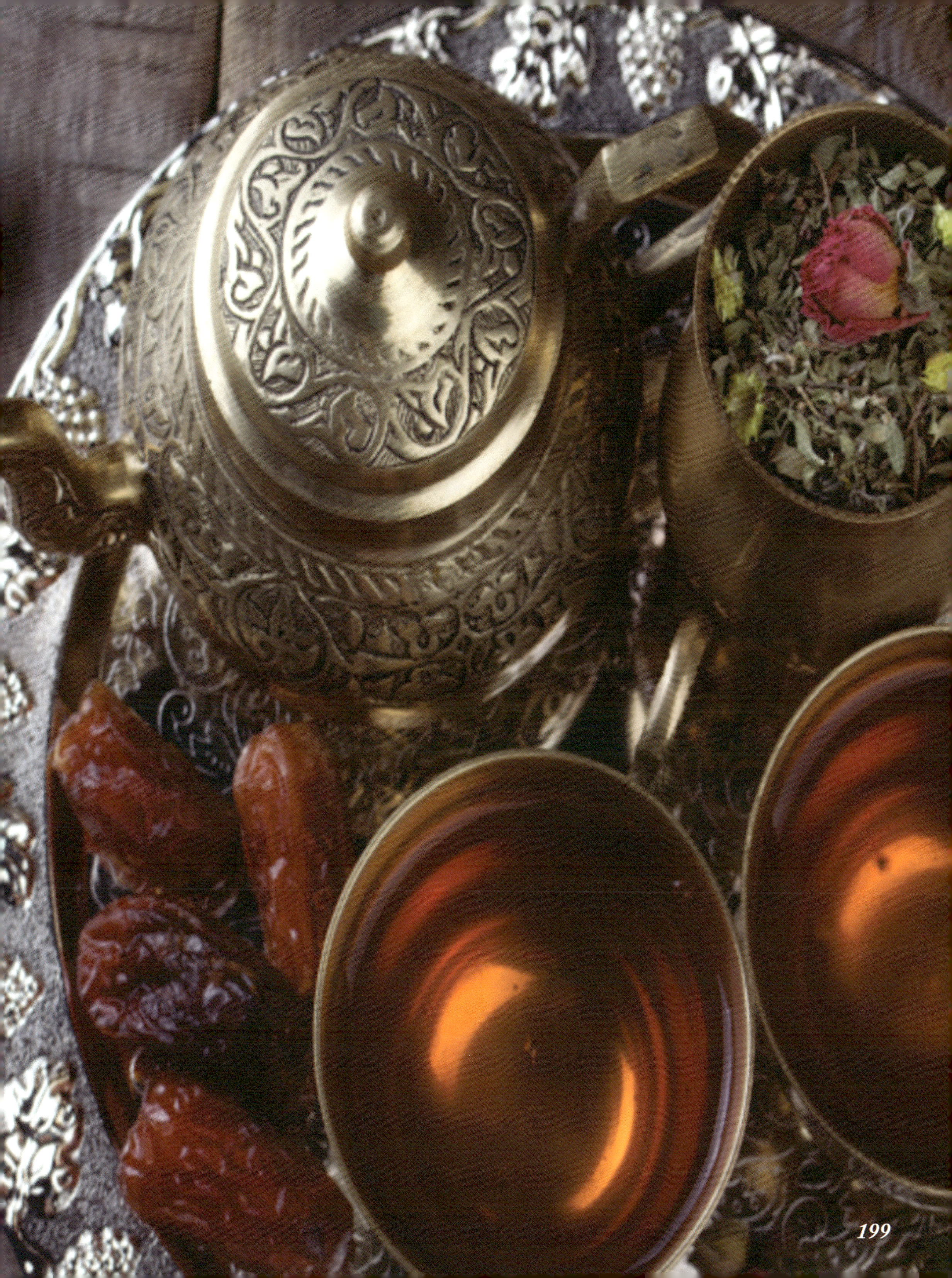

TEAS

CINNAMON TEA

For longevity

2 Medium cinnamon sticks (from Ceylon or Viet Nam)
Filtered water

Place the cinnamon sticks in a teapot and pour boiling water into it. Let it brew for 10 to 15 minutes.

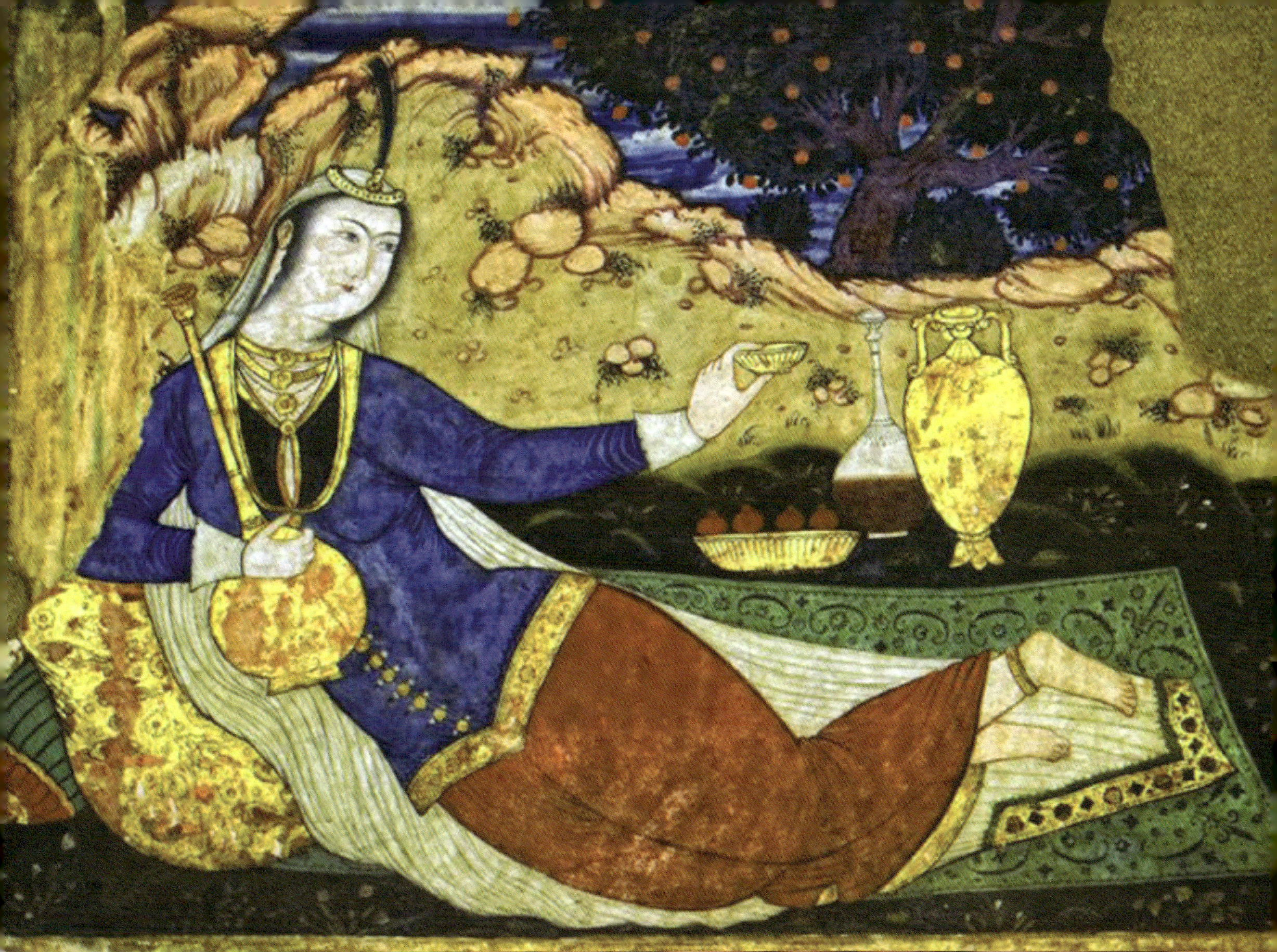

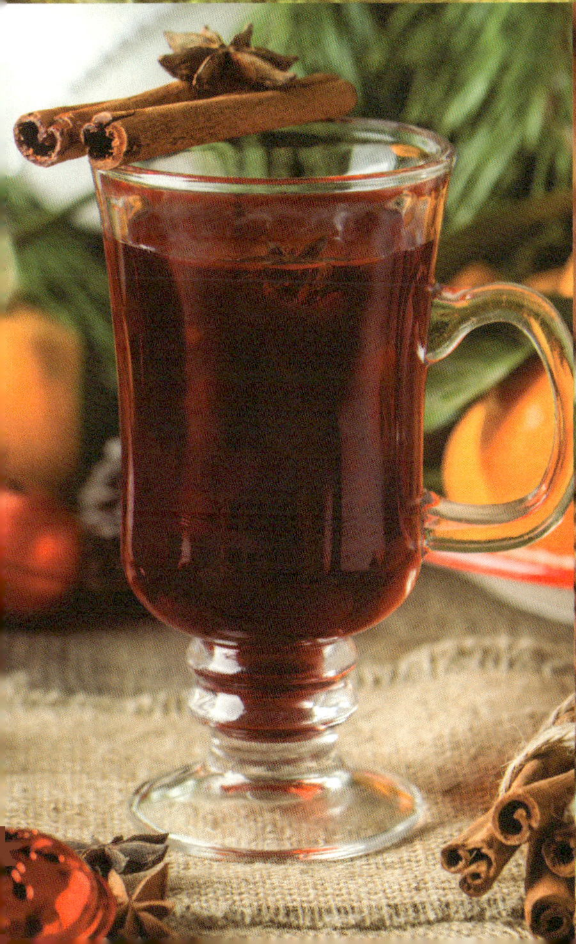

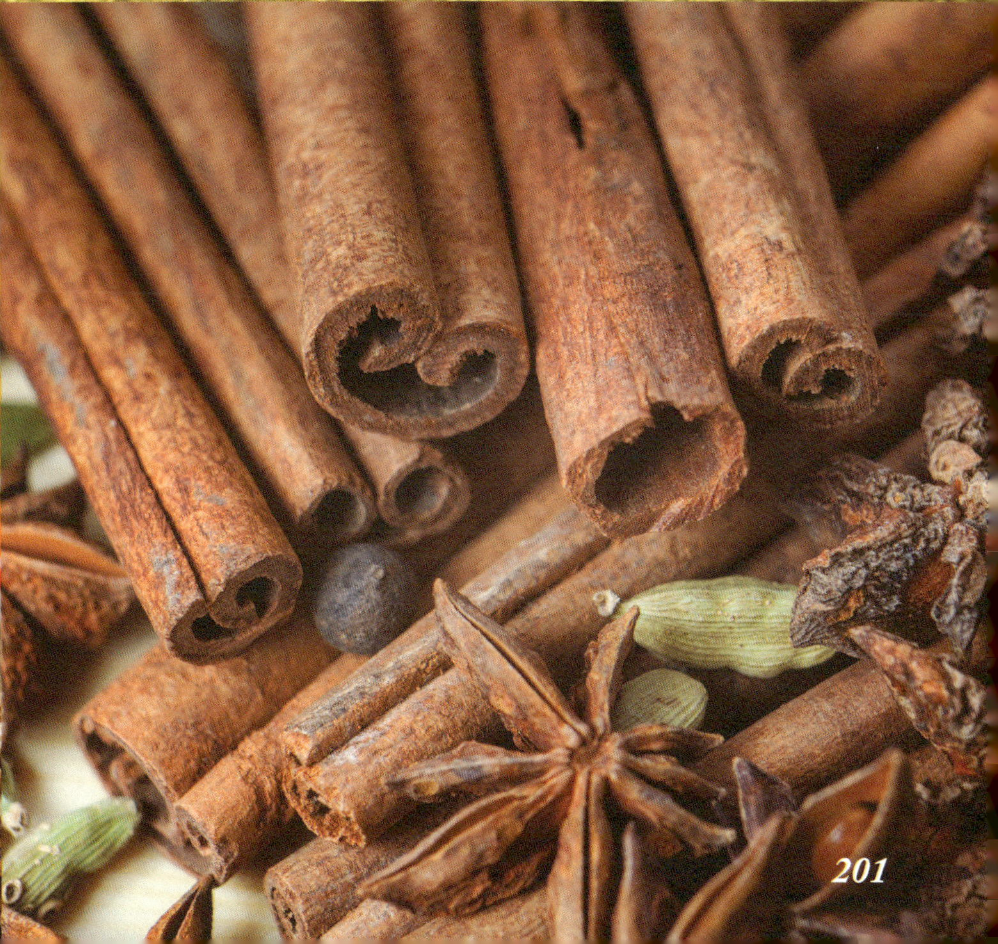

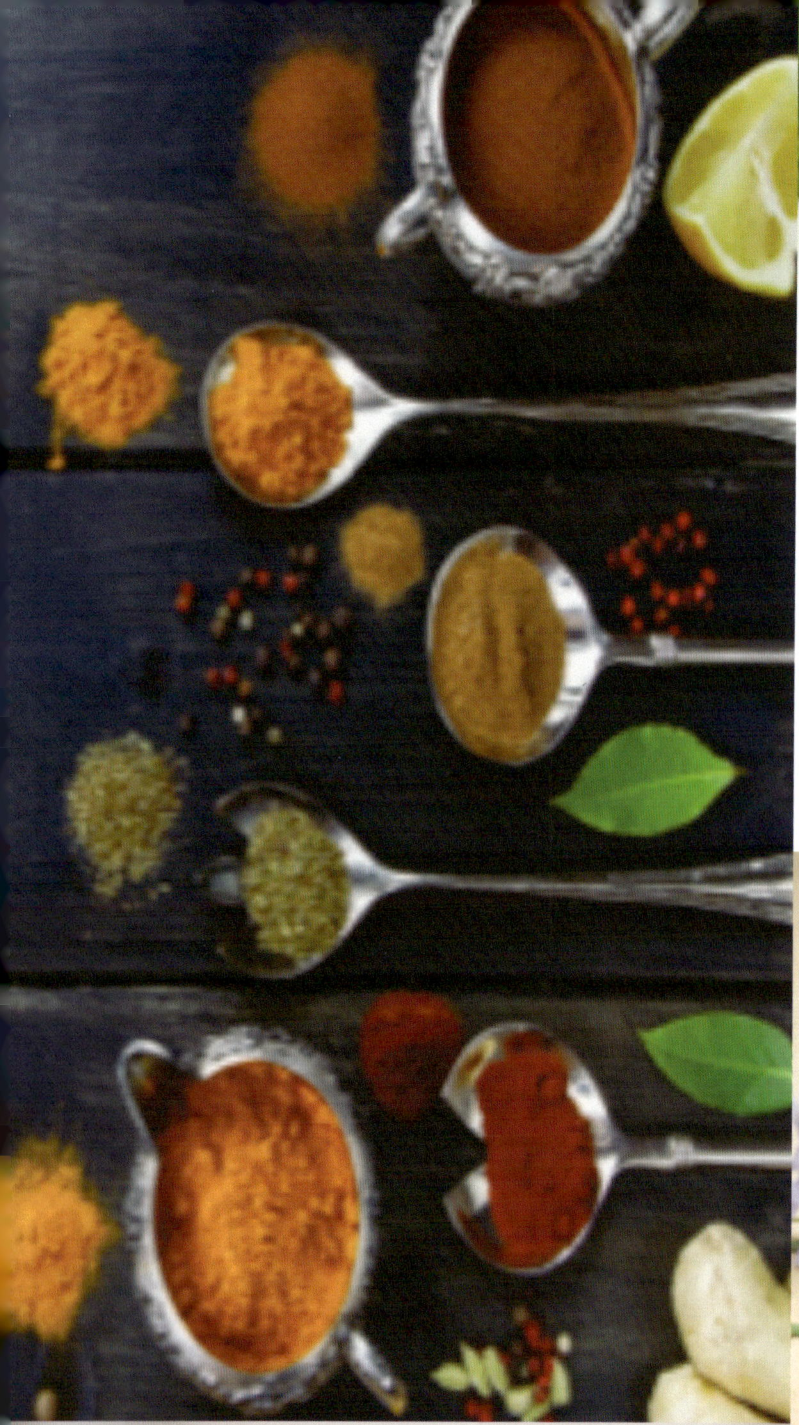

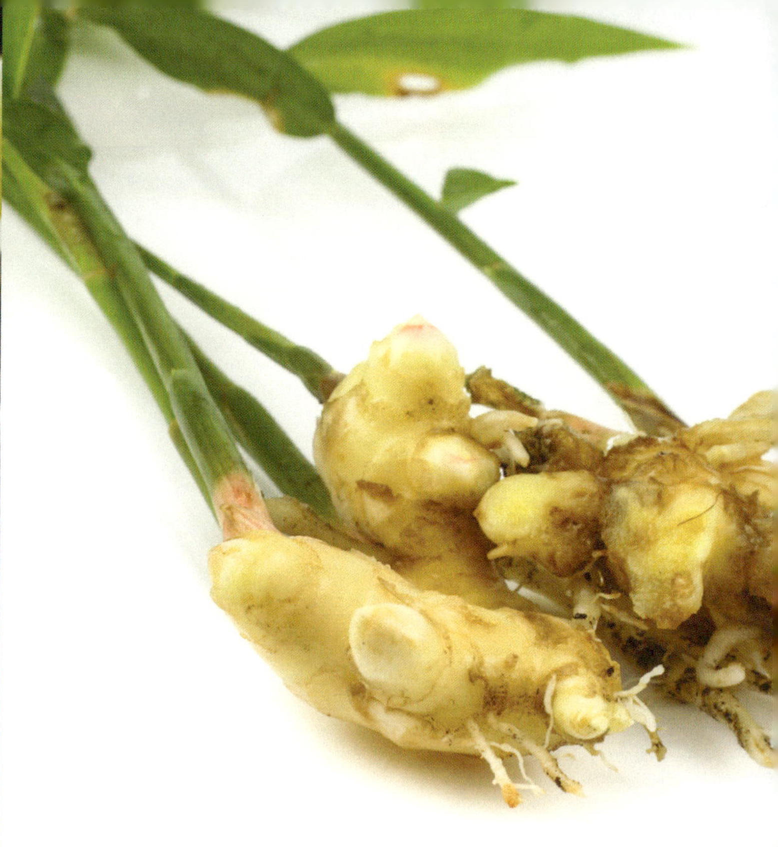

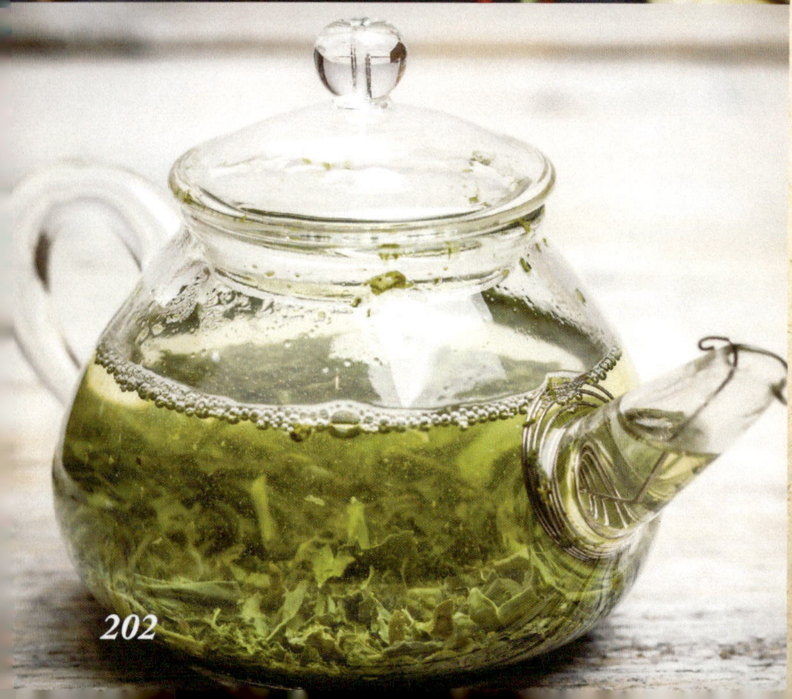

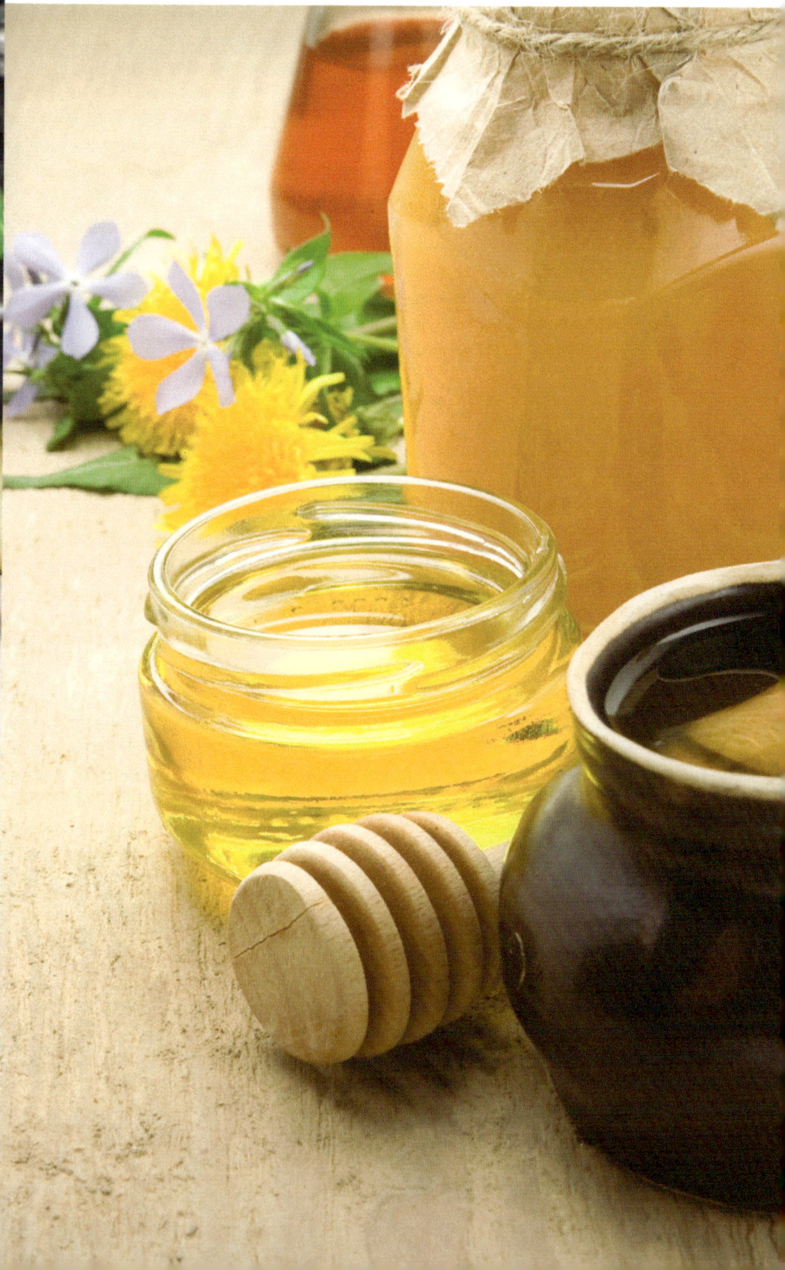

TURMERIC TEA

Pot of black or green tea
1 Teaspoon ground turmeric
1 Teaspoon raw honey or Manuka honey
3 Slices ginger root
3 peppercorns

Stir last three ingredients into black or green tea. Drink 3 or 4 times a day for relief of flu, cold and to detox.

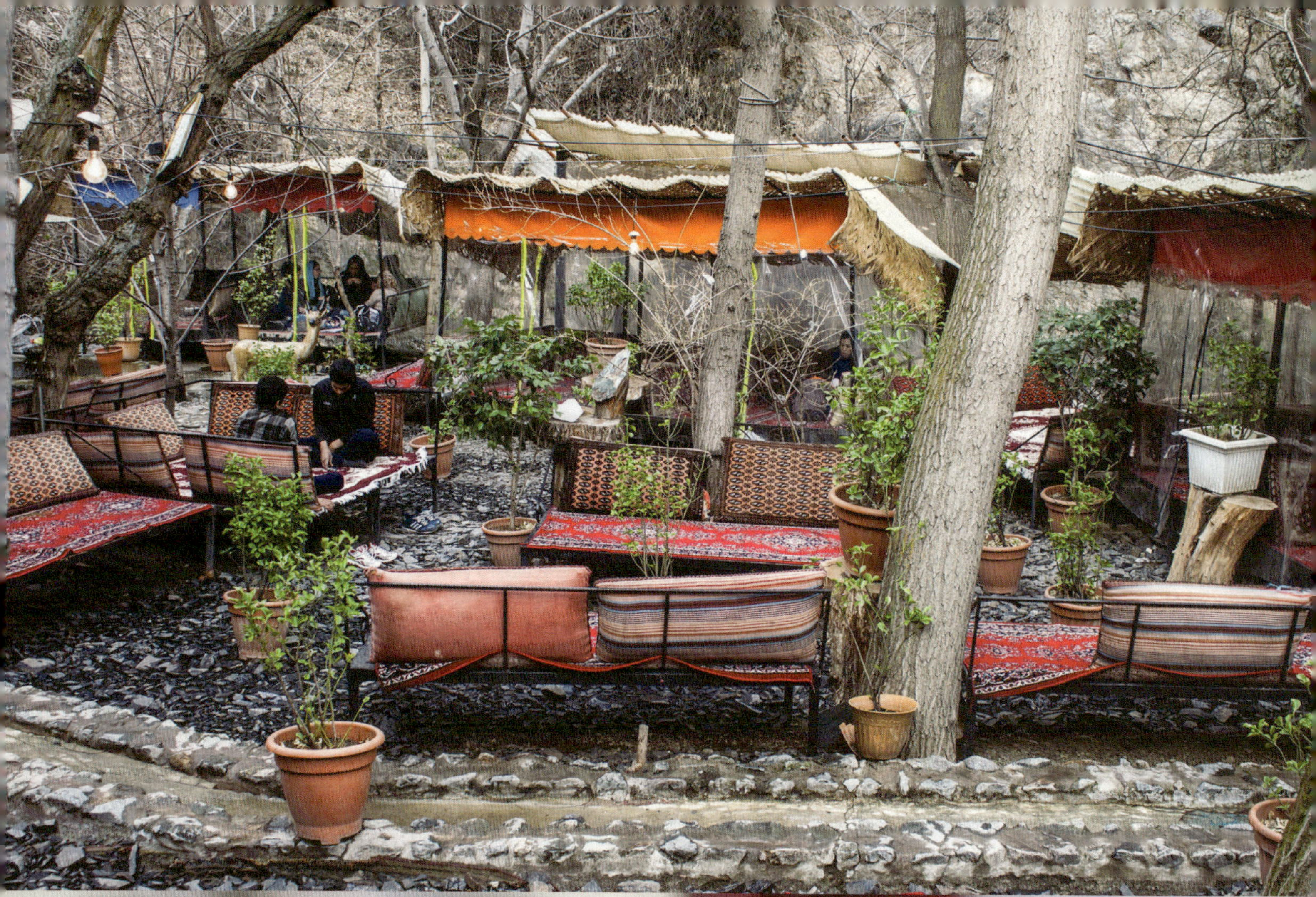

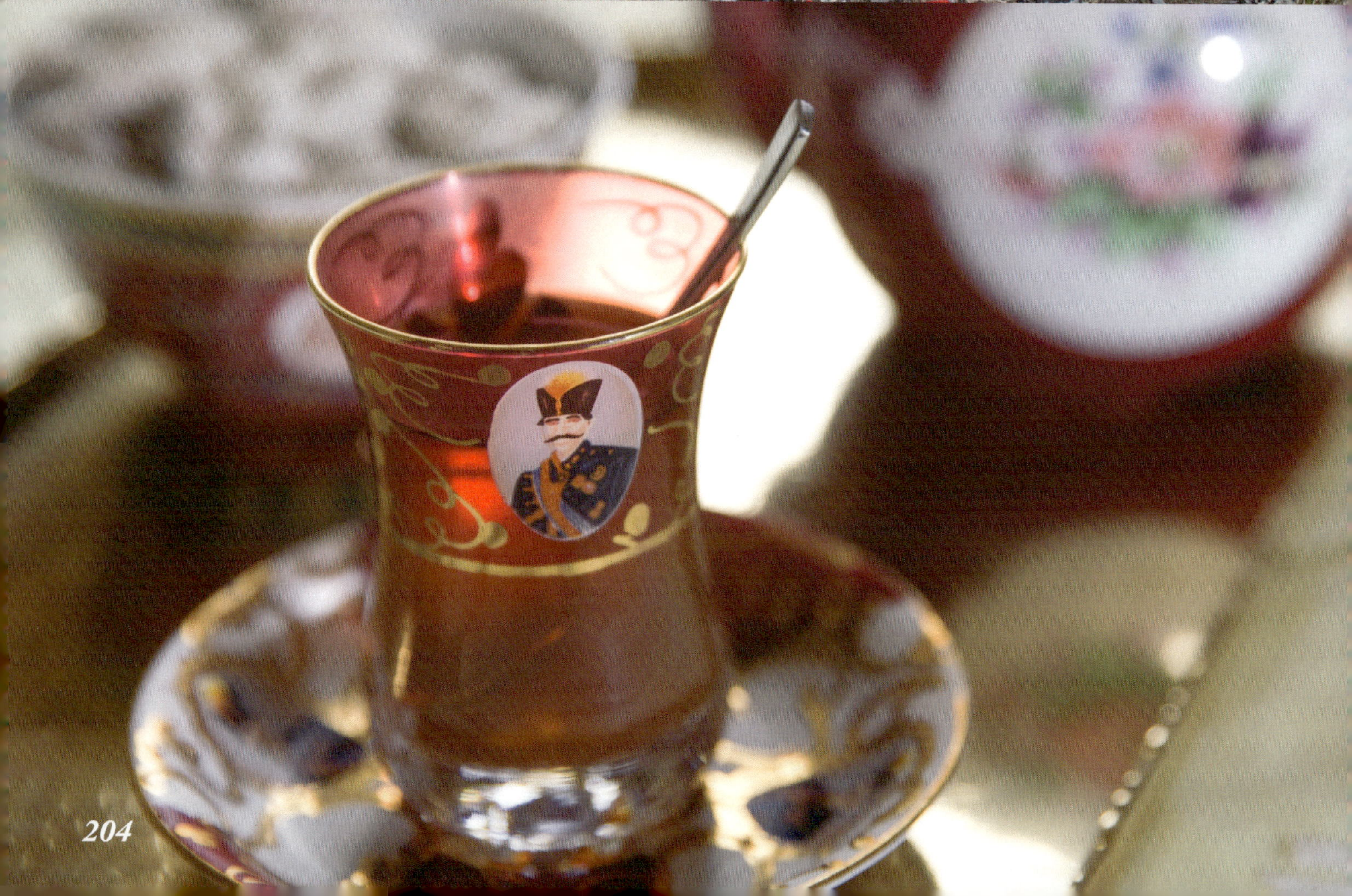

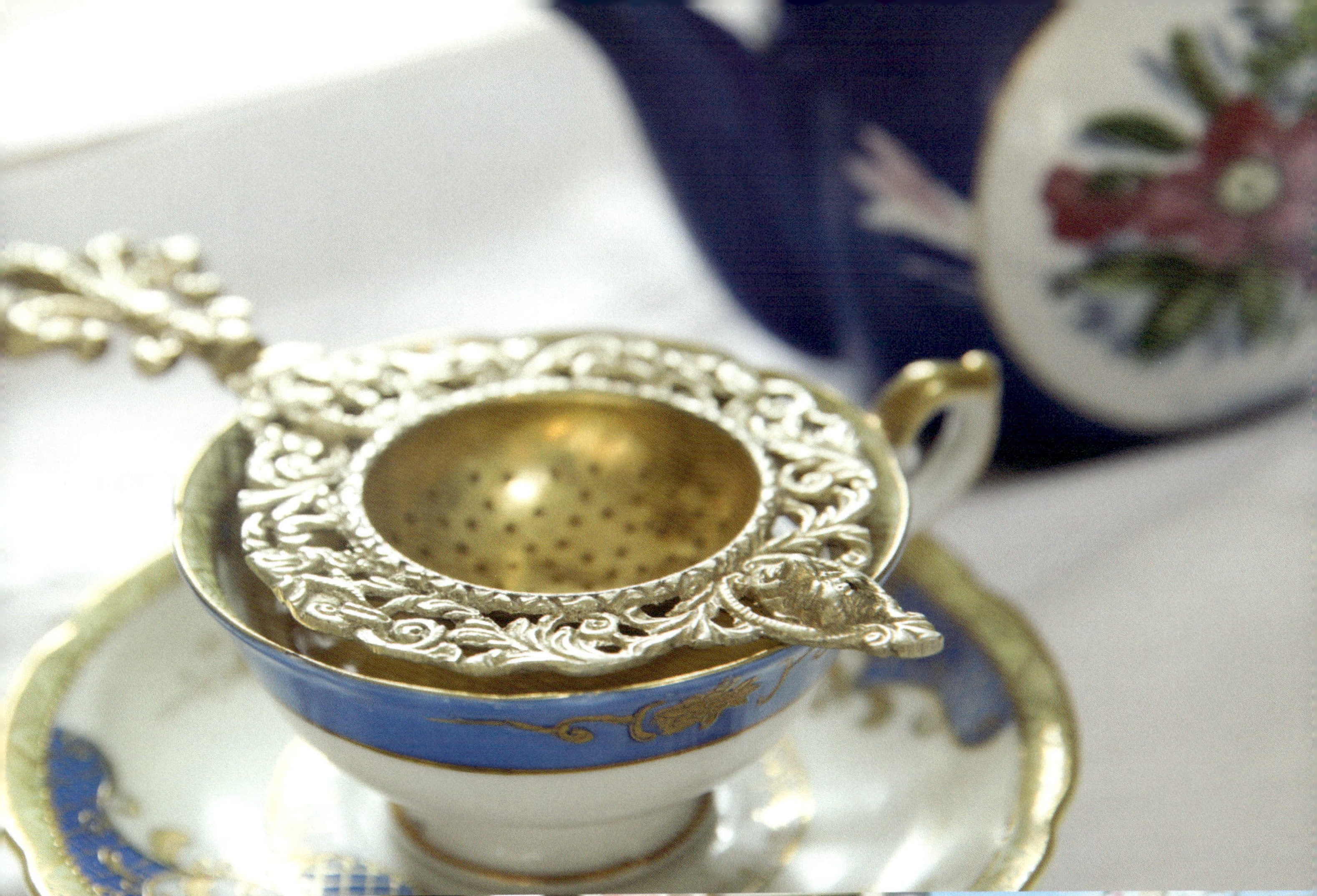

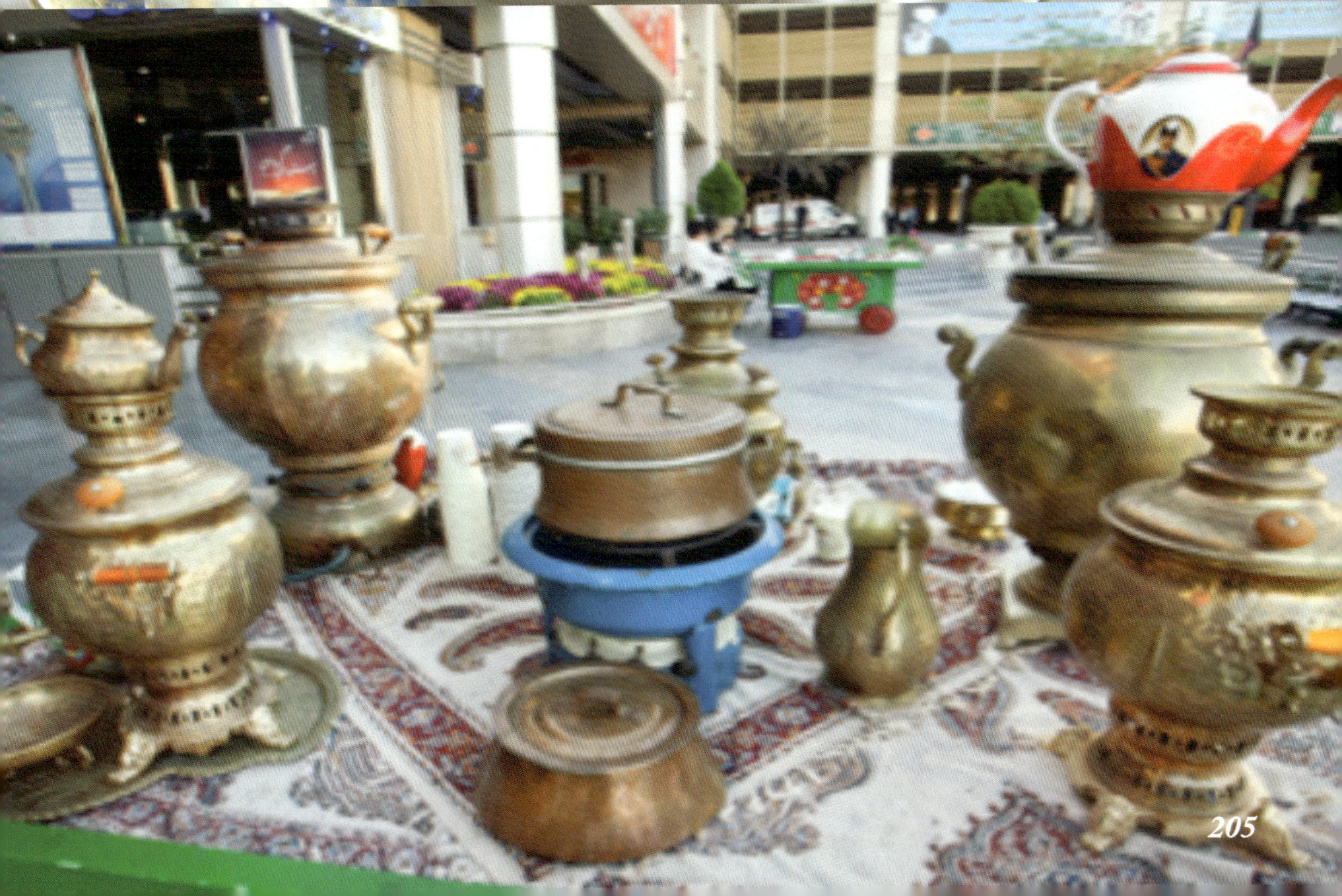

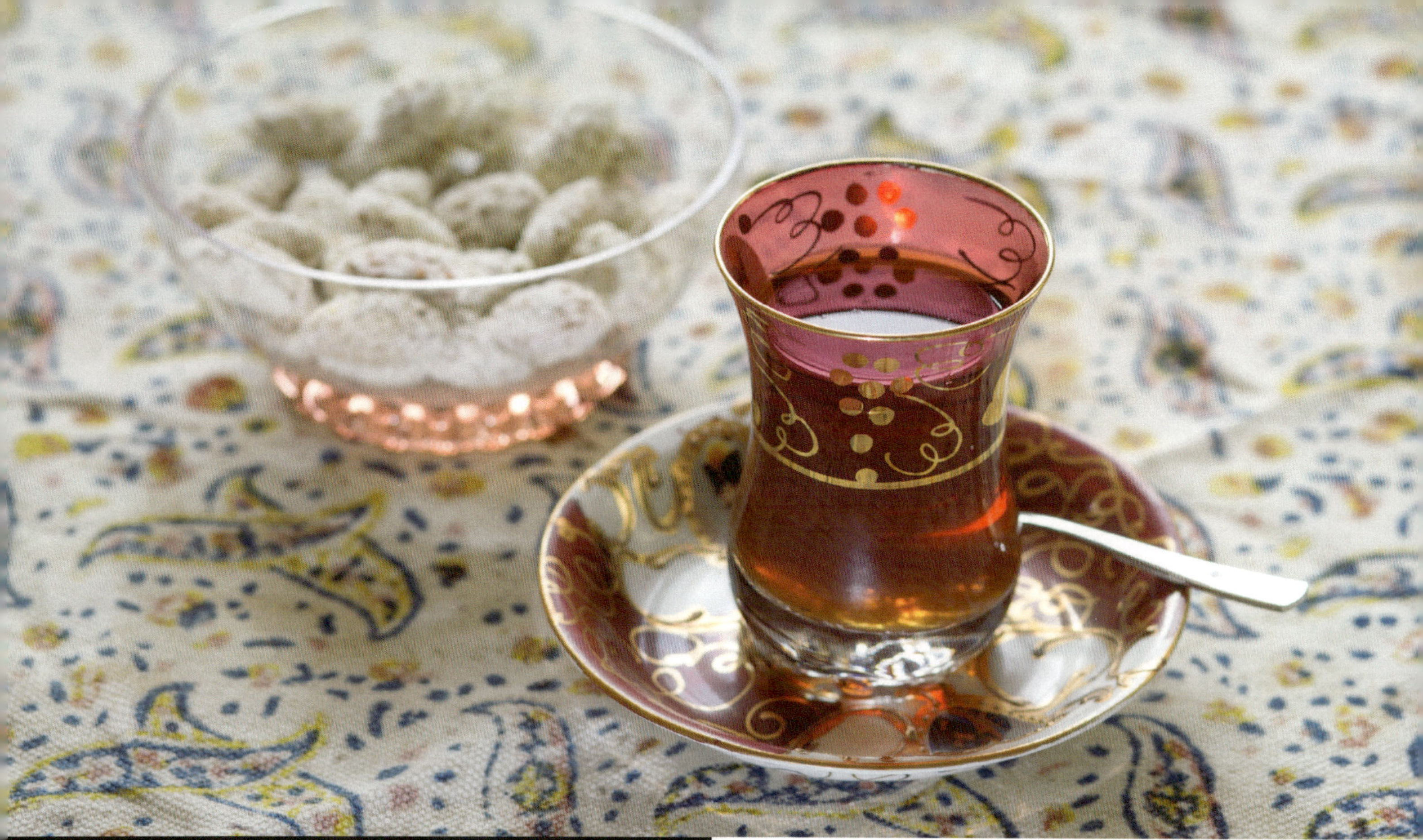

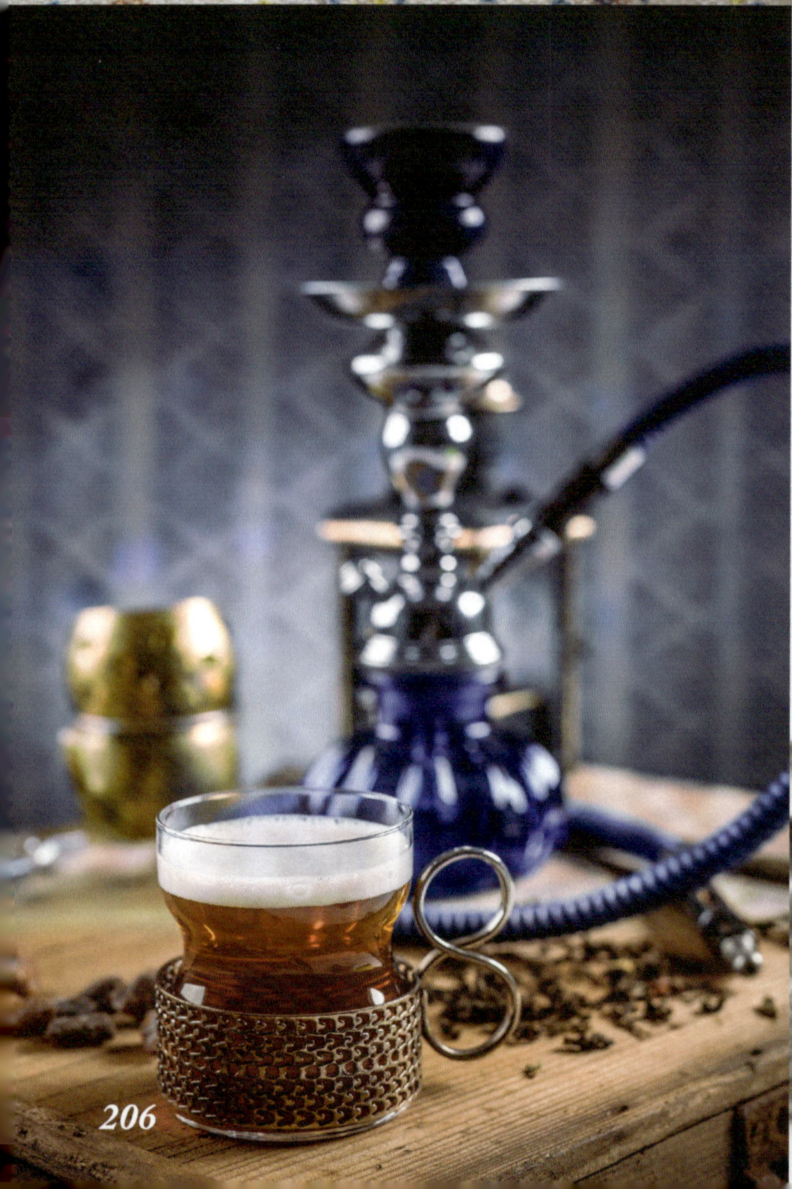

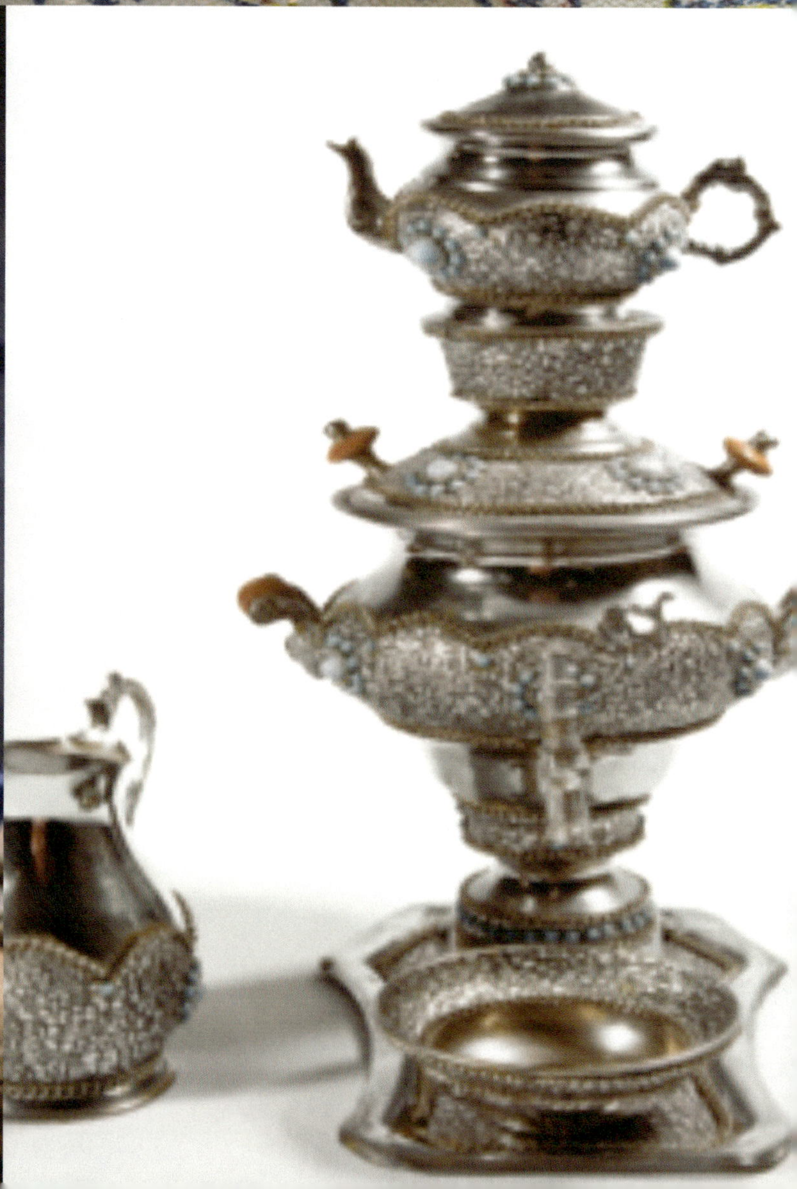

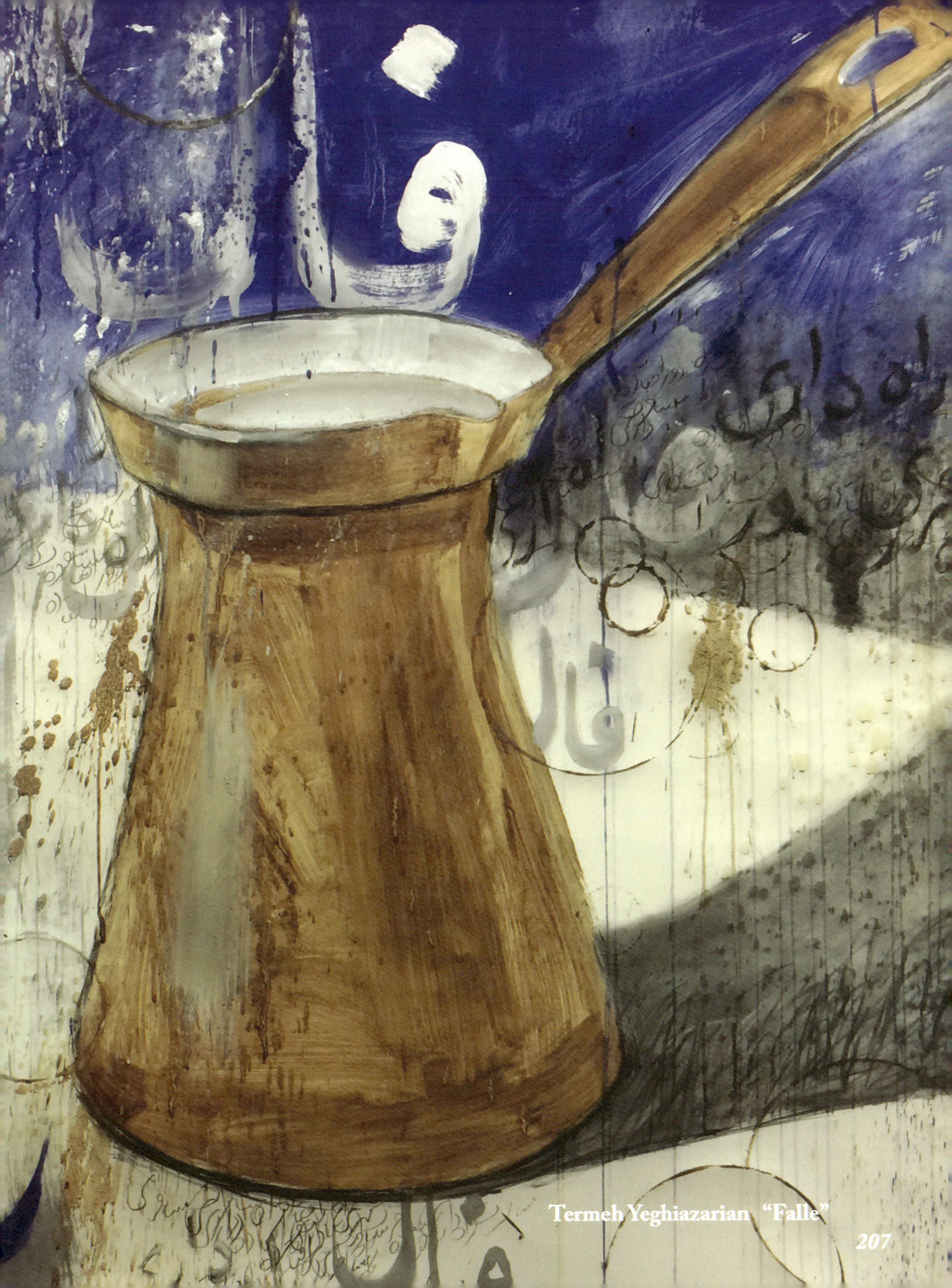

Termeh Yeghiazarian "Falle"

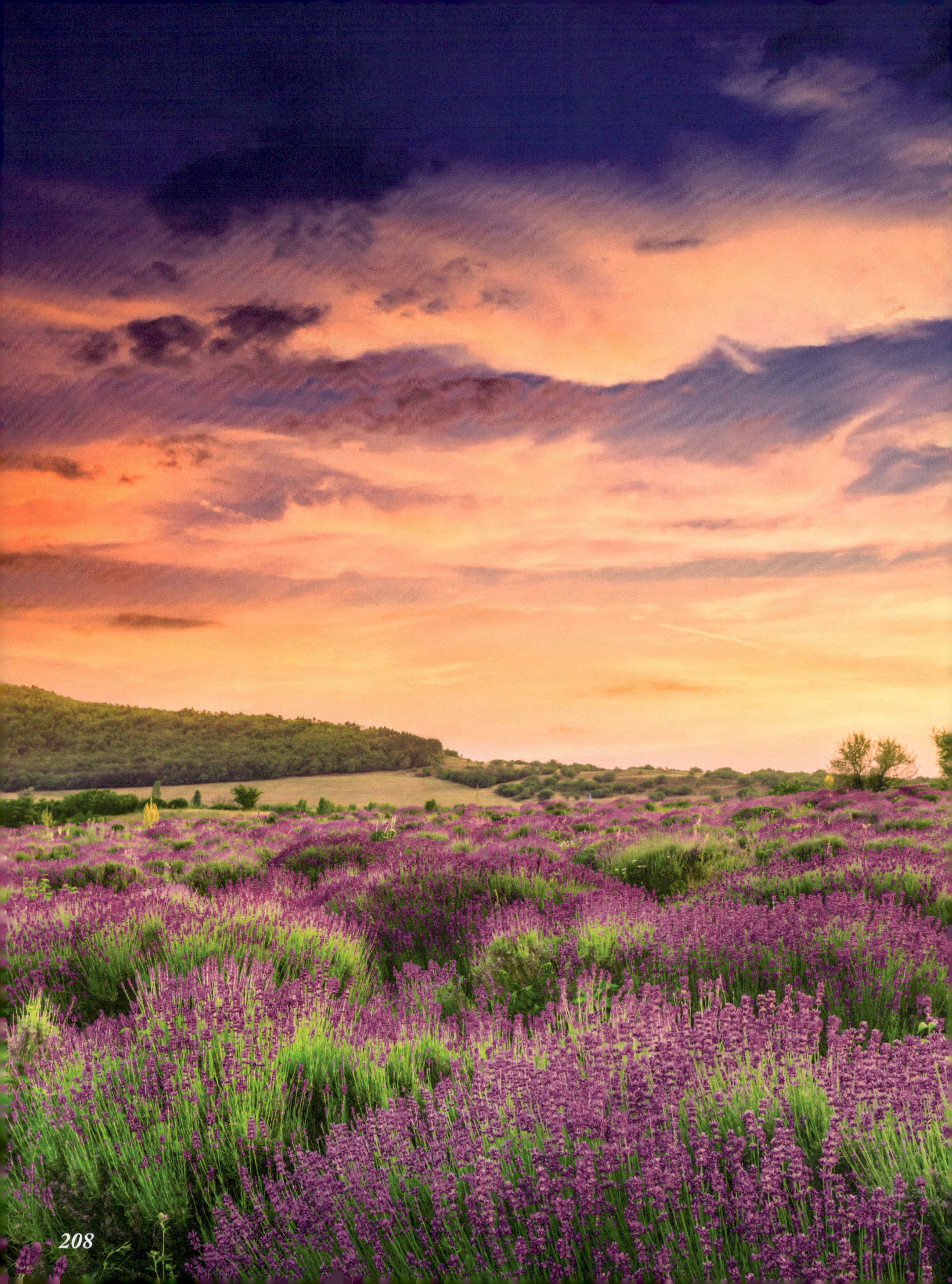

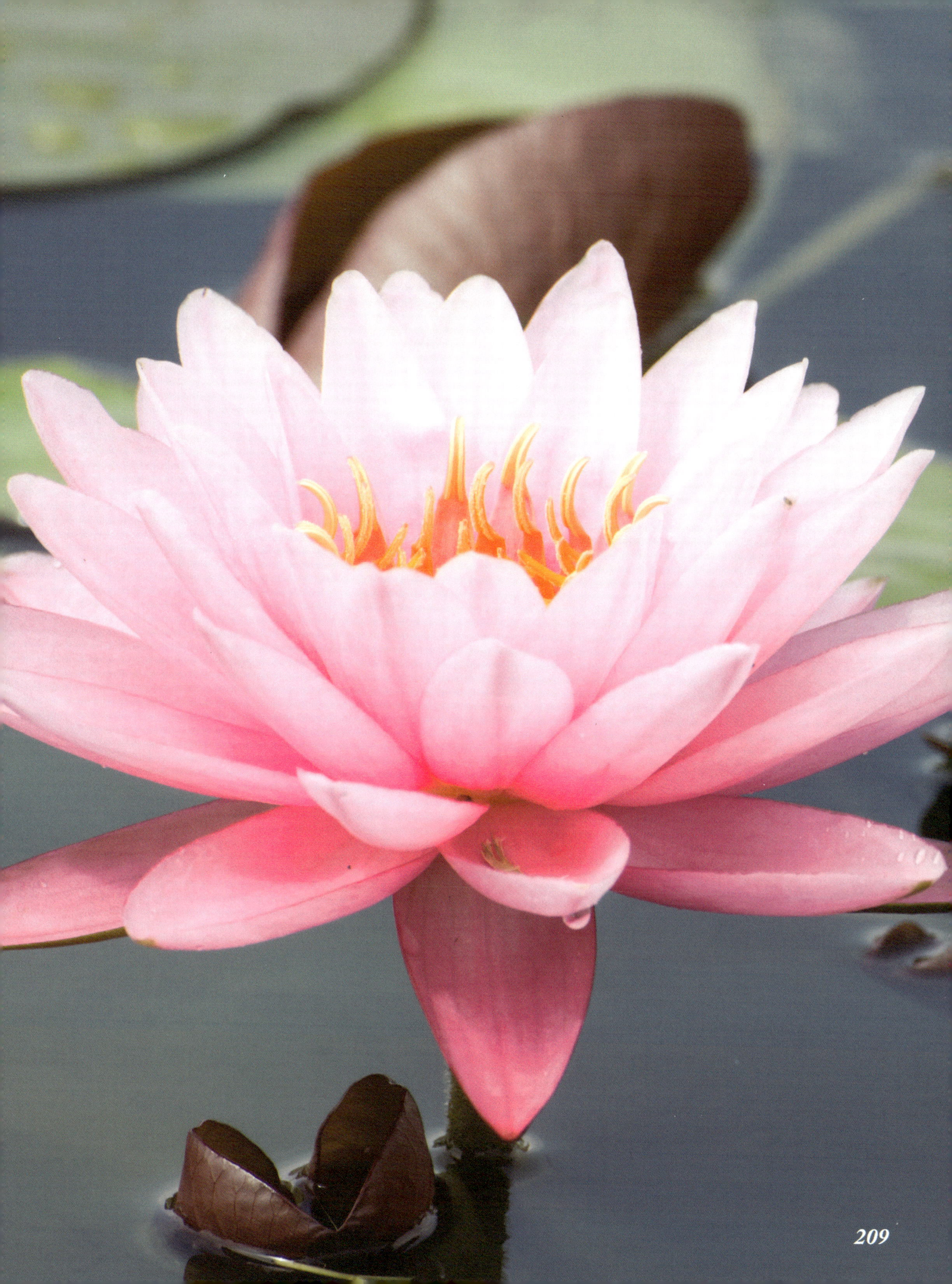

MAMANJOON'S NEAR DEATH STORY

When she was a young girl Mamanjoon's temperature was 104. Regardless of cold compresses, baths and medication her doctor could not bring it down and she had fallen into a coma. At the time her wise and stern grandmother, who was very gifted in the art of herbs, was away visiting her distant family in Tabriz, which was a one or two-day journey from Tehran.

Mamanjoon (her name was Soghra) was her grandmother's favorite and everyone knew that if – God forbid! – something was to happen to Soghra her grandmother would hit the roof. So one of the houseboys was sent to Tabriz on the first day she fell sick to notify Gamar Saltaneh of her granddaughter's ailment.

By the fifth day the doctor's diagnosis was that Soghra had water in her lungs and brain. To save her life he would have to perform surgery. It was a matter of life and death. But no one dared to do anything until Gamar Saltaneh arrived. Thankfully by the sixth day Sograh's temperature had gone down one degree and Gamar Saltaneh arrived early that morning having been driven to Tehran by her brother's chauffeur.

She entered the room shouting at the top of her lungs, "What have you done to my child!" And swept everyone away like dust. She cradled her hand around Soghra's forehead and pulled her eyelids wide open to check her condition. She signed with her hand to the maid to fetch her special treasure box filled with a multitude of herbs.

She instructed the maid to brew her special lavender tea and proceeded to place Mamanjoon's head over her knee and patiently trickle the lavender tea into her mouth with a tiny spoon, closing her mouth and nose every few seconds to make sure she swallowed the tea. There she stayed for hours with Mamanjoon's head in her lap feeding her like a mama chick. By midday Mamanjoon's complexion appeared rosier and by later that afternoon, she opened her eyes and gradually sat up in bed. Everyone was relieved, especially the family doctor who no longer had to perform major surgery on Mamanjoon's brain. By the following day Soghra was talking, making jokes and laughing, no longer burning from high temperature and induced sleep.

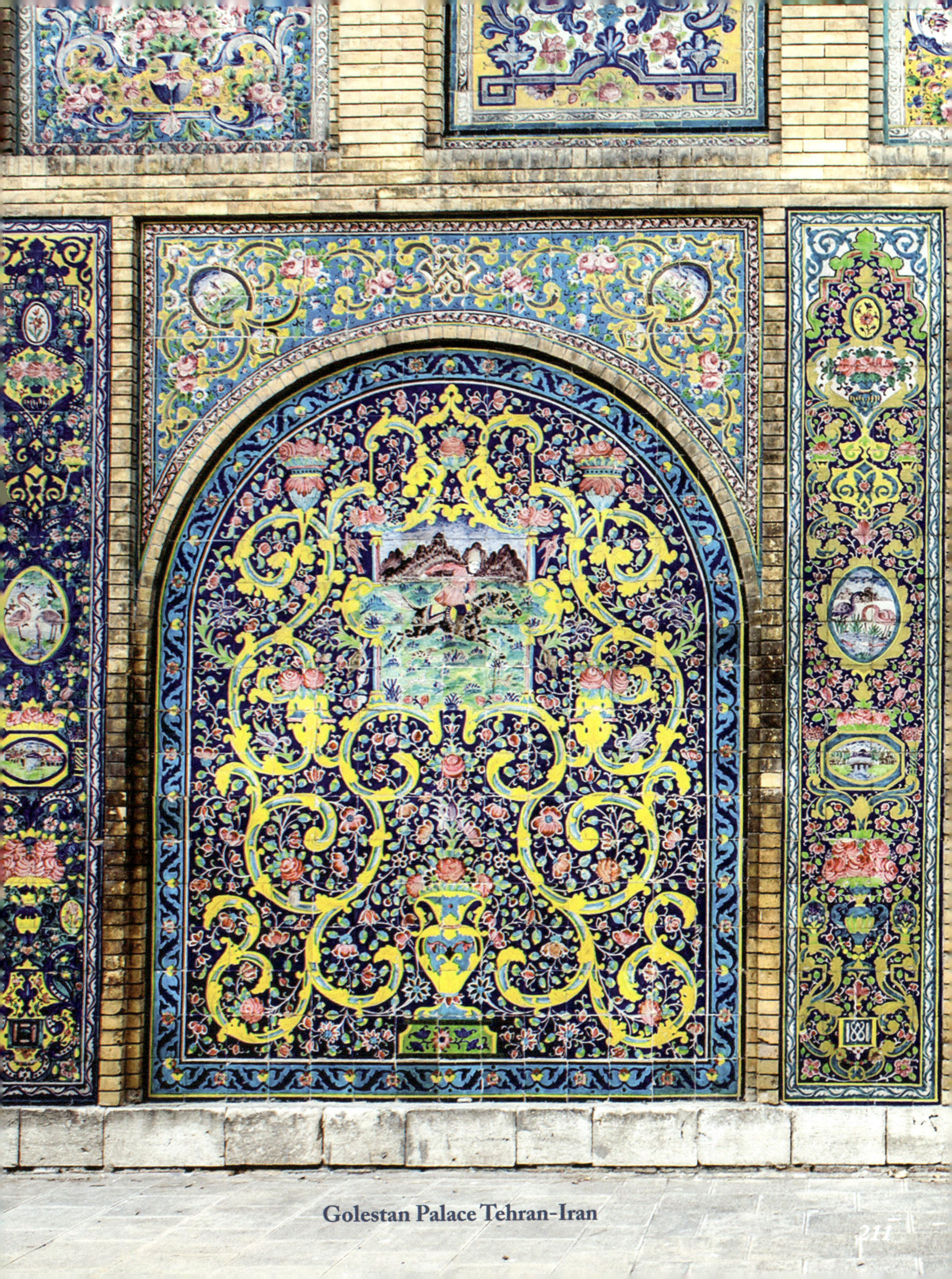

Golestan Palace Tehran-Iran

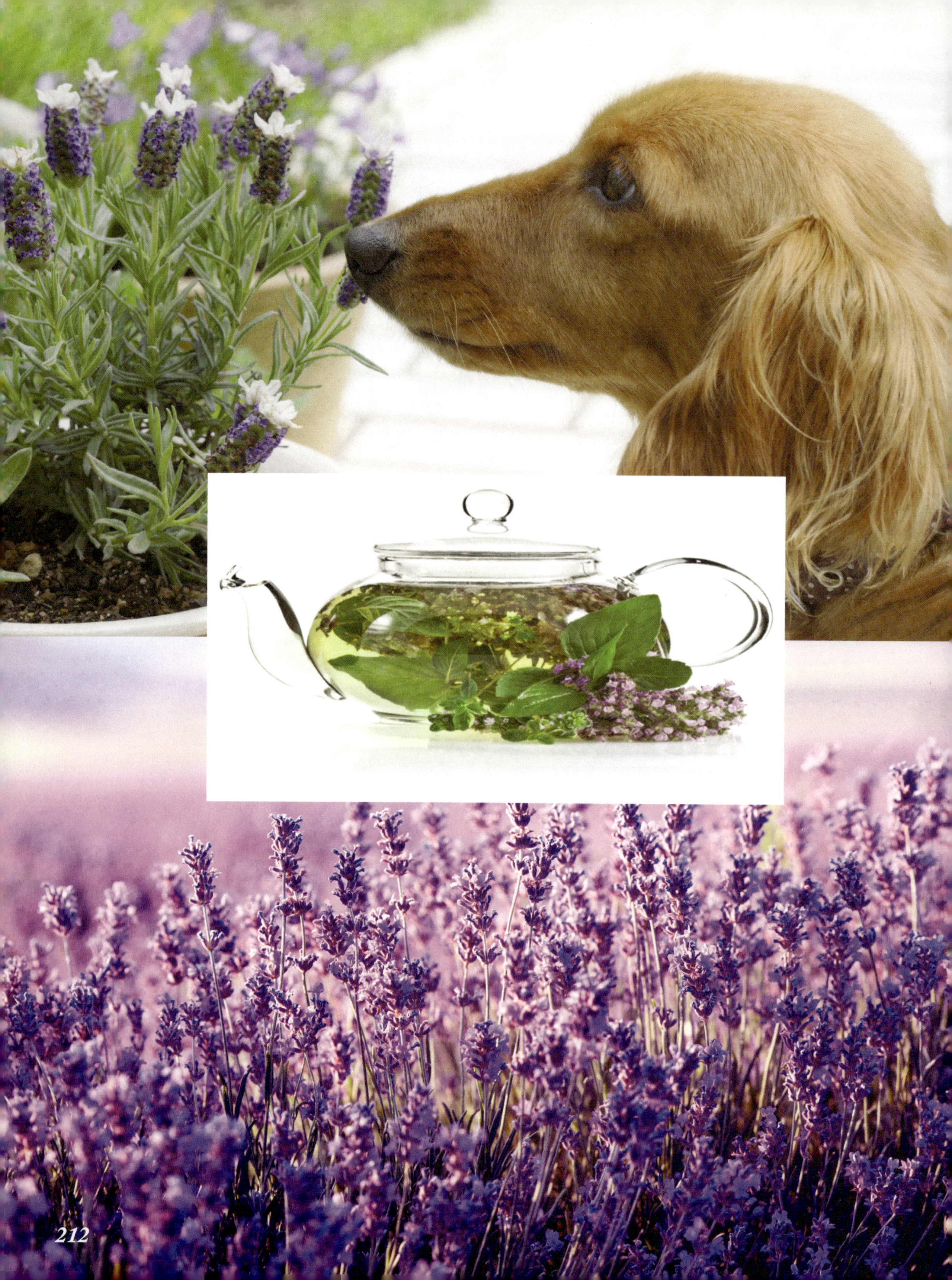

LAVENDER TEA

For flu, cold, pneumonia, bronchitis

Lavender has a great deal of healing and soothing properties. It contains compounds that help to relieve pain, build new tissues and reduce inflammation. It's great for relief of bronchitis and pneumonia, is known to diminish stress and have a sleep inducing effect, and to aid with digestion.

2 6-inch Stalks fresh lavender with flowers (avoid the woody stems near the base)
3 Cups water

Cover lavender with boiling water and let it simmer on very low heat to brew.

LETTUCE TEA INSOMNIA CURE

Bunch organic Romaine lettuce
2 Cups distilled water

Cut lettuce in 3 pieces and place in a small pan with 2 cups of distilled water. Simmer on low heat for 25 minutes. When cool store in glass bottle in the fridge. Drink a cup every night 30 minutes before bedtime. It will help you sleep soundly until morning!

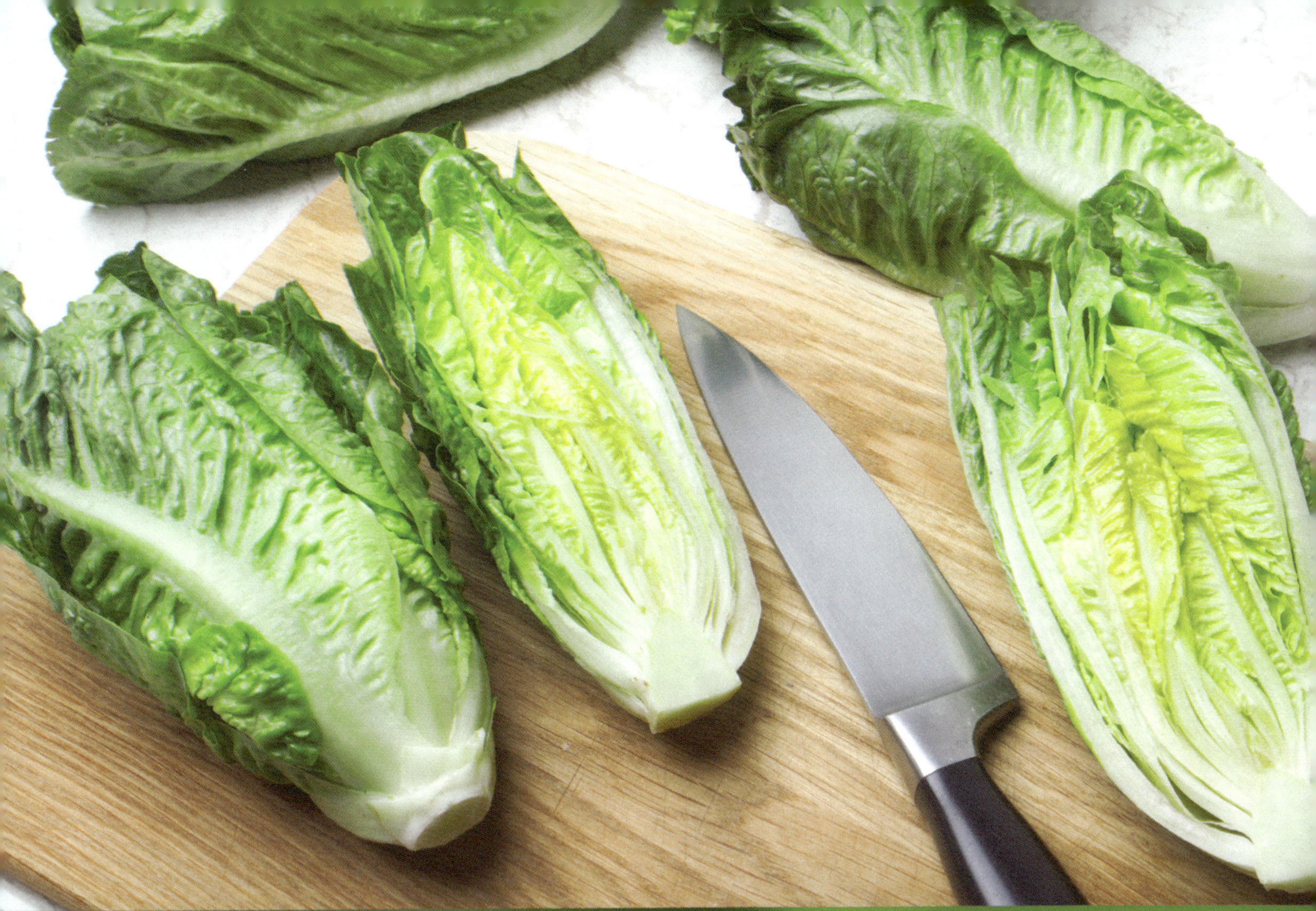

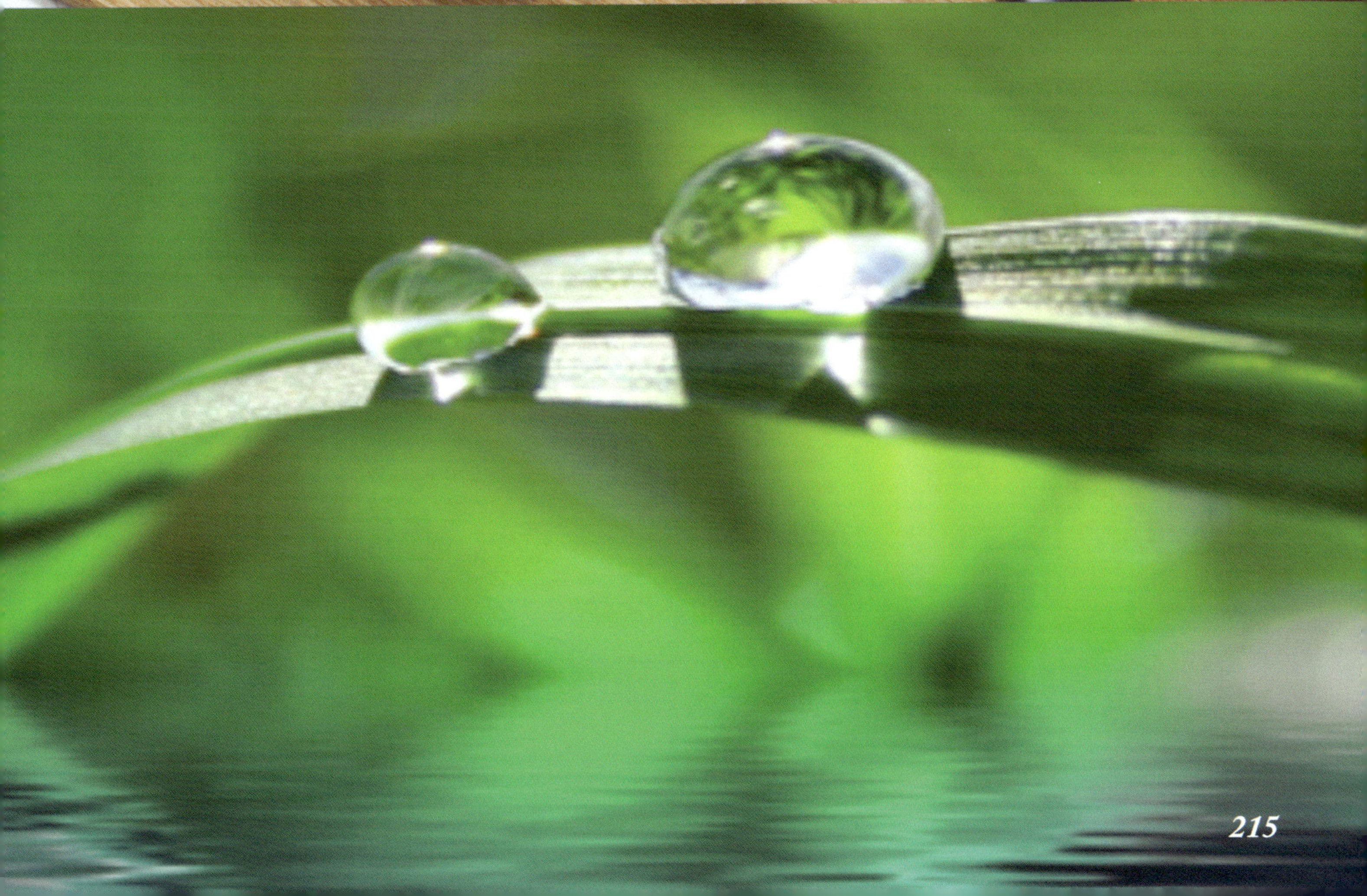

MAMANJOON'S SLEEPY TEA

10 oz Filtered water
1/2 Medium white cabbage
½ Pomegranate
1 Medium celery root
1/4 Teaspoon of cinnamon (Ceylonese or Vietnamese)
1/4 Medium fresh ginger (peeled)

Chop cabbage and celery root and boil in filtered water for 15 minutes. Fork test to see the celery root is cooked (soft in the middle). Set aside to cool. When cool add pomegranate and ginger to the liquid, put in a blender. Strain it in a muslin or cloth drink as is. Drink every night one hour prior to bed.

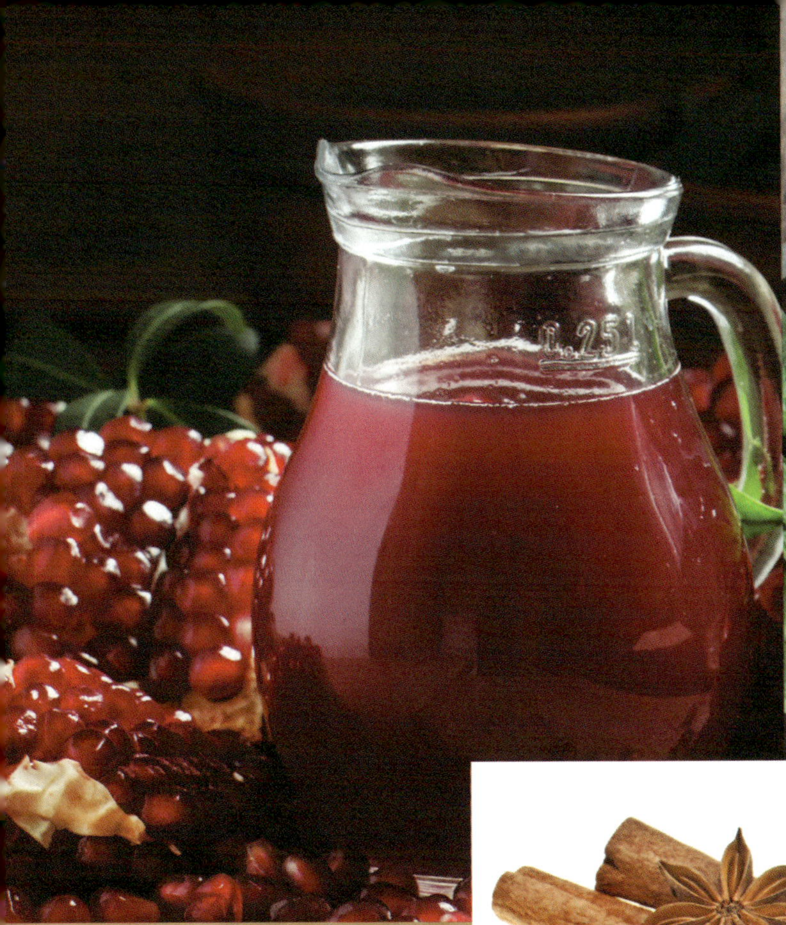
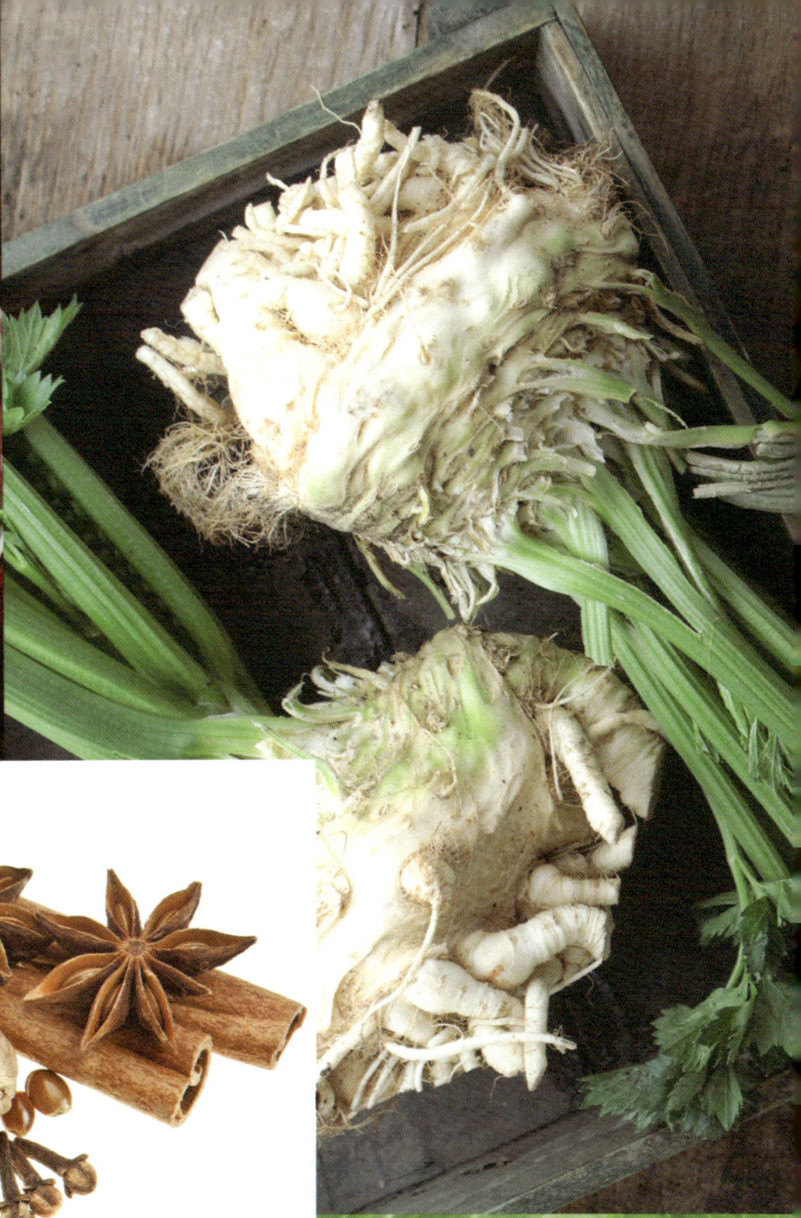
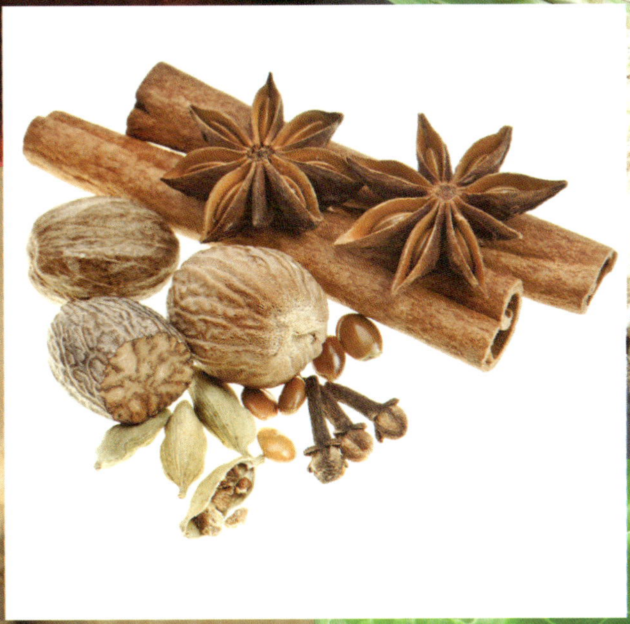
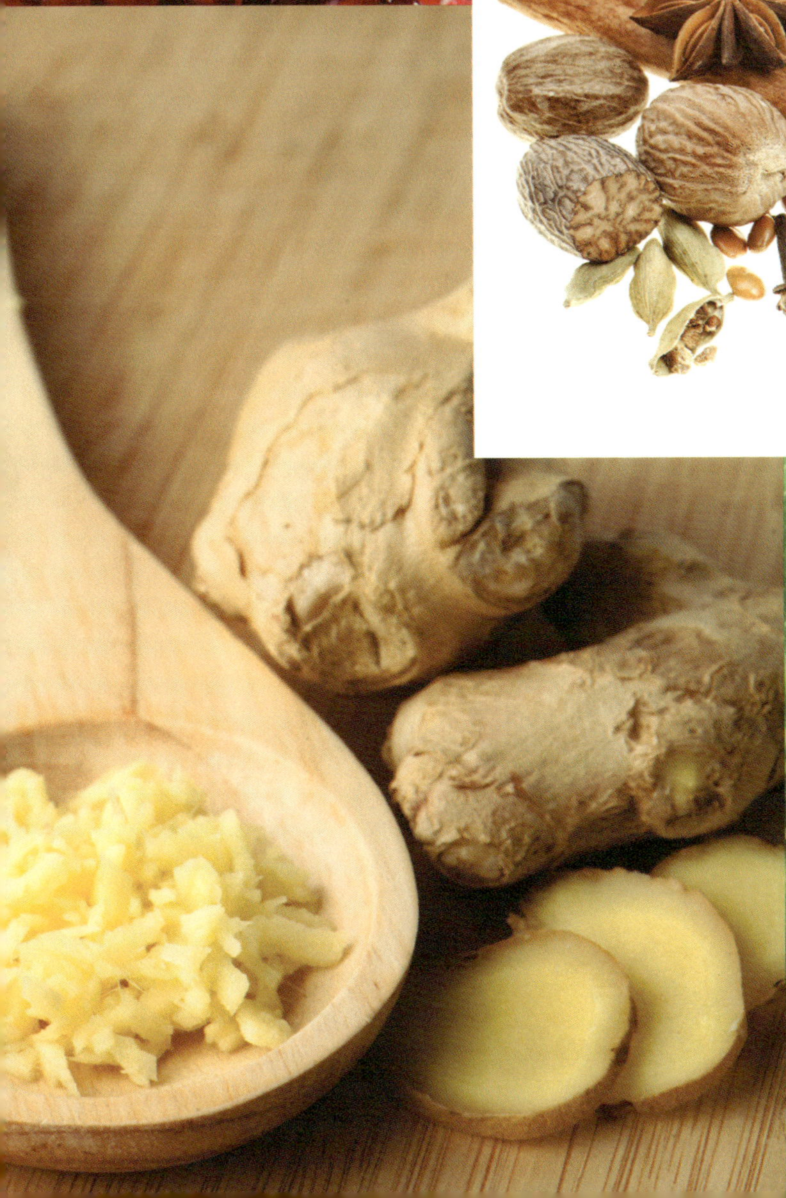
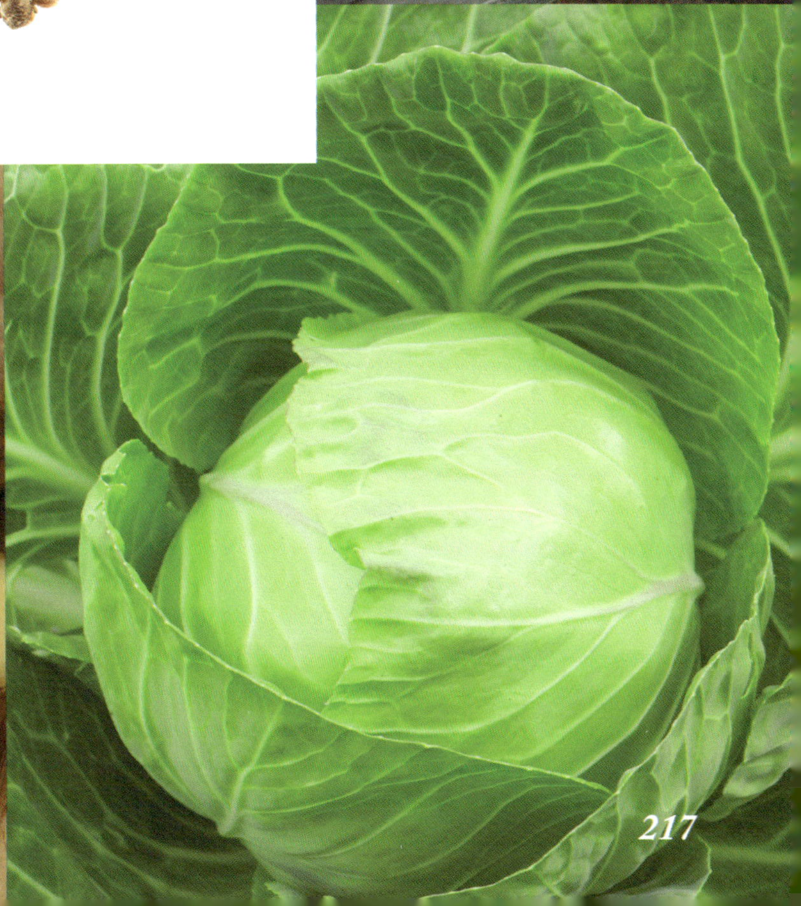

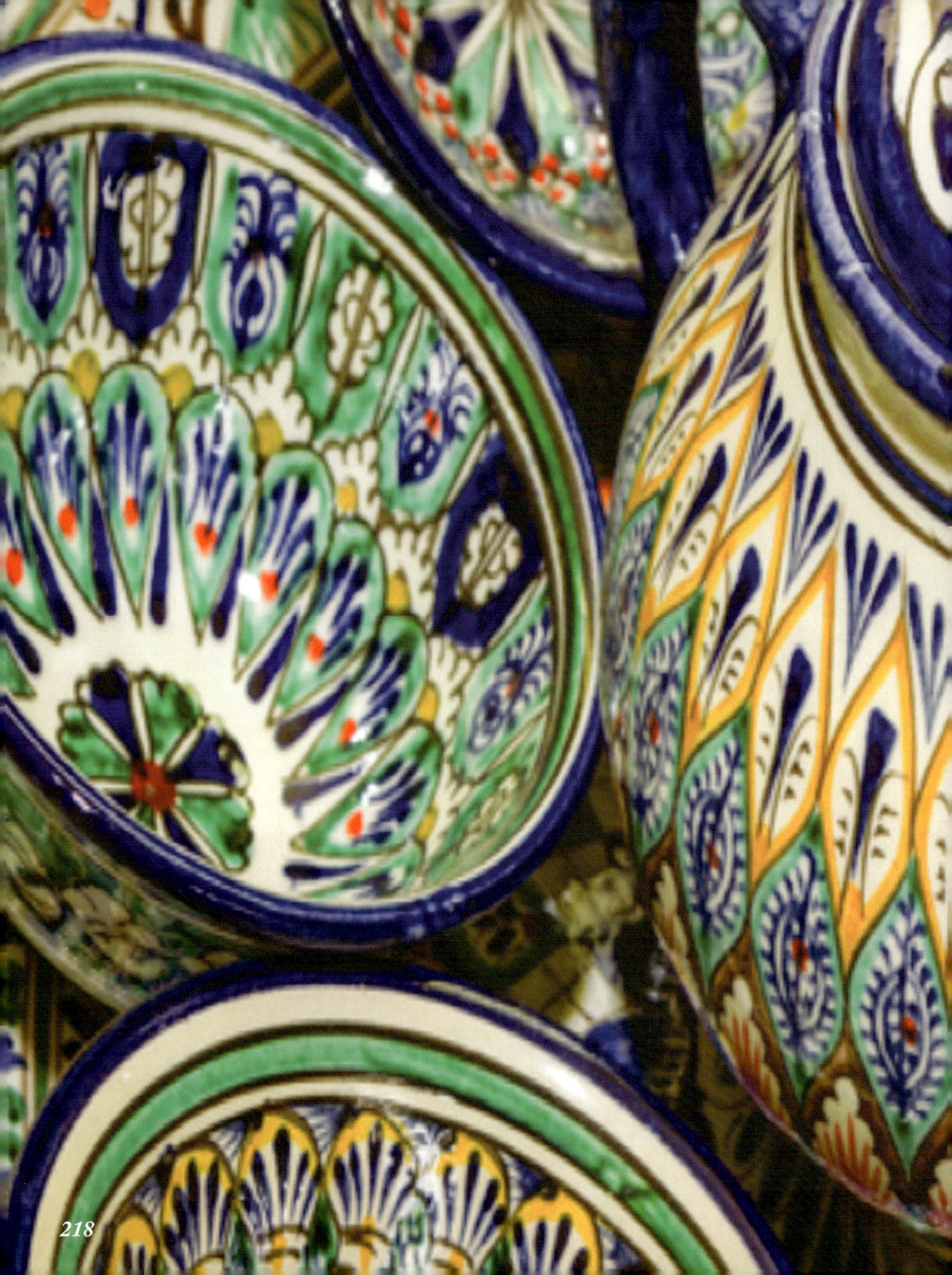

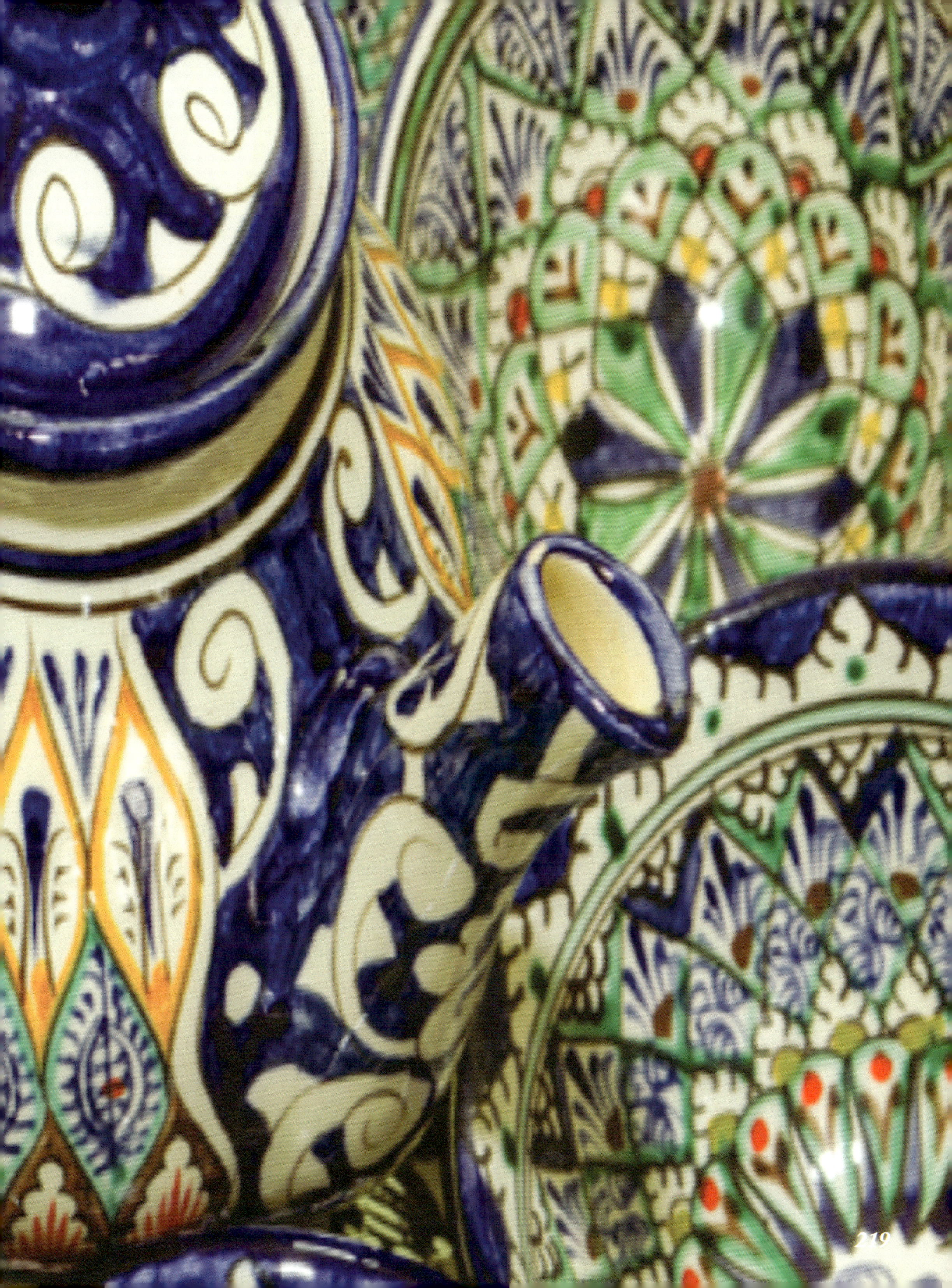

POMEGRANATE SYRUP

Charbat Anar

5 large sour pomegranates
5 large sweet pomegranates
1/2 lb raw sugar or raw honey

You can either buy pure pomegranate juice or use a fresh pomegranate. To get the juice of pomegranate fruit, cut it in half around the midline deep enough to pierce the skin, but shallow enough that you don't cut into the seeds inside. Pull apart the two halves with your thumbs. Gently submerge the two halves in a deep bowl of water and gently push the edges down and away to open the fruit. The water will soften the pith (the white tissue under the skin of the fruit). Turn each half upside down and tap it gently with the back of a spoon. Seeds will tumble out into your hand and the bowl of water below. Look at the pomegranate half and release any stragglers with your hands or another whack of the spoon. Seeds will sink to the bottom. Scoop any floating pith out of the water with a slotted spoon or sieve and drain the water. Now you have pomegranate seeds ready to place in a blender to juice!

Mix juice and honey and cook on low flame until the consistency of thick syrup. Cool and keep until needed.

Pomegranate syrup will keep without refrigeration for a very long time. To serve, dilute one part of syrup in 3 to 6 parts (to taste) of hot or cool water (in summer).

Pomegranate has been shown to benefit the heart and blood vessels, reverse atherosclerotic plaque, relieve and protect against depression and osteoporosis, and reduce fevers.

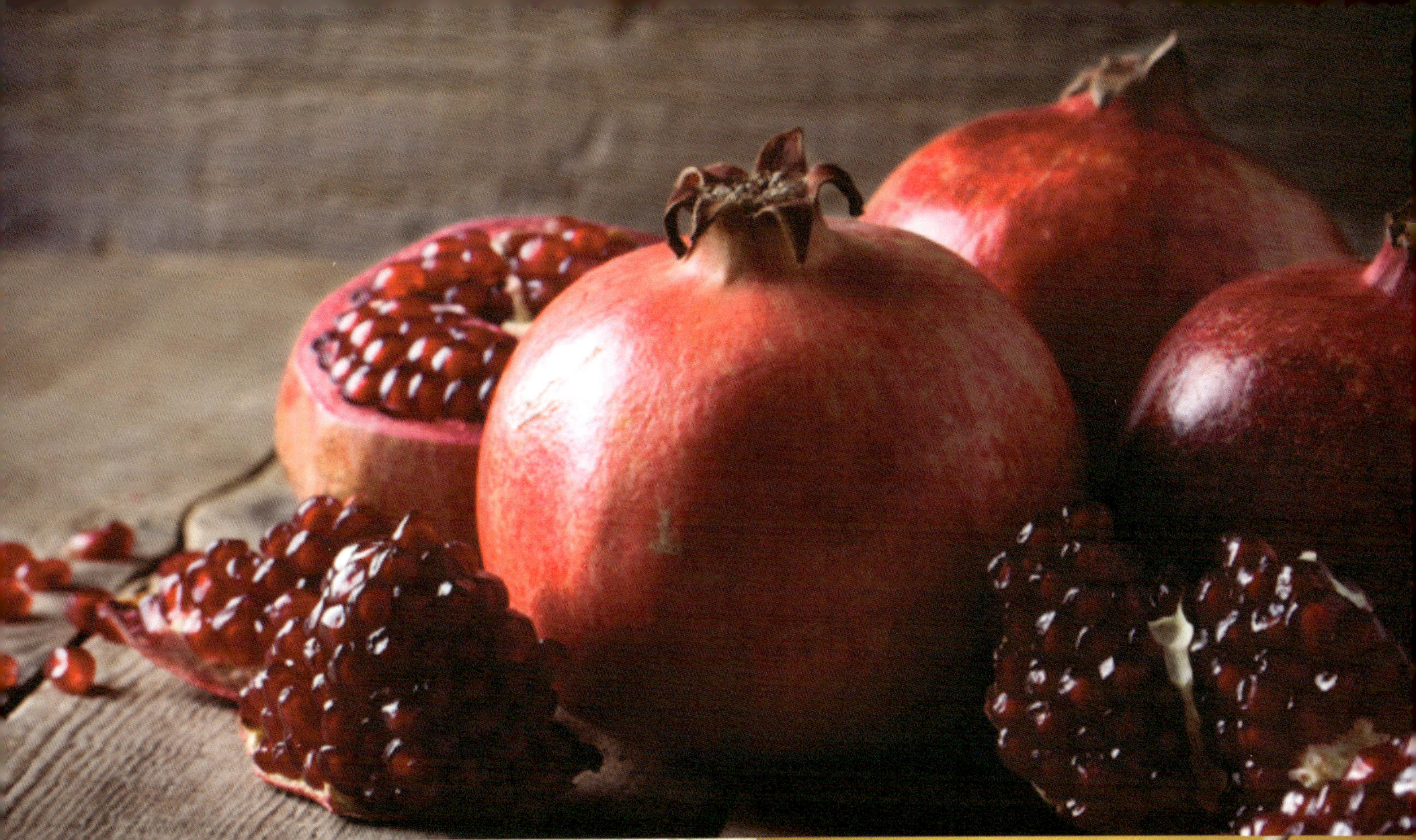

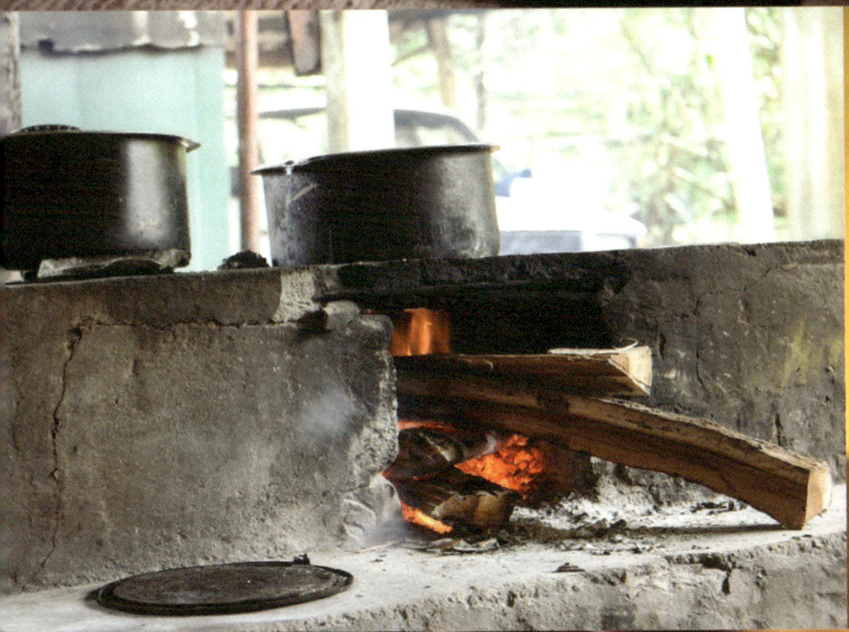

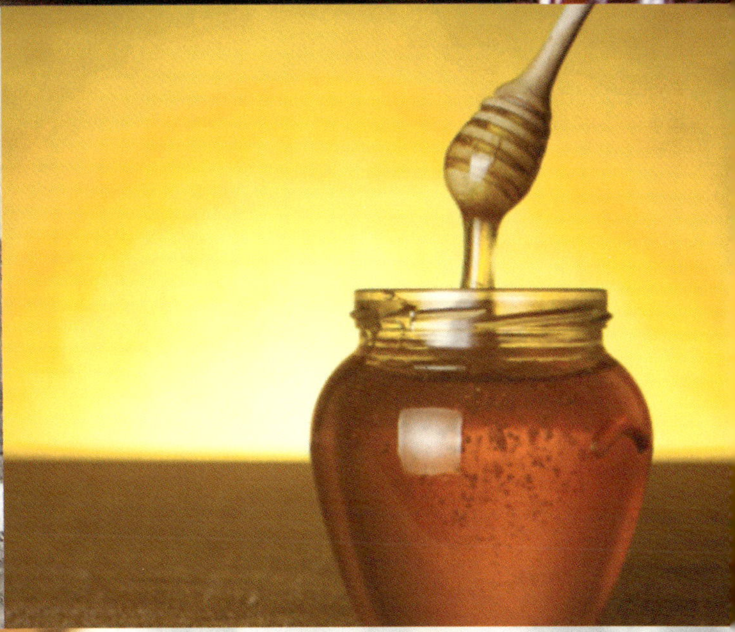

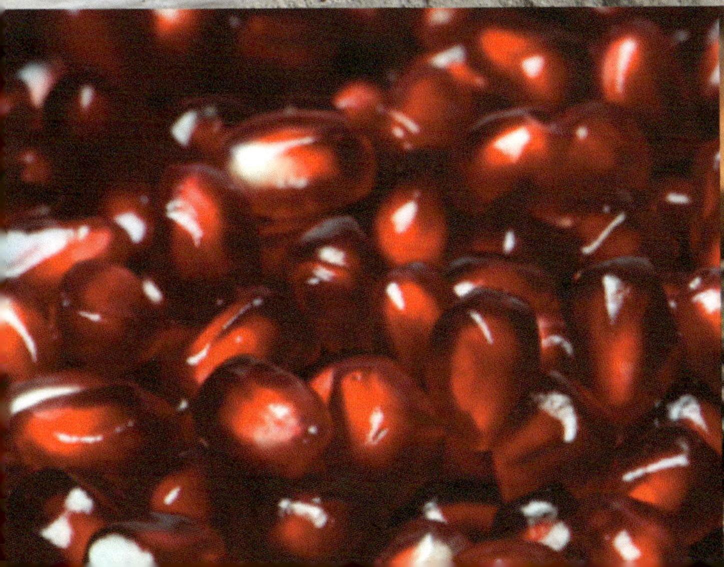

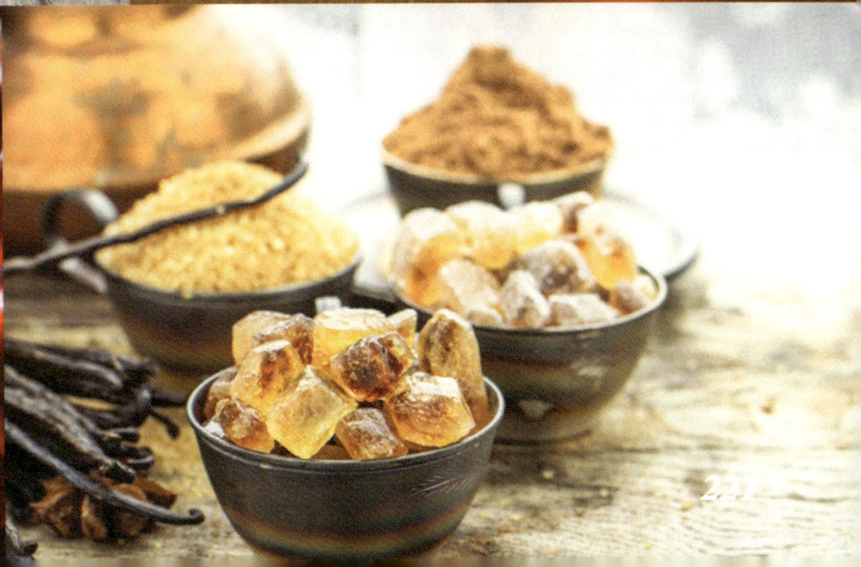

BLADDER FLUSH

To heal, fortify and strengthen your bladder

This natural antibiotic gets rid of UTI symptoms and inflammation, which affect about half of women over the course of a lifetime and happen to be the reason for about 8 million doctors' visits each year.

4 oz Raw Parsley root (they look like white carrots)
4 oz Lemon peel
4 oz Raw honey
1 Tablespoon coconut oil
1 Tablespoon virgin olive oil

Chop parsley root and put in a blender with other ingredients until all ingredients are liquefied, refrigerate.

Take ½ Tablespoon every morning.

Reminder: You need to make sure the honey and the lemon are organic and pesticide free.

Avoid consuming caffeine and chocolate because these will stimulate if there is bacteria or infection present.

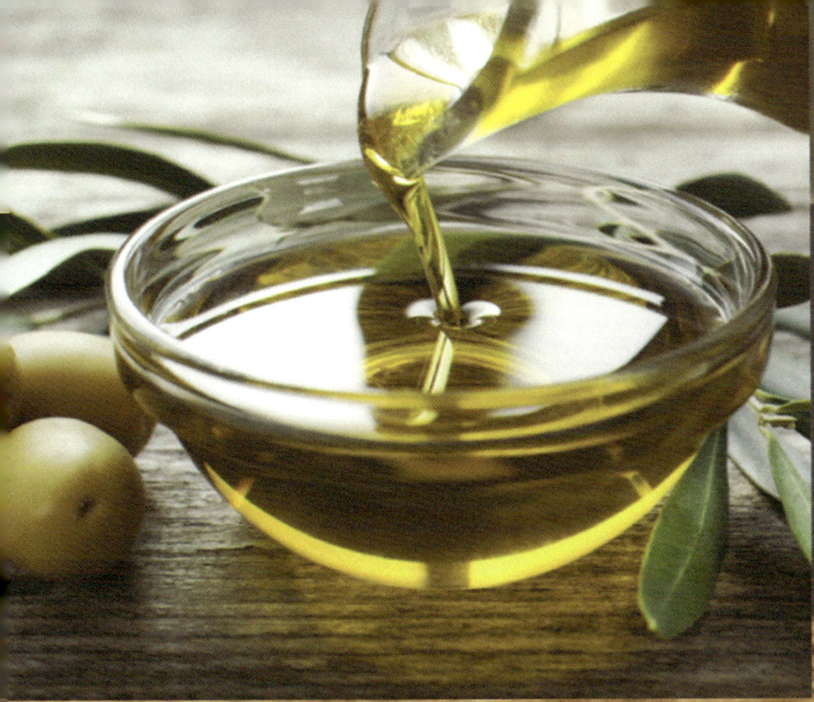
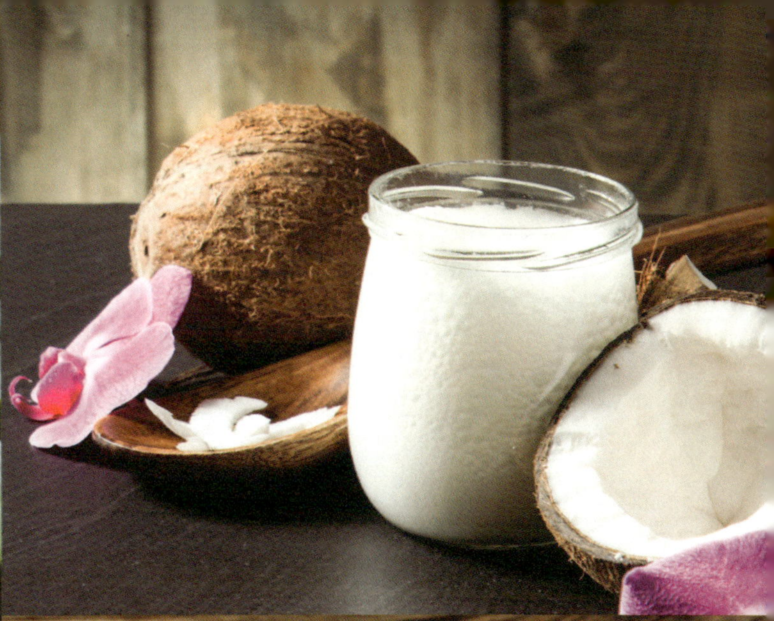
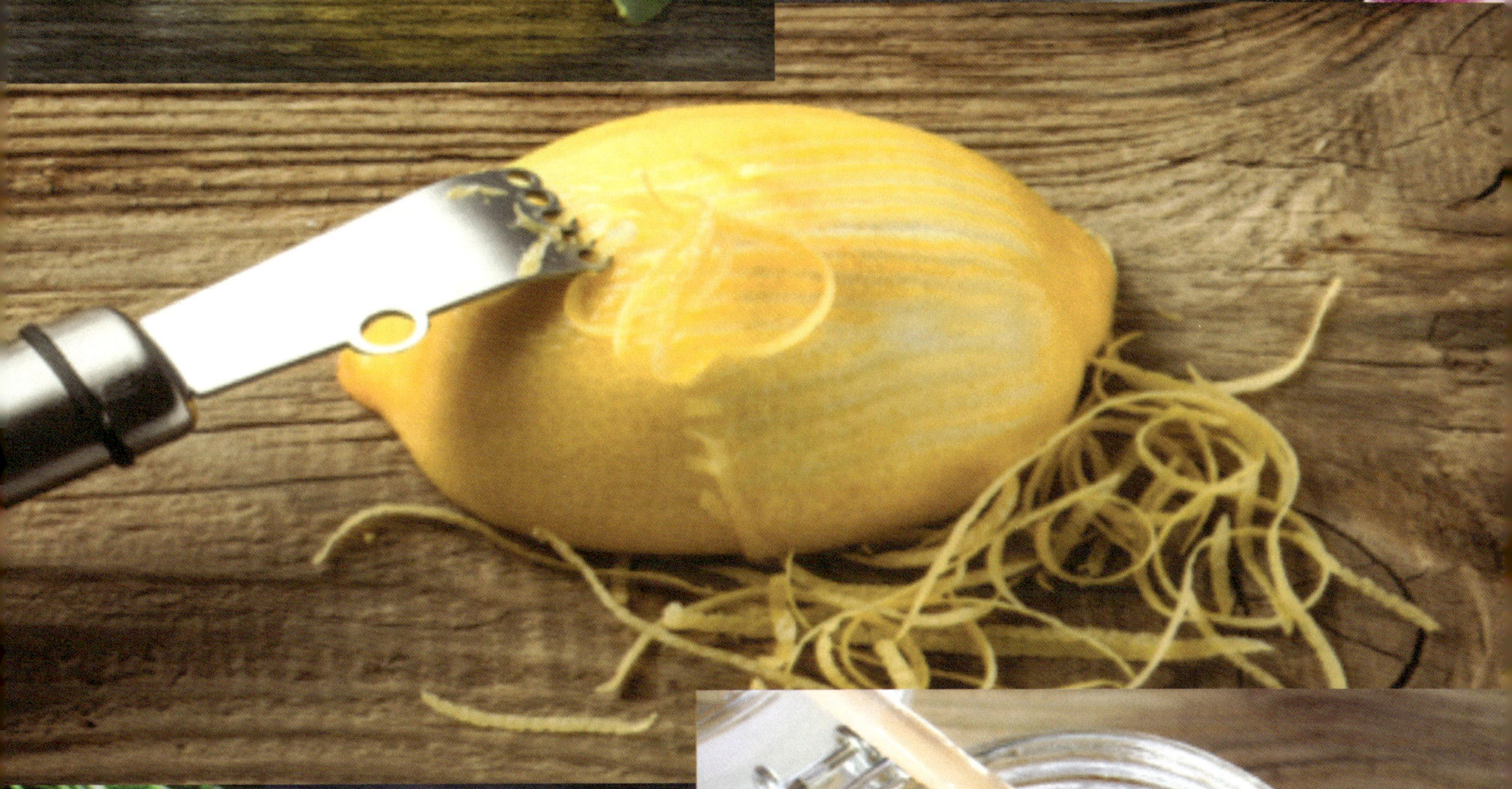
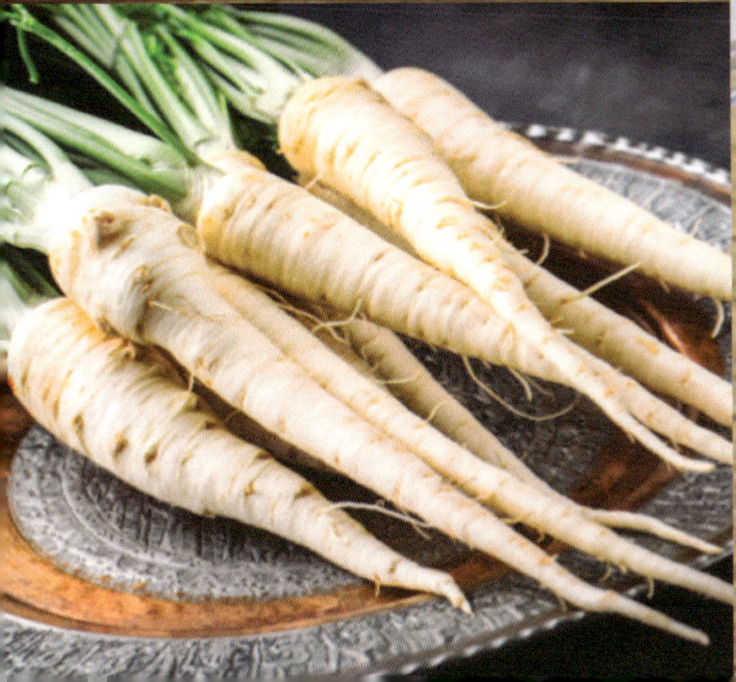
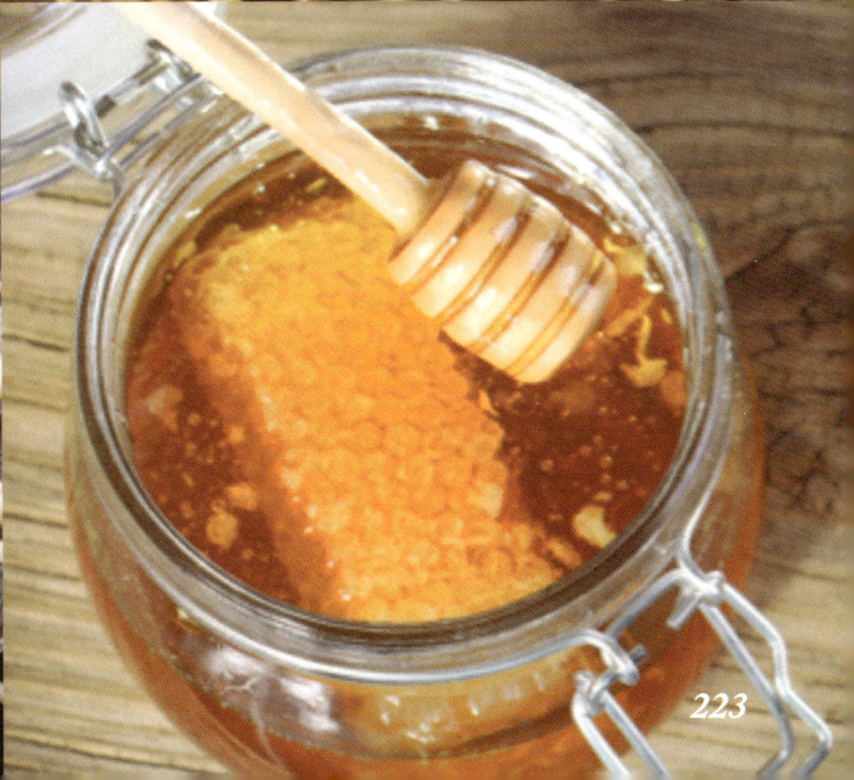

HOT FLASH ERASE AWAY POTION

Many women young and old suffer from night sweats and hot flashes. Different women experience different symptoms, depending mostly on hormonal makeup, diet and lifestyle. A high percentage of women experience them within the first year or two of menopause. Now we have a cure!

7 Tablespoons of raw or Manuka honey
1 Tablespoons licorice root powder
2 Tablespoons turmeric
4 Tablespoons coconut oil
2 Tablespoons fresh cherry juice
1 Teaspoon fresh organic lemon juice

Add turmeric and licorice powder to raw or Manuka honey, mix slowly then add coconut oil, lemon juice and cherry juice. Mix well and place the mixture in a jar for 24 hours at room temperature. One teaspoon three times a day.

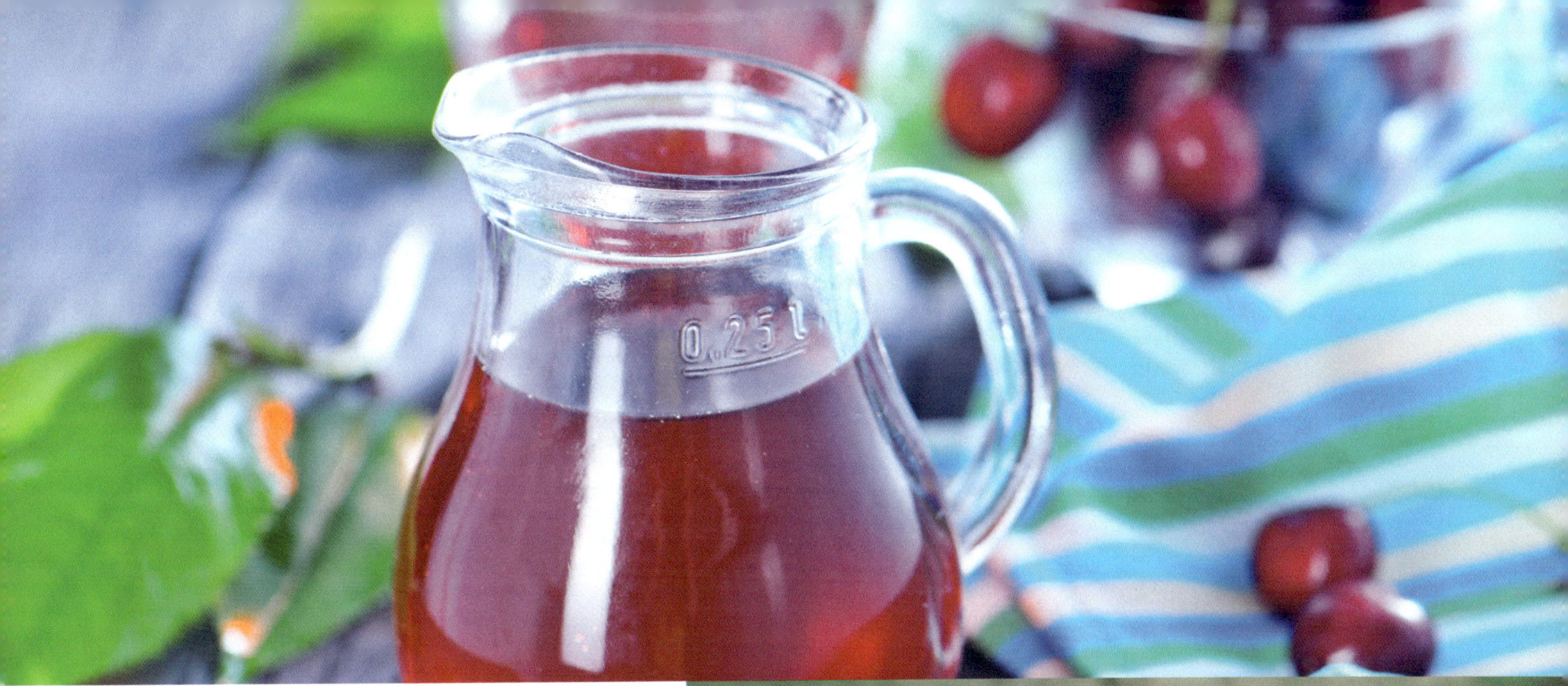
0,25 l
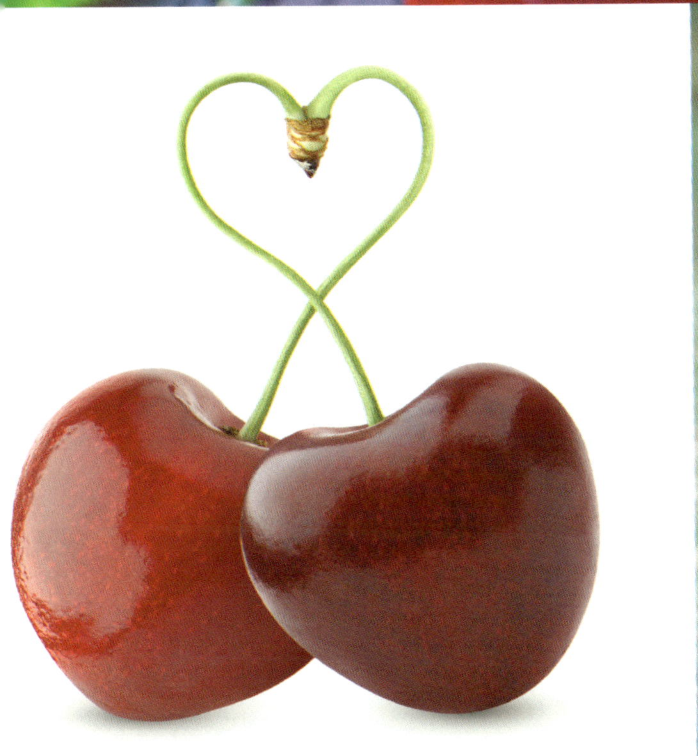
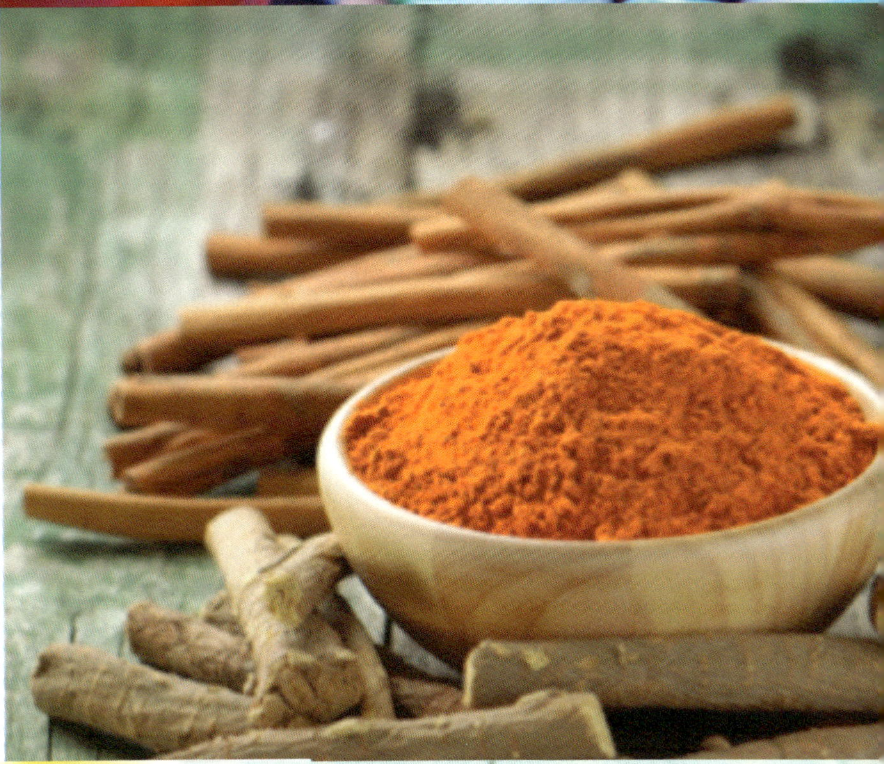
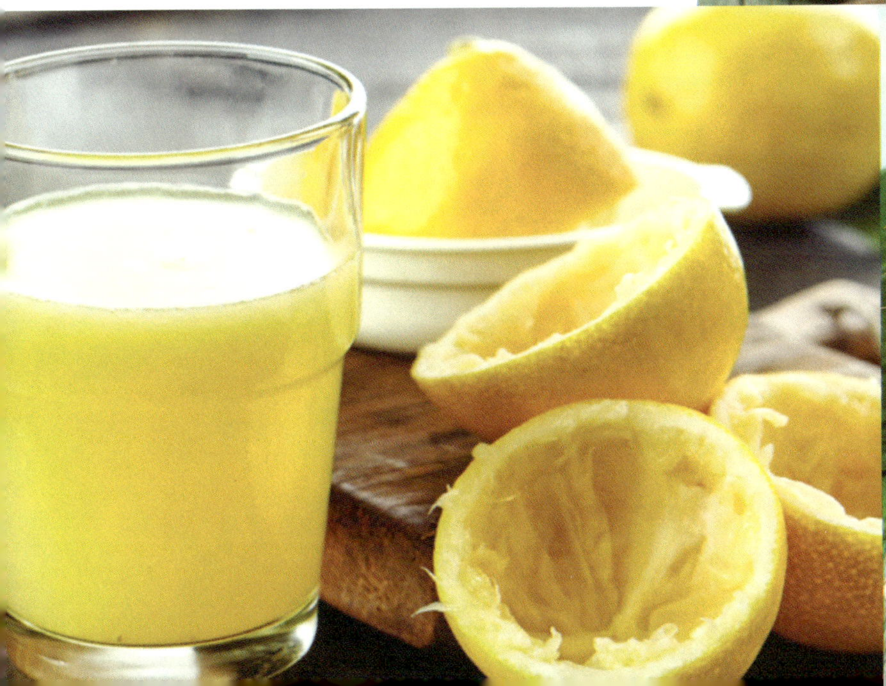
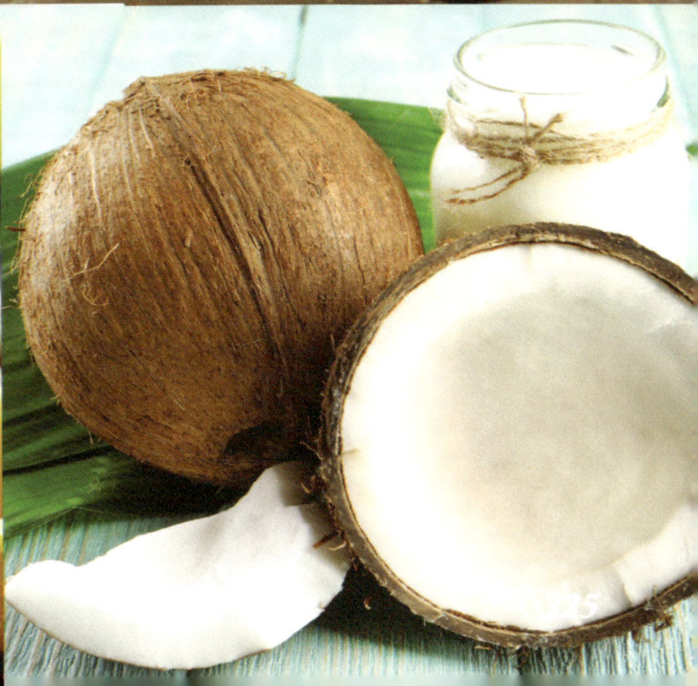

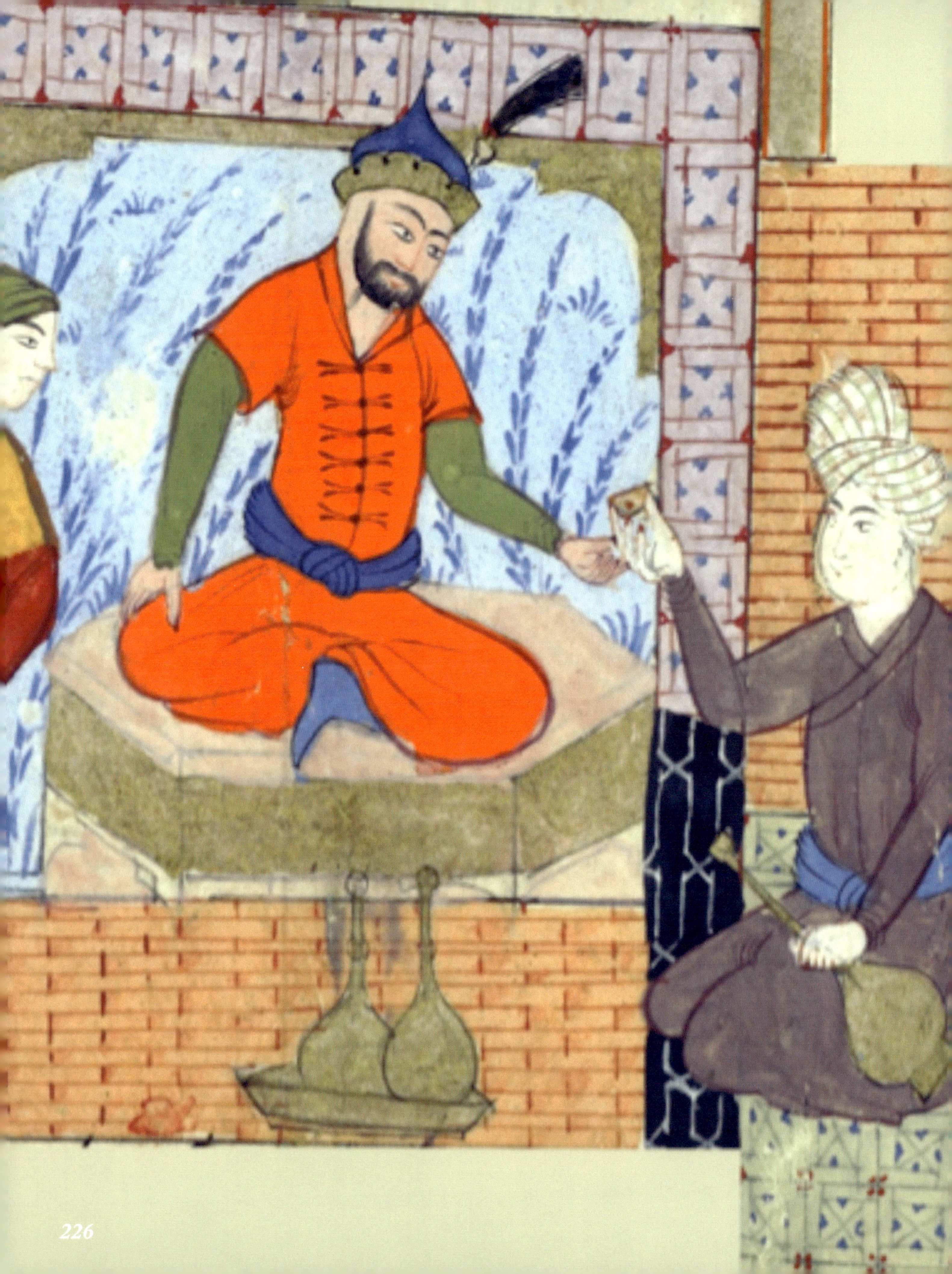

NATURAL VIAGRA

For men with prostate problems

Watermelon is high in the amino acids citrulline and arginine that help the circulation of blood and other aspects of our cardiovascular health.

Medium organic yellow watermelon with seeds
1/2 Lemon (organic)
5 Stalks cilantro

Cut watermelon in small pieces with skin, add lemon, put in a blender, then add cilantro. Blend till liquefied. Drink every day.

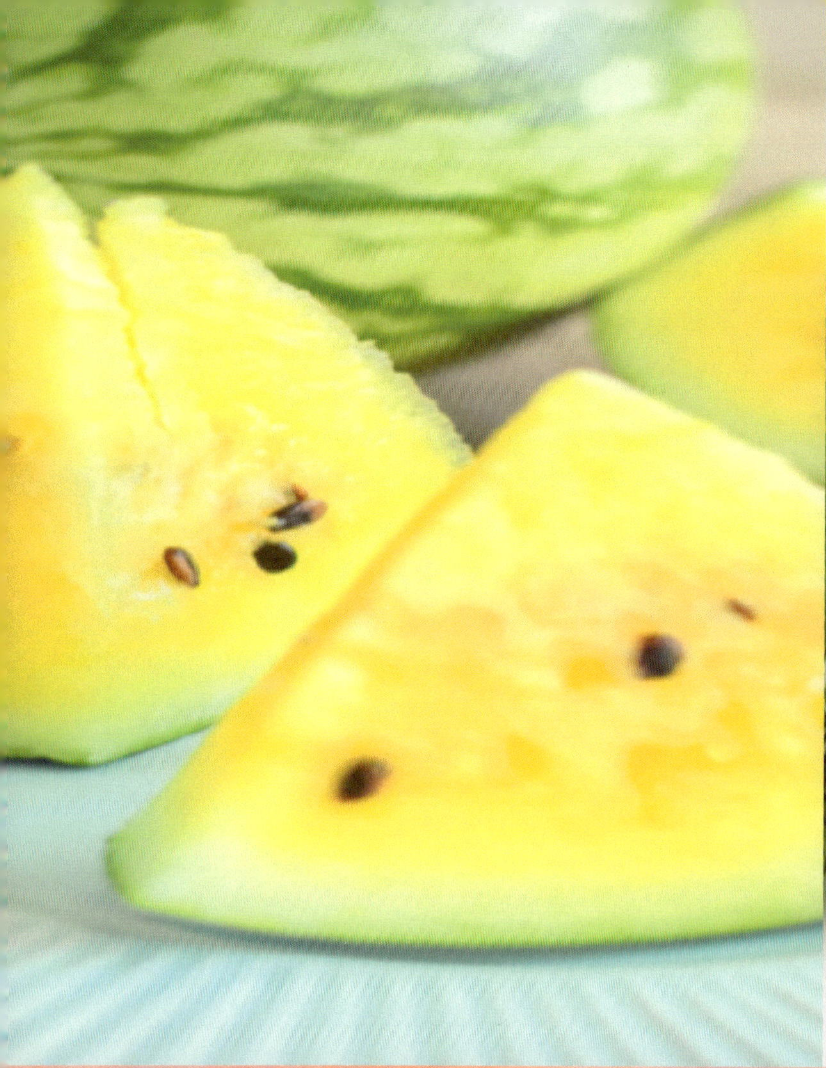
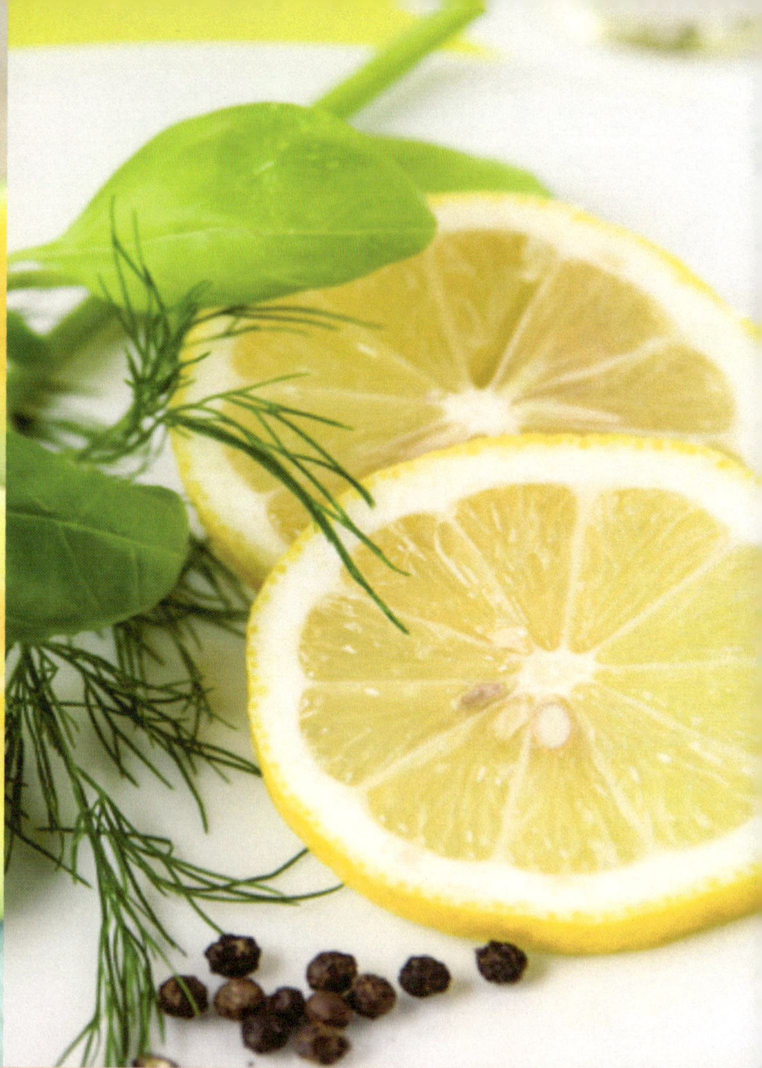
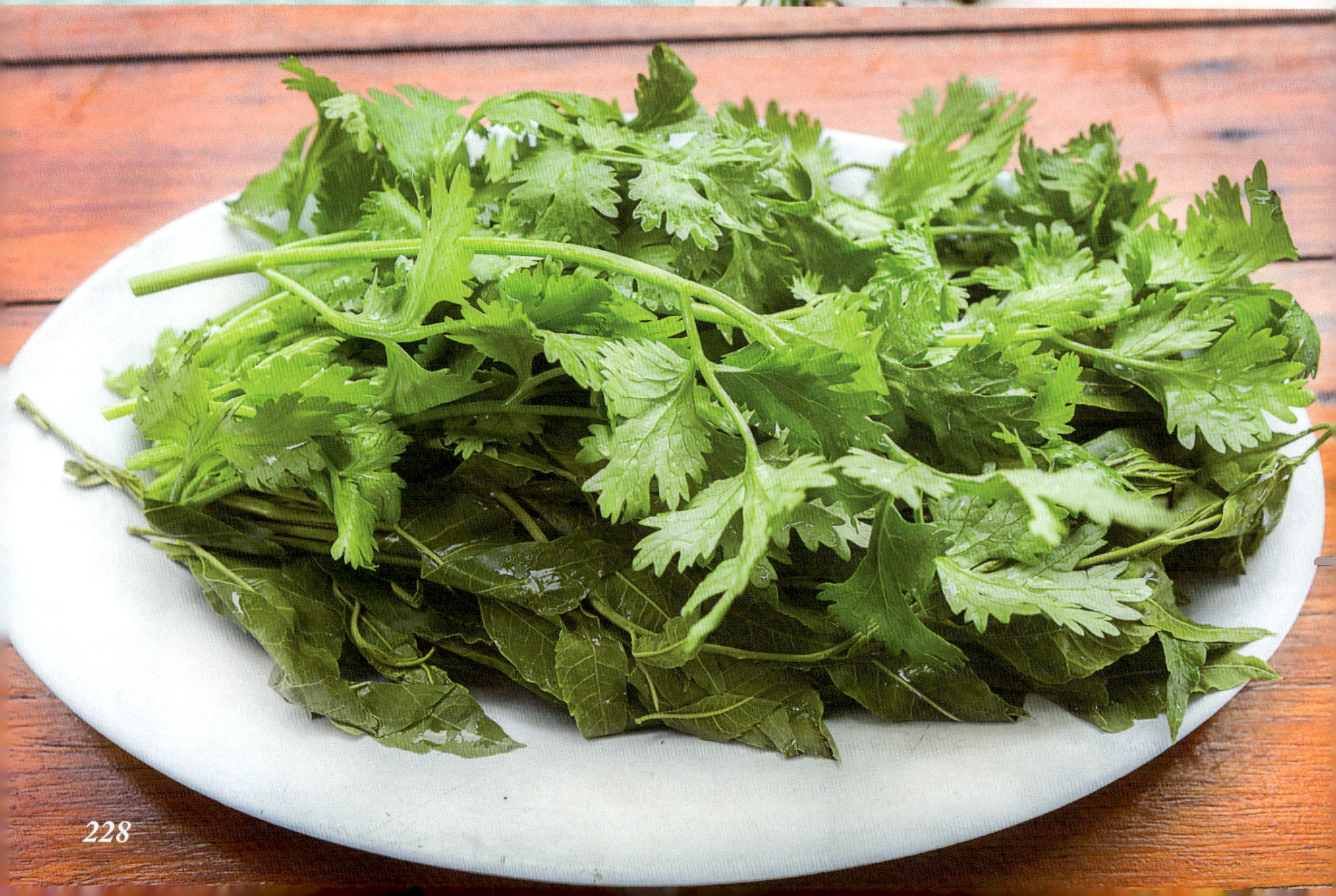

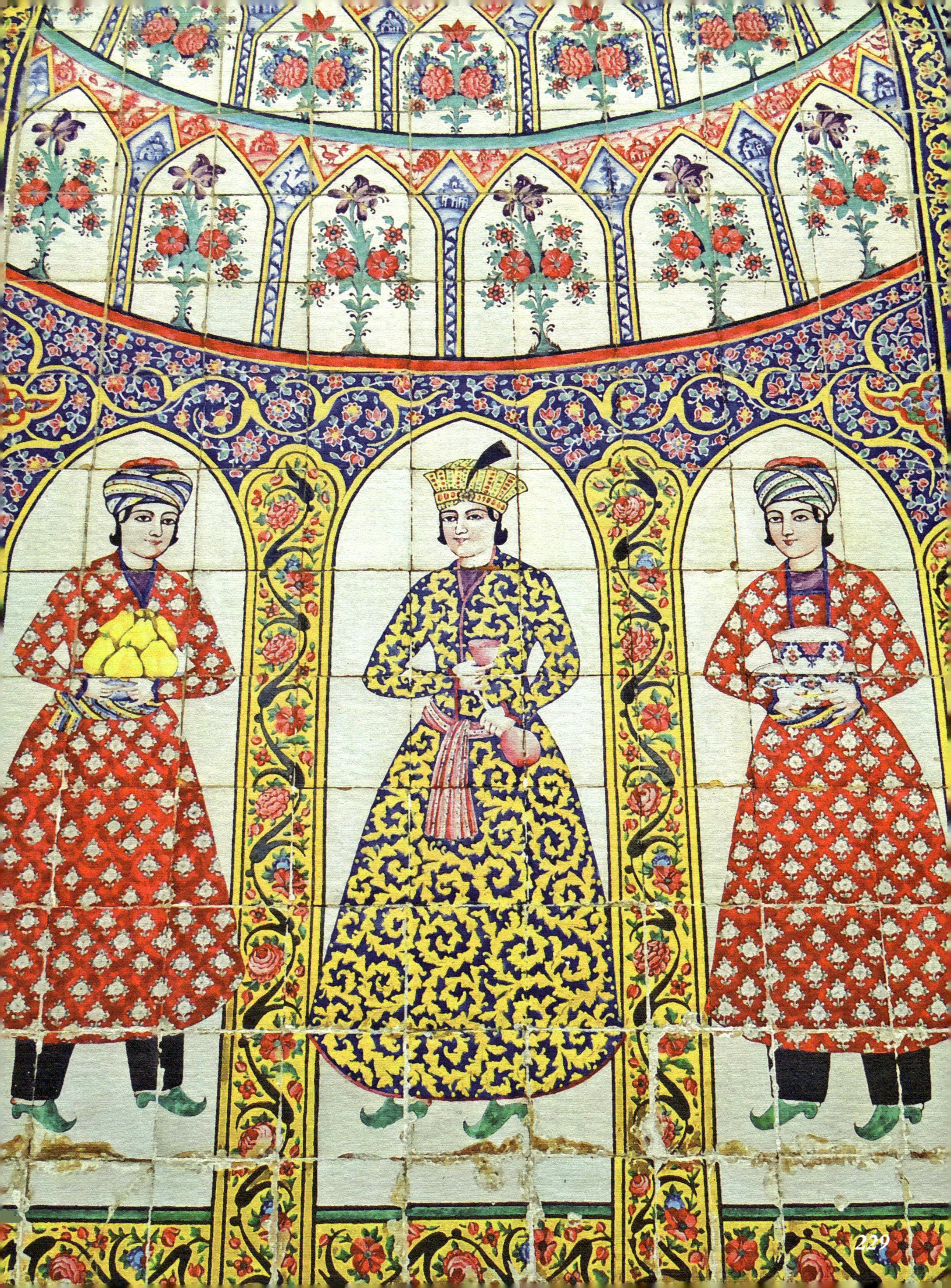

KAMA SUTRA ELIXIR FOR WOMEN

Many ancient practices for boosting libido and metabolism are about increasing the heat of your organs. Nutmeg and cinnamon are warming herbs that increase blood flow in the abdominal and pelvic regions. Dates are known in Persian mythology to be the fruit from the heavens. They are said to stimulate your appetite for sex. The blood-pumping effects of these delicious spices increase vaginal moisture and intensify sexual pleasure.

8 Oz goat, coconut or almond milk
2 Dates
1 Teaspoon powdered nutmeg
2 Sticks cinnamon or 2 Teaspoons cinnamon powder

Liquefy all ingredients in a food processor. Drink cold or heat up for a comforting evening drink to heat up your desire and invoke passion!

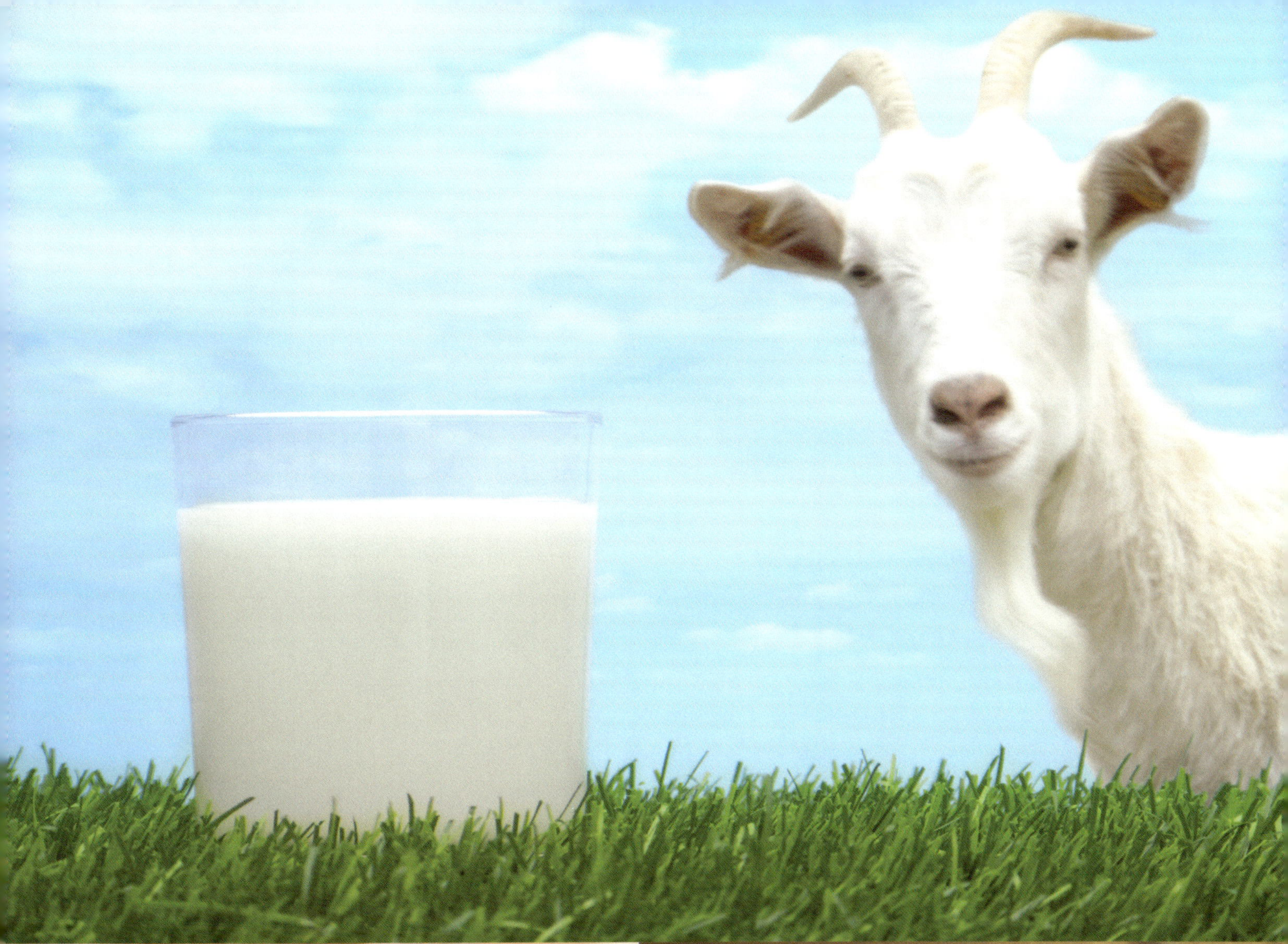

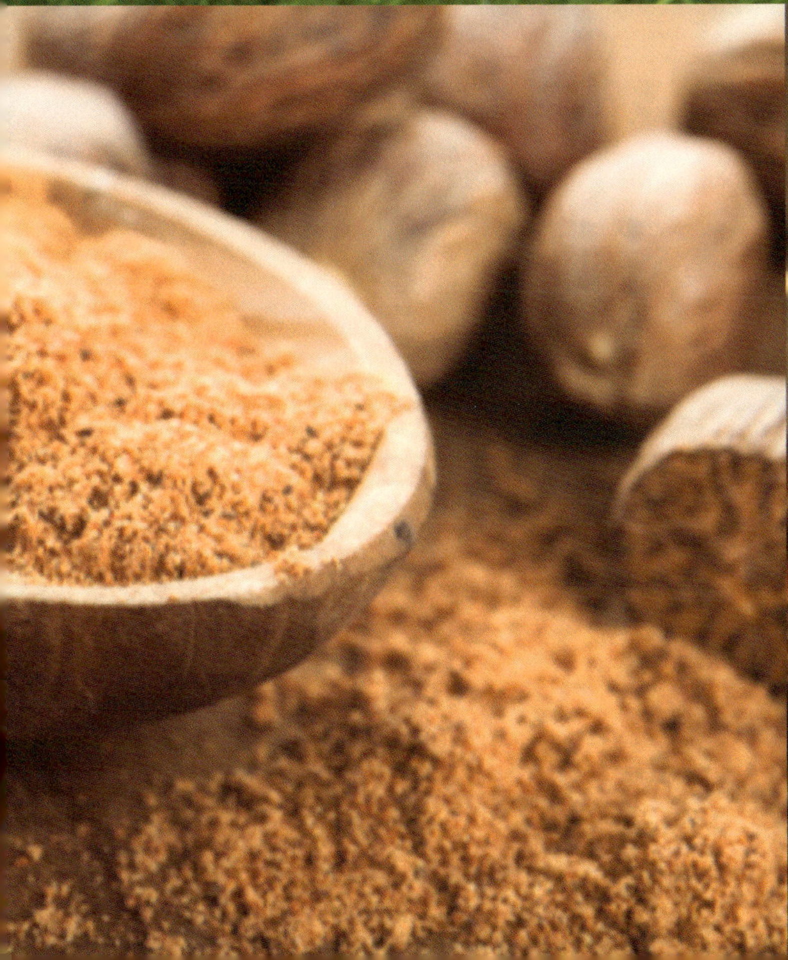

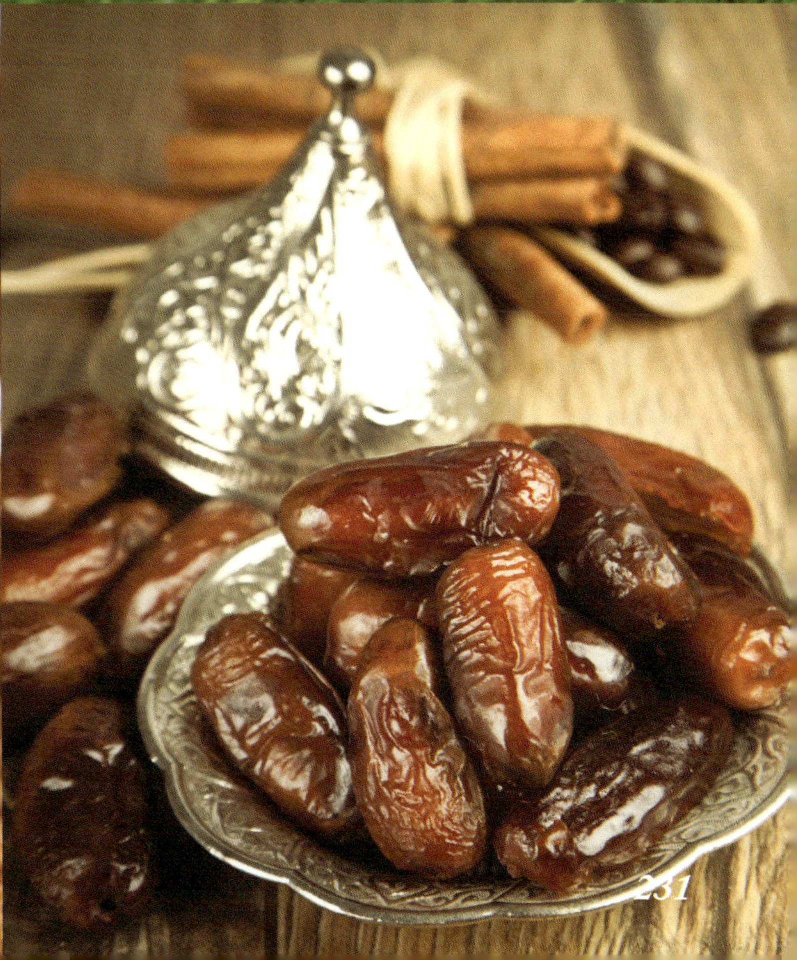

KAMA SUTRA ELIXIR FOR MEN

Cinnamon, cardamom and cloves are spices considered useful for producing "heat" within the body, and cinnamon has been measured to increase appetite, both physical and sexual. Since ancient times cloves have been used as an aphrodisiac for the treatment of male sexual disorders, erectile dysfunction, enhancing the libido and sperm potency.

It is even said that a drop of cinnamon oil rubbed onto the genitals is surprisingly useful in producing powerful sexual stimulation.

8 Oz Coconut or almond milk
2 pods of cardamom (pierced)
2 sticks of cinnamon or 2 Teaspoons cinnamon powder
1 Teaspoon raw honey
2 cloves

Put the spices in the milk of your choice and let soak for an hour or two. Warm over the heat add your organic raw honey.

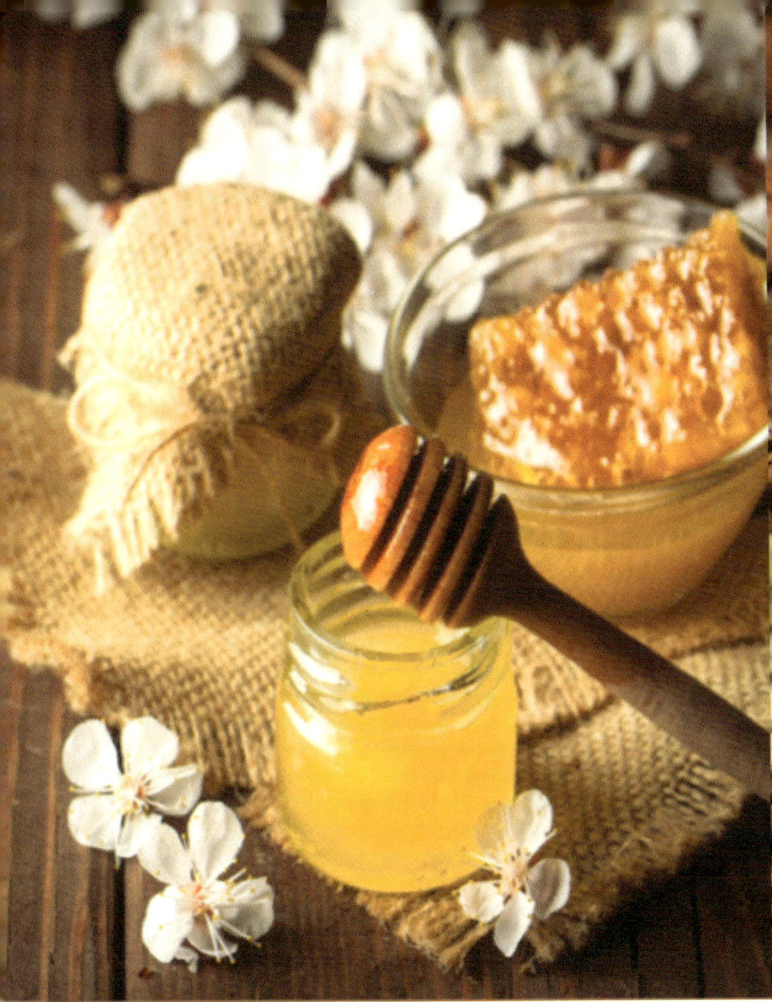
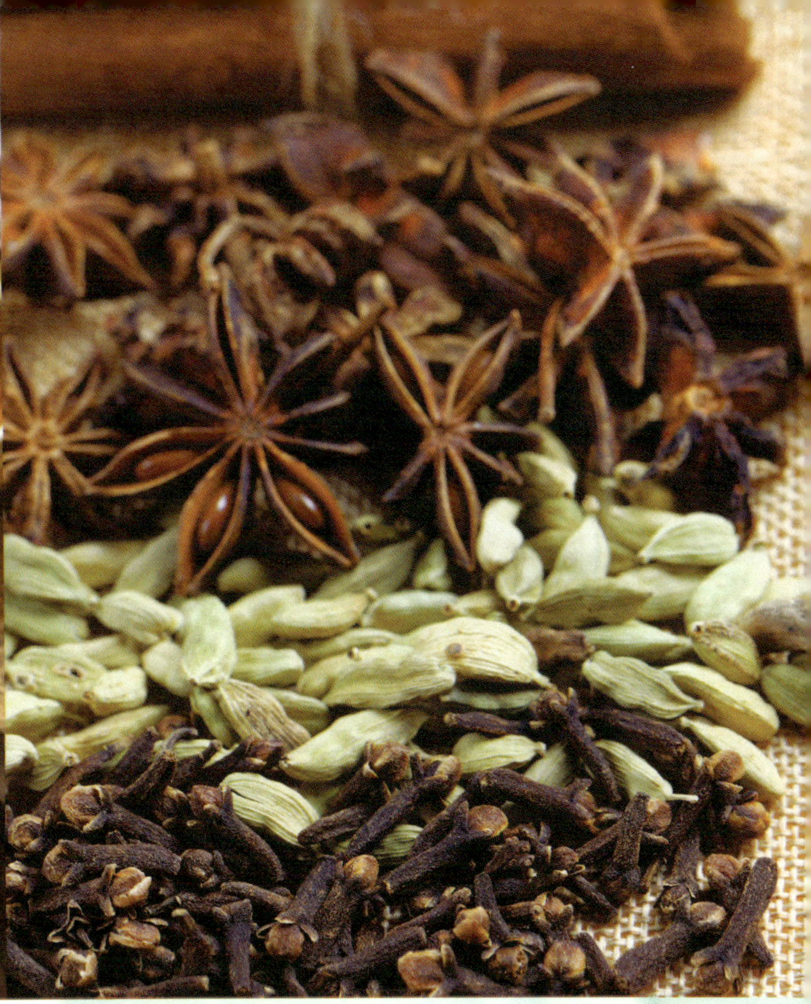
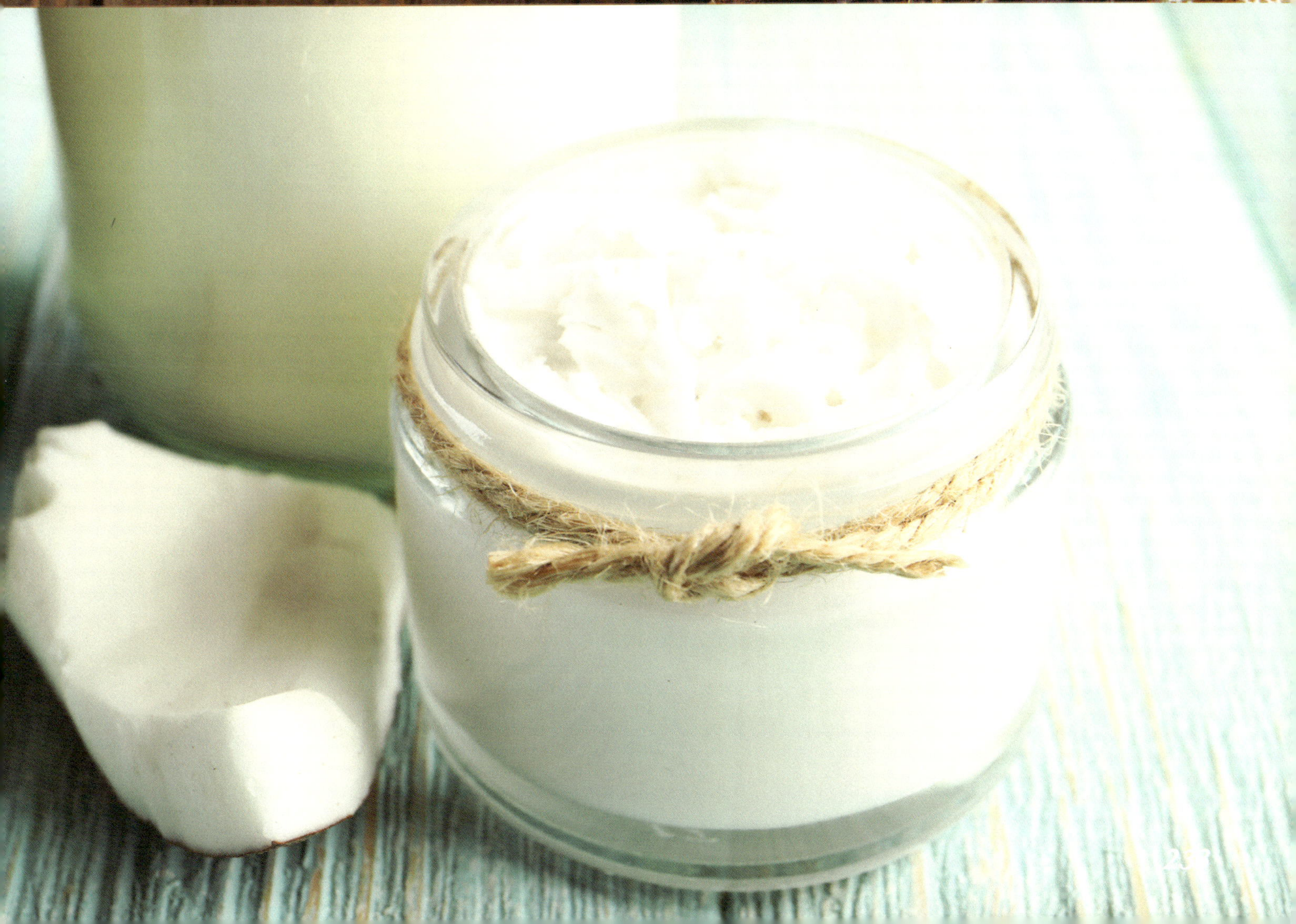

HOW TO REMOVE PESTICIDES FROM FRUITS AND VEGETABLES

Fill a large bowl with 4 parts water to 1 part white vinegar. Soak the fruit or vegetables you'd like to clean in the mixture for 20 minutes. Rinse well.

بسوی سپد کوه بنهاد روی | چنان چون بود مردم جنگجوی
چنین گفت شاه جوان با تخوار | که آمد بسوی یکی نامدار
نگه کن به بین تا ورا نام چیست | بدین مرد جنگی که خواهد گریست

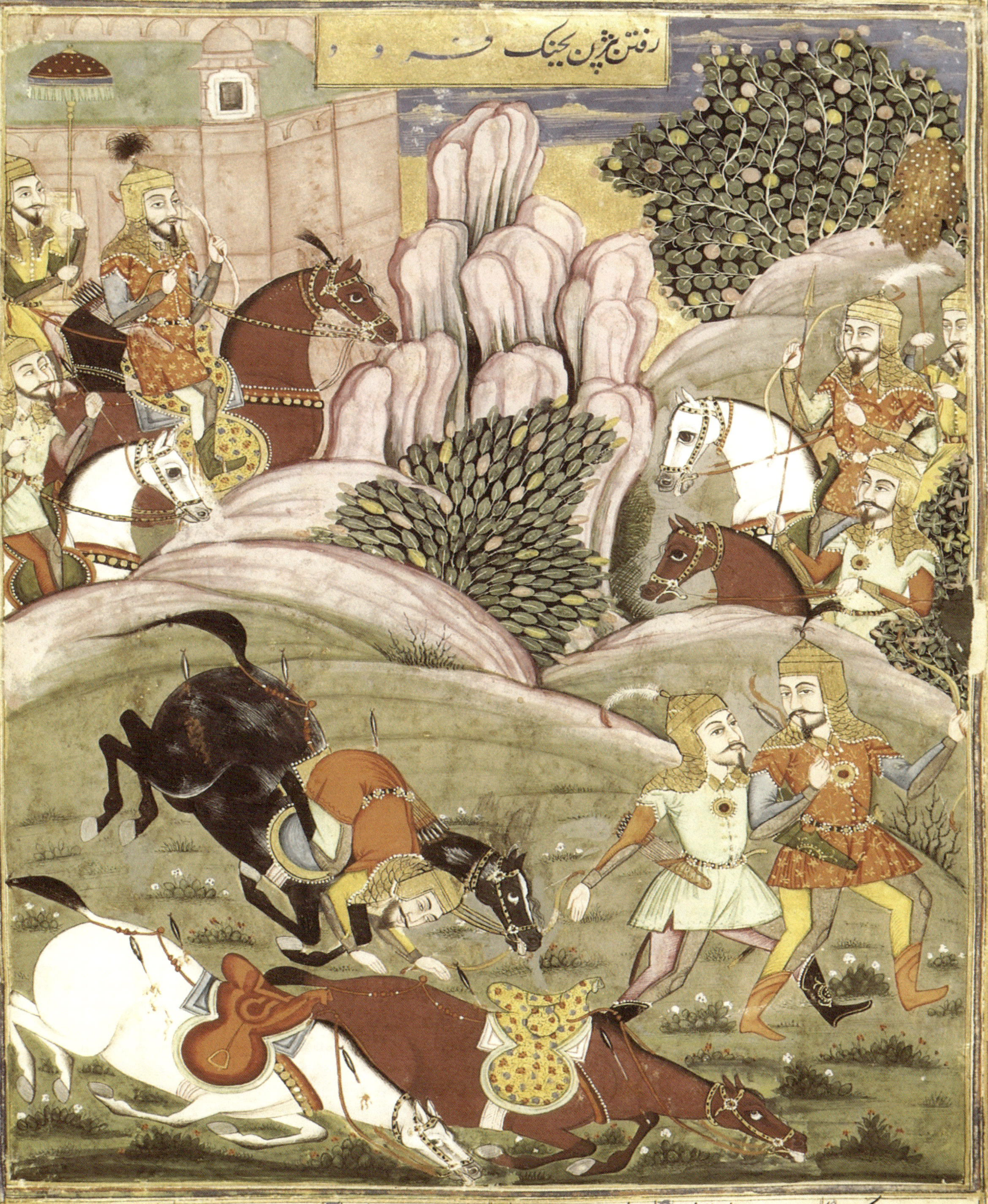

بخسرو تخوار پراینده گفت | که این راز ایران کسی نیست جفت
که فرزند گیوست و مرد دلیر | بهر جنگ پیروز باشد چو شیر
گرامی ترست او ز جان عزیز | ندارد جز او گیو فرزند نیز

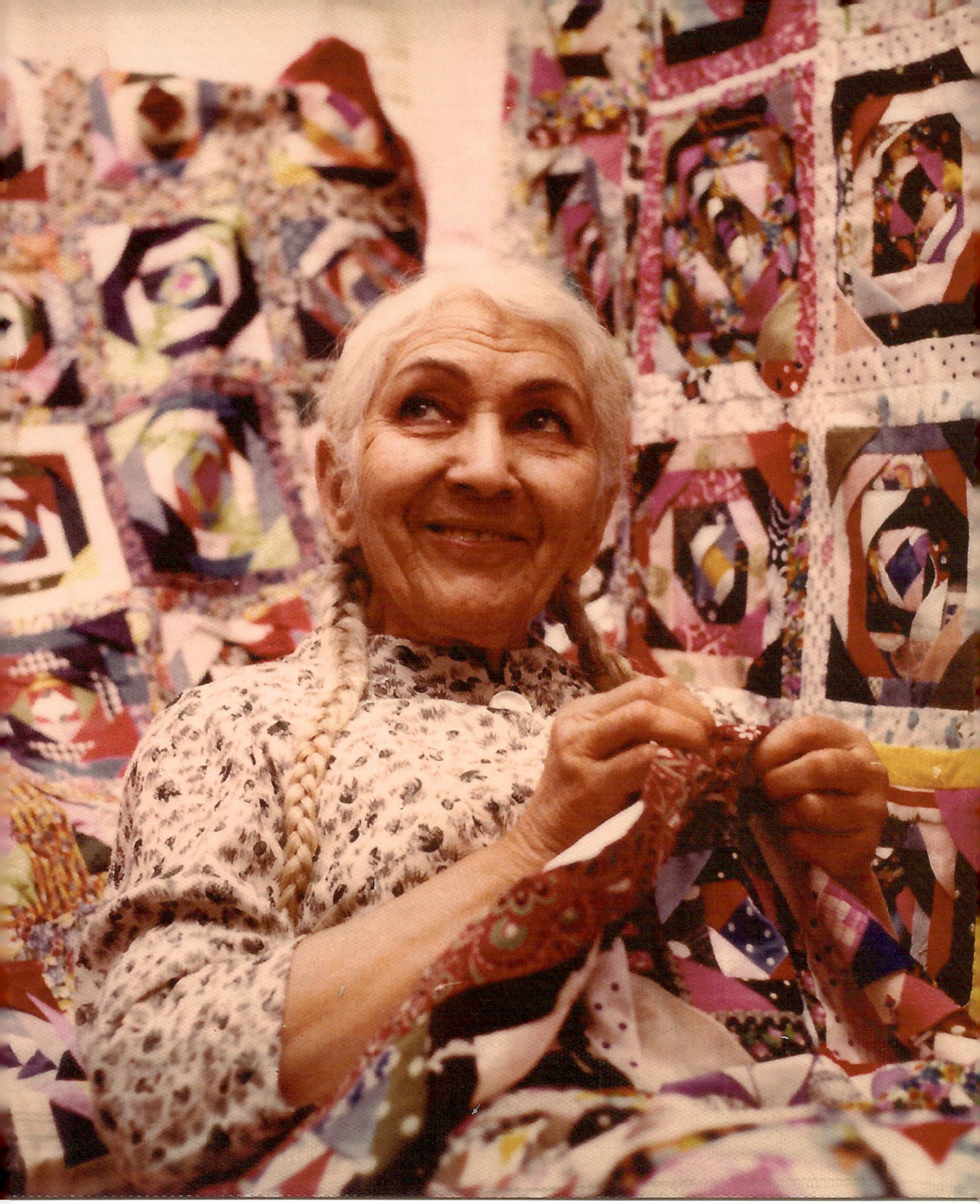

Mamanjoon at the age 92 with her quilt creations behind her

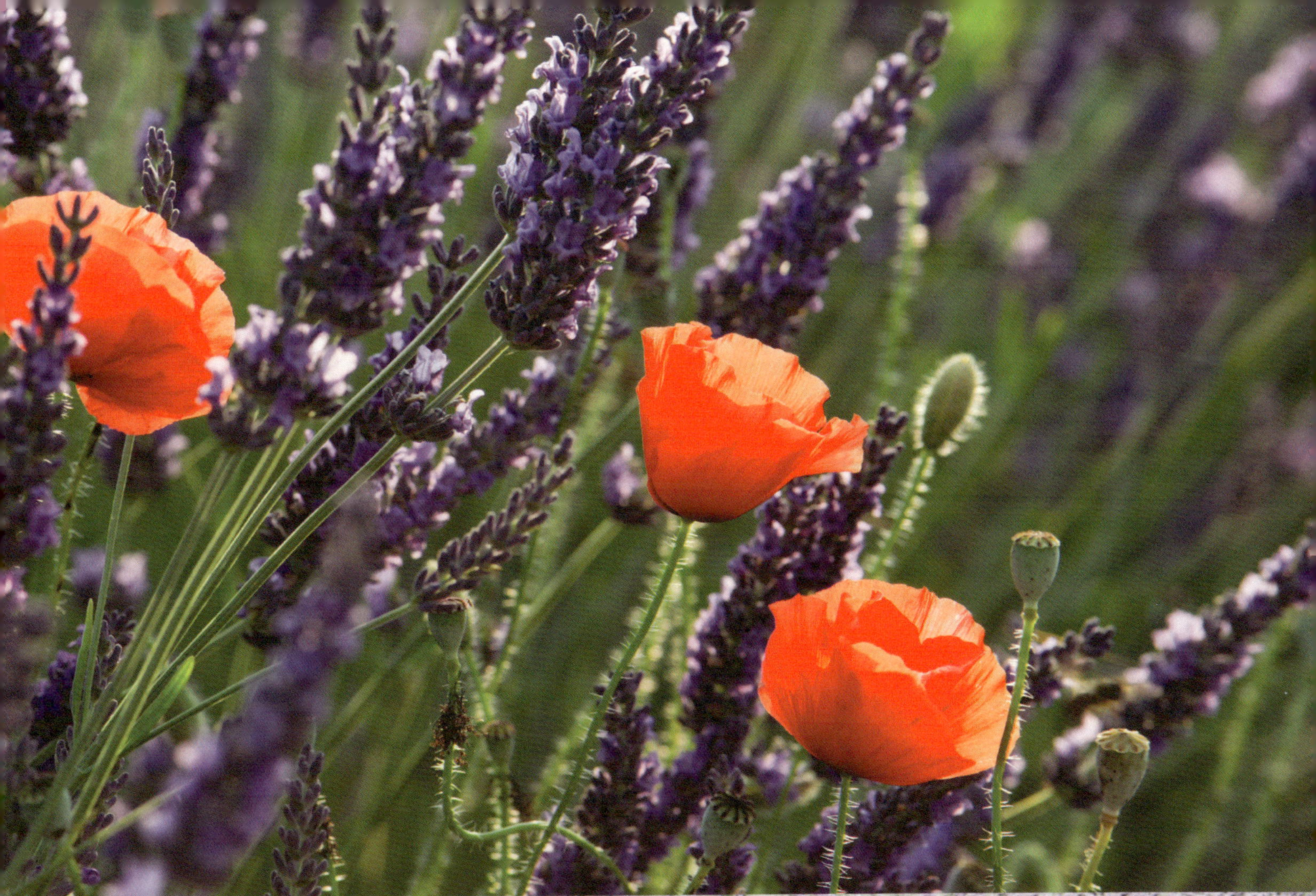

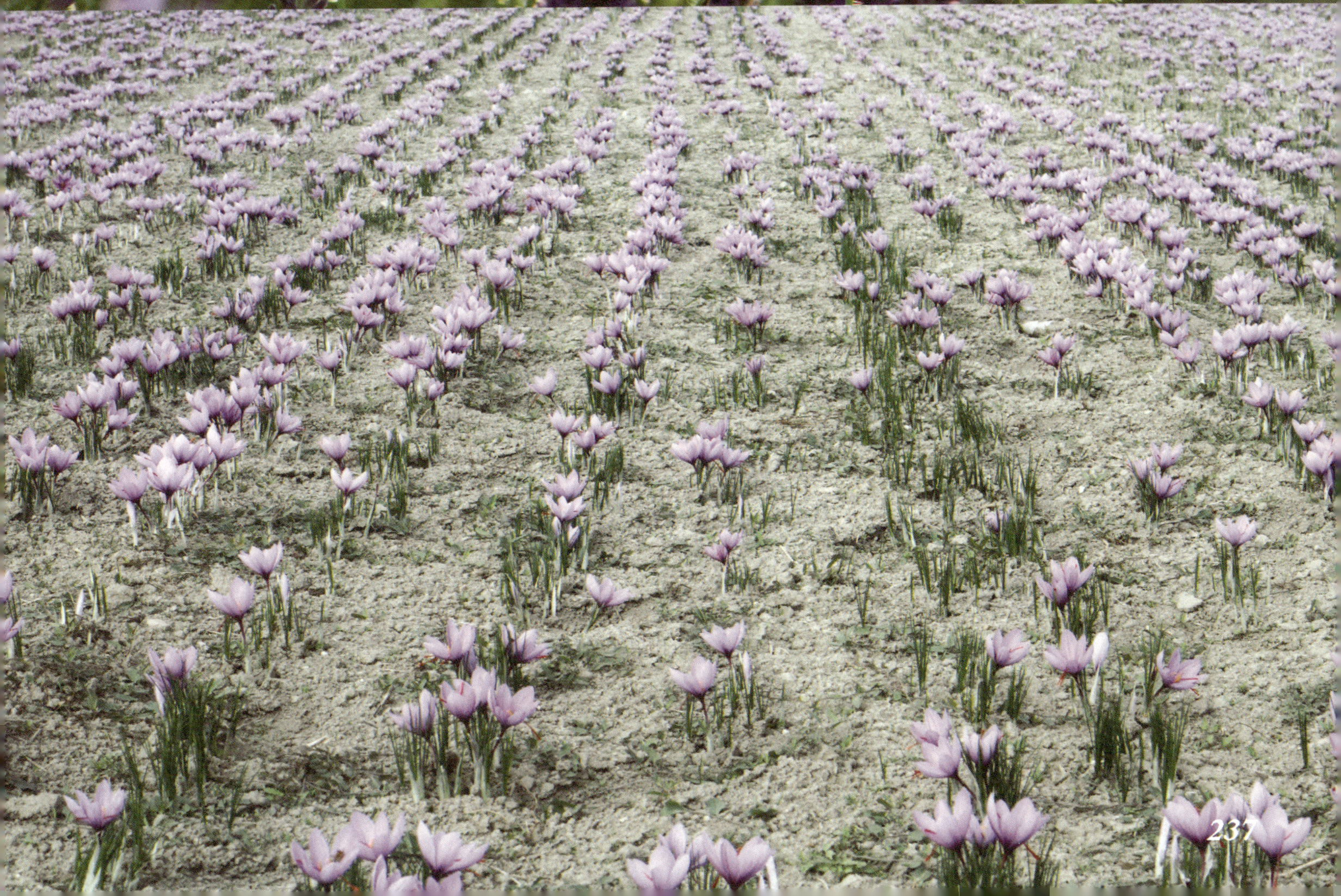

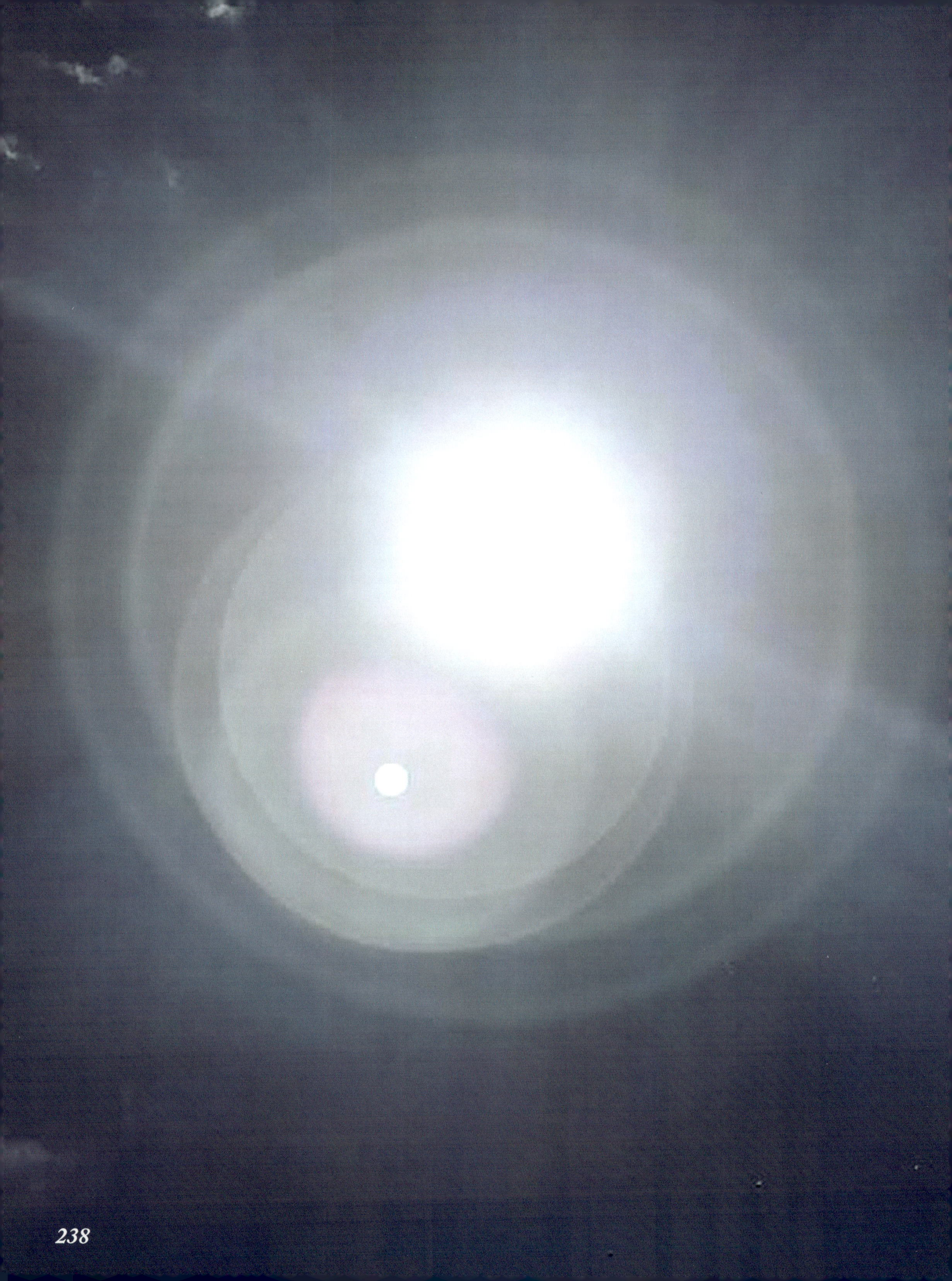

MamanJoon's Secret Potions

The information and recipes presented in this book should be in no way interpreted as a substitute for diagnosis and/or treatment by health care professionals. Although the information and the recipes presented in this book are based on hundreds of years of documented result, we do not presume to give medical advice.

Anyone wishing to use this information should consult with his or her health care provider prior to embarking on any therapeutic program.

Cover Art Design: Sue Climpson
Interior Design: Lorraine Hansen
Edited by: Debra Scott
Models: Ava O'Hara
Paintings: Hayedeh Daftari
Mandana Dalaie
Sevada Younesian
Termeh Yeghiazarian

Library of Congress Control Number: 2016918930
ISBN# 978-0-9976499-2-5 ebook- MamanJoon's Secret Potions
ISBN# 978-0-9976499-3-2 paperback-MamanJoon's Secret Potions
ISBN# 978-0-9976499-1-8 hard copy-MamanJoon's Secret Potions
Version: 2016.12.14

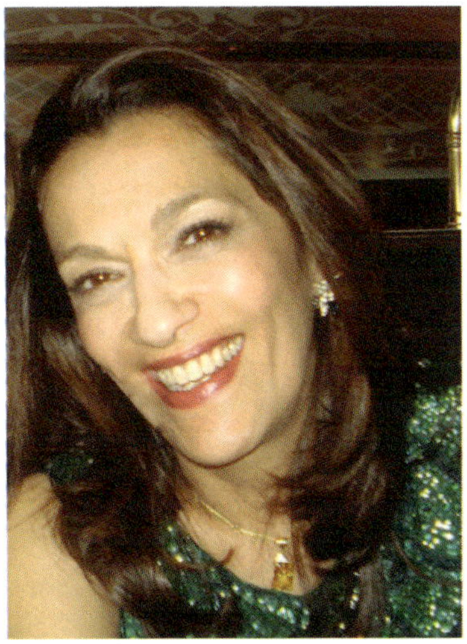

Visit the author website:
www.mamanjoonssecretpotions.com

Copyrigt Photo ID:
386801689, 390671944, 54675028, 459747304, 137373755, 197704085, 275791019, 260590877, 260590877, 260254718, 352177772, 464784476, 299373746, 475271158, 399784162, 376118449, 296414711, 144014848, 410218546, 160775306, 108625742, 77026618, 369768824, 261906719, 401577994, 405233449, 333265097, 95019640, 106550492, 327318794, 326861648, 217254727, 202361062, 428885989, 252802516, 462221638, 462932968, 319292966, 156202382, 71148712, 2777502, 282115907, 84988150, 183283202, 133164701, 185592344, 132742097, 138048434, 317037515, 305158262, 299849987, 122248753, 288949205, 288908288, 320299067, 142628674, 144058621, 175797077, 87915037, 322976672, 54675040, 440974321, 130286066, 107327777, 109391732, 223985104, 86807791, 429138232, 138639686, 402635986, 99899009, 82560304, 388995481, 446384455, 151513970, 111769100, 284085503, 418222717, 423103282, 77300020, 316149275, 136688048, 327177479, 186560807, 179857913, 309026411, 193671185, 277009871, 394716478, 230825536, 301572848, 327128258, 192366527, 10669171, 100255673, 412447219, 172688360, 371386885, 322976657, 345871676, 44600743, 315644969, 425546467, 83534995, 49177633, 153298814, 330469679, 119129767, 465583277, 394354153, 157983245, 255442270, 215455975, 361668680, 70685983, 110008847, 361077272, 154042517, 253044214, 125429075, 437804839, 463330757, 410969572, 78853978, 79213555, 427308088, 358656386, 287304434, 227214283, 386801689, 390671944, 54675028, 228187063, 228187087, 118761841, 205915768, 397925281, 397925287, 210141136, 443716600, 270596975, 140598805, 78853972, 370125116 , 286562549, 218616265, 195408770, 108674084, 247566094, 237891415, 365997176, 203256163, 458803921, 207619867, 207619867, 41498802, 4363088796, 262155599, 111769100, 277009871, 428894956, 291445157, 291445163, 354628184, 68524612, 110150702, 124287346, 261562829, 368119763, 169792445, 232054723, 138875666, 219830731, 24284095, 112518428, 206432569, 213319438, 184815377, 183542060, 305903018, 188307800, 159810950, 310505864, 484670413,

Copyright Photo ID (continued):
287304431, 90912671, 231526351, 350750582, 84913084, 84913084, 130921997, 65089477, 62300530, 240791833, 330122795, 189324212, 279193442, 287414318, 285091961, 278728763, 102876086, 143935909, 474458677, 429160420, 416176651, 235419391, 196119239, 163961957, 394765957, 390669631, 240923182, 148020260, 143704672, 134433038, 173929679, 182074403, 127603379, 381323761, 171480209, 337966187, 199762937, 199760480, 199760522, 377642452, 321031562, 254235883, 425248438, 60627880, 167843159, 151007150, 203292037, 162979526, 376829452, 35095761, 324332015, 302363219, 324332015, 294782978, 73493227, 207058639, 257388970, 260887604, 4025101, 3191610, 127425236, 93325624, 93325612, 411846892, 284375393, 378681250, 363403886, 24767458, 348504728, 356874338, 350179640, 327260912, 286474160, 420211612, 478892755, 289036913, 350083064, 124882783, 296002607, 330511979, 410561743, 416825002, 392968396, 392968393, 391044931, 418922173, 365962679, 356874341, 467803589, 315818615, 319388792, 238616341, 260246189, 371213212, 453284932, 453285040, 410218546, 160775306, 108625742, 77026618, 369768824, 261906719, 401577994, 405233449, 333265097, 95019640, 106550492, 327318794, 326861648, 217254727, 202361062, 428885989, 252802516, 413733400, 201822853, 202715689, 424008031, 274203017, 383712088, 348658046, 368193263, 68549756, 105191090, 423806893, 423808072, 296297186, 301761605, 304439030, 86208019, 62183665, 410218546, 160775306, 108625742, 77026618, 369768824, 261906719 , 401577994, 405233449, 333265097, 95019640, 106550492, 327318794, 32686164, 217254727, 202361062, 428885989, 252802516, 413733400, 201822853, 202715689, 424008031, 274203017, 383712088, 348658046, 68549756, 105191090, 423806893, 423808072, 296297186, 301761605, 304439030, 422294329, 86208019, 62183665, 309452699, 354281054, 362526863, 114526555, 159810950, 146183111, 294970319, 377609446, 476898529, 54675040, 259543400, 259221500, 395872, 269976092, 395872, 395872, 294782978, 282553499, 446431585, 446443840, 415322512, 139540037, 453295243, 409308655, 208321783, 208321801, 266455283, 260262620, 401295787, 401294695, 399345772, 290087615, 353472722, 216349768, 334557314, 108813458, 264133136, 196333577, 176110283 , 230773984, 220416622, 161565866, 426079267, 316271612, 335808896, 179830214, 196282229, 332253026, 112059833, 76260622, 415104073, 377733145, 255598918, 275691188 , 215898847, 246230038, 415155178, 141729409, 200945726, 449441371, 203943361, 439919338, 162692921, 423354253, 132989957, 229035097, 310996580, 79232101, 345469454, 476577451, f165c59917847d326d5f369119b61f65

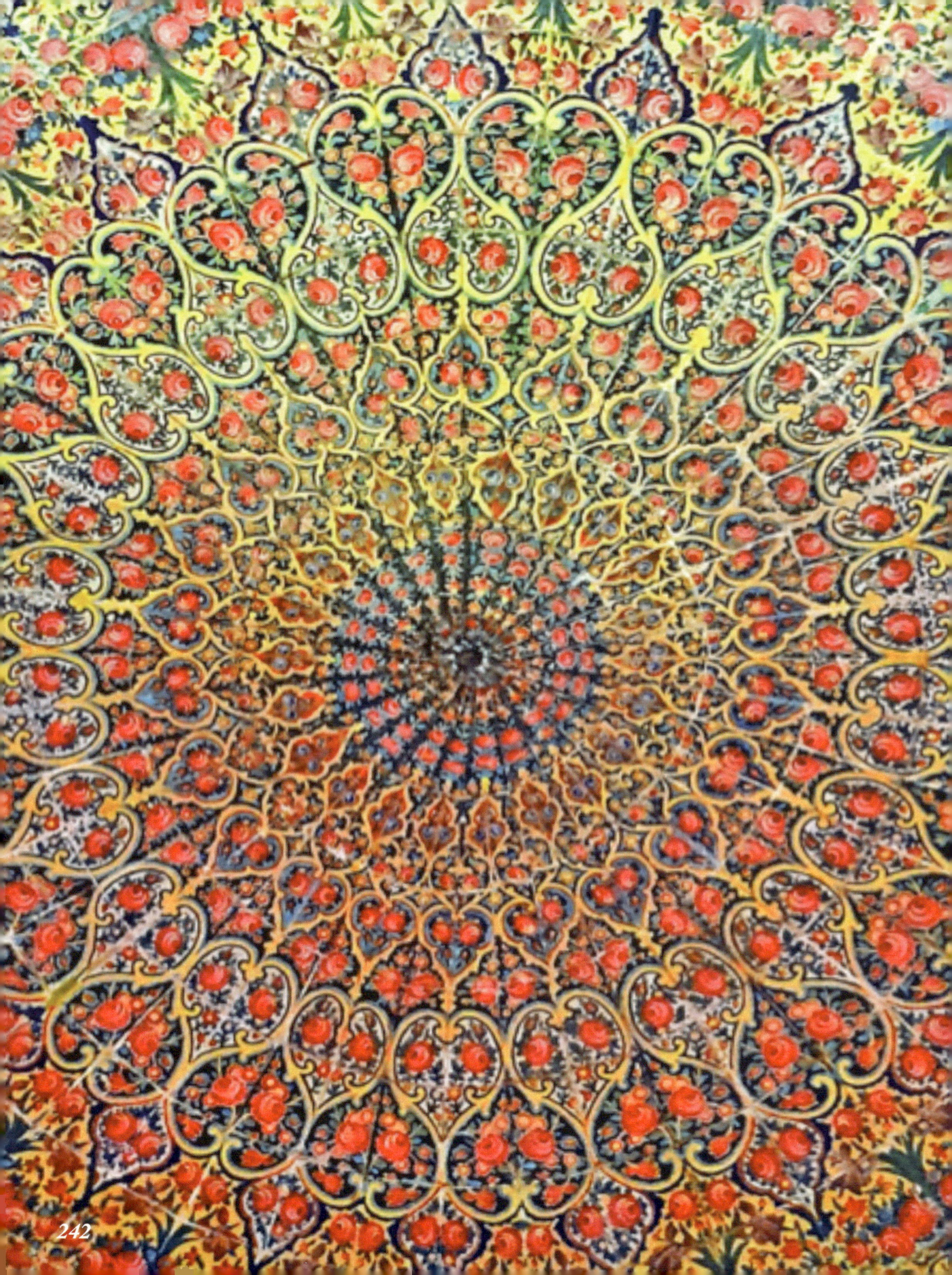

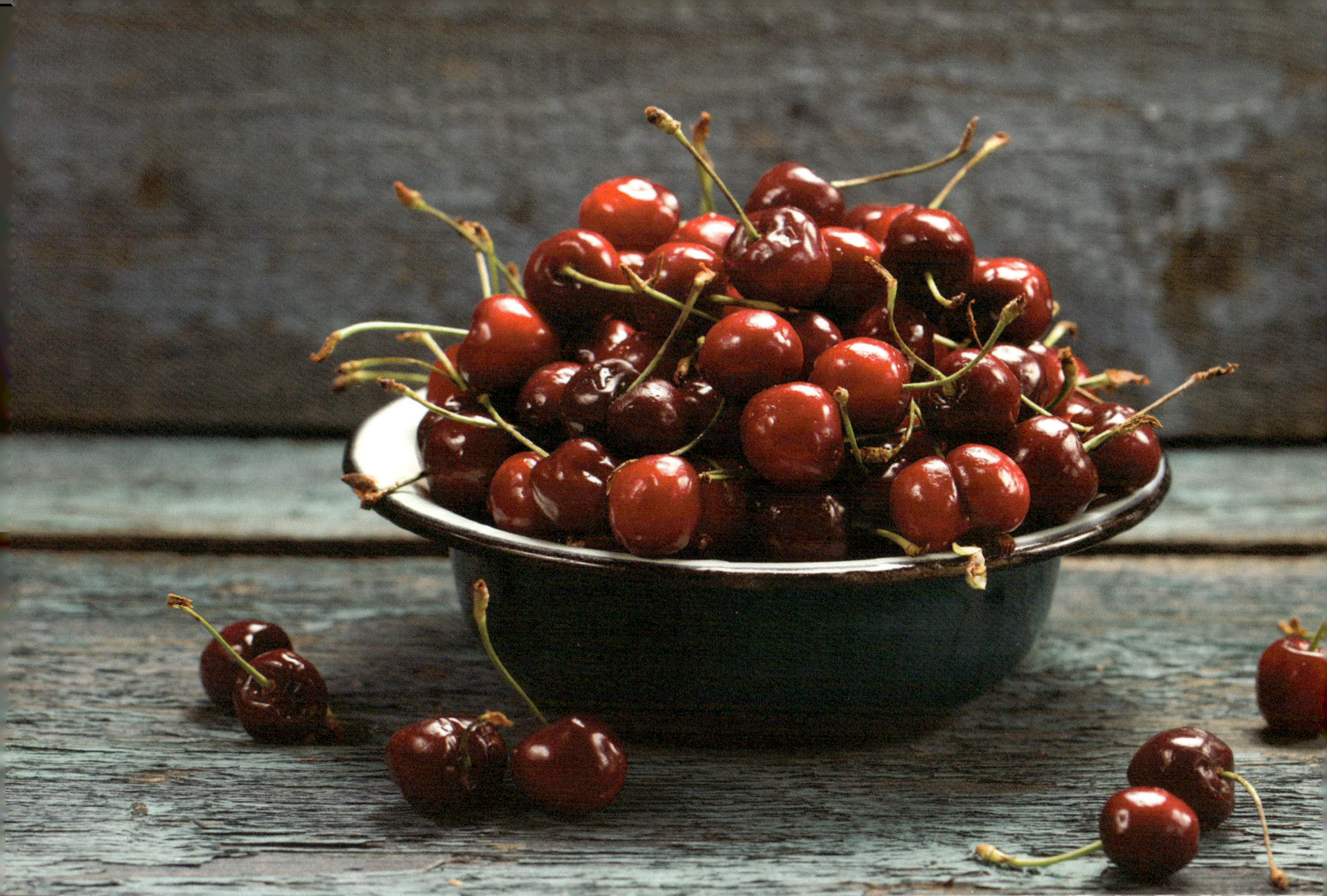
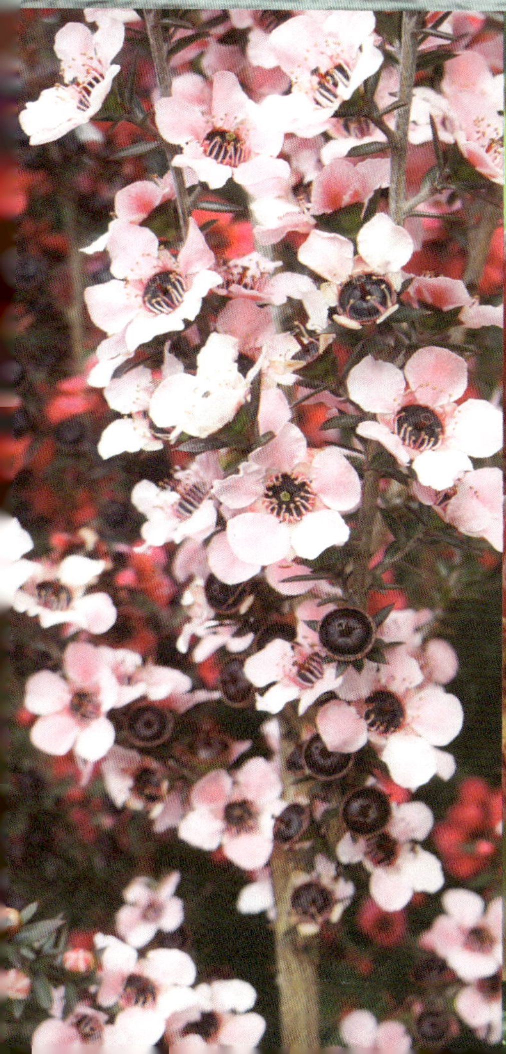
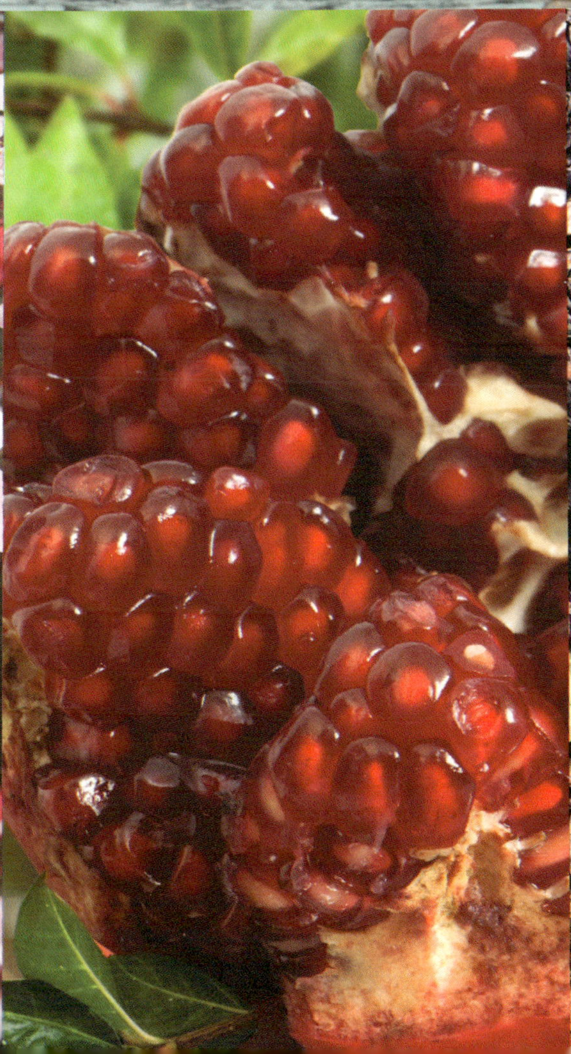
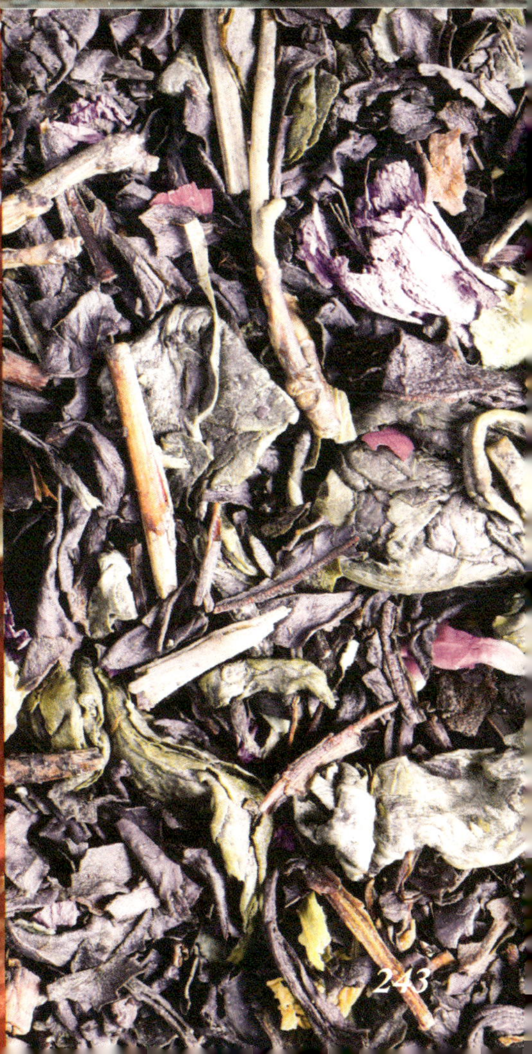

CPSIA information can be obtained at www.ICGtesting.com
Printed in the USA
BVIW12n2146270717
490468BV00007B/18

* 9 7 8 0 9 9 7 6 4 9 9 1 8 *